THE CLINICAL INTERVIEW USING DSM-IV

VOLUME 2:
THE DIFFICULT PATIENT

THE CLINICAL INTERVIEW USING DSM-IV

VOLUME 2:
THE DIFFICULT PATIENT

Ekkehard Othmer, M.D., Ph.D.
Sieglinde C. Othmer, Ph.D.

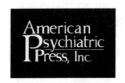

1400 K Street, N.W.
Washington, DC 20005

Copyright © 1994 Ekkehard Othmer and Sieglinde C. Othmer
ALL RIGHTS RESERVED
Manufactured in the United States of America on acid-free paper
97 96 95 94   4 3 2 1
First Edition

American Psychiatric Press, Inc.
1400 K Street, N.W., Washington, DC   20005

Library of Congress Cataloging-in-Publication Data
(Revised for vol. 2)
Othmer, Ekkehard.
    The clinical interview using DSM-IV.

    Rev. ed. of: The clinical interview using DSM-III-R. c1989.
    Includes bibliographical references and index.
    Contents: — v. 2. The difficult patient.
    1. Interviewing in psychiatry. 2. Diagnostic
and statistical manual of mental disorders.
    I. Othmer, Sieglinde C. II. Othmer, Ekkehard.
    Clinical interview using DSM-III-R. III. Title.
    [DNLM: 1. Interview, Psychological.   WM 141 087c 1994]
    RC480.7.O743 1994   516.89′14   94-2525
    ISBN 0-88048-520-5

British Library Cataloguing in Publication Data
A CIP record is available from the British Library.

To our children

Konstantin
Johann Philipp
Julia Christie

Contents

PART I
SYMPTOM LANGUAGE

CHAPTER 1
CONVERSION

CHAPTER 2
DISSOCIATION

PART II
PSYCHOTIC COMMUNICATION

PART III
COGNITIVE IMPAIRMENT:
THE LANGUAGE OF THE FAILING BRAIN

CHAPTER 7
INATTENTION AND HYPERACTIVITY 227

CHAPTER 8
AMNESIA 241

PART IV
SELF-PROTECTIVE AND DECEPTIVE BEHAVIOR

CHAPTER 12
CONCEALING 319

CHAPTER 13
FALSIFYING AND LYING 349

LIST OF TABLES

ABOUT THE AUTHORS

Ekkehard Othmer, M.D., Ph.D., is Clinical Professor of Psychiatry at the University of Kansas Medical Center and Medical Director at a freestanding psychiatric hospital in Kansas City. He is a Diplomate of the American Board of Psychiatry and Neurology and one of its examiners. He is a fellow of the American Psychiatric Association and a member of the American Medical Association, Society of Biological Psychiatry, and other organizations. He is a member of the psychiatric hospital surveyor panel of the Health Care Financing Administration (HCFA) of the Department of Health and Human Services, Baltimore, Maryland. Dr. Othmer graduated from the Department of Psychology (Ph.D.) and the Medical School (M.D.) of the University of Hamburg, Germany, and trained in psychoanalysis at the Psychoanalytical Institute in Hamburg, Germany. He completed his residency in psychiatry at Renard Hospital, Washington University Medical School in St. Louis, Missouri.

Sieglinde C. Othmer, Ph.D., is a member of the Society for Clinical Trials. Dr. Othmer studied Romance languages at the Sorbonne in Paris, France, and history at the Social Sciences Department of the University of Hamburg, Germany. She earned her Ph.D. in the social sciences at the University of Hamburg. Her thesis on the expansion of human rights in Europe in the prerevolution era was selected for publication as a book by the Berlin Historical Commission at the Friedrich-Meinecke Institut of the Free University of Berlin, Germany. She completed a postdoctoral fellowship in genetics at Renard Hospital, Department of Psychiatry at Washington University, St. Louis, Missouri. As Research Assistant Professor, she conducted investigational drug studies at the University of Kansas Medical School, Department of Psychiatry, Kansas City, Kansas.

Drs. Ekkehard Othmer and Sieglinde C. Othmer are married to each other.

FOREWORD

The success of *The Clinical Interview Using DSM-IV, Volume 1: Fundamentals* by Ekkehard Othmer, M.D., and Sieglinde C. Othmer, Ph.D., indicated a significant need in the mental health field. The Othmers perceived that need and have now followed up with *The Clinical Interview Using DSM-IV, Volume 2: The Difficult Patient.*

From my perspective, before DSM-III, interviewing by mental health workers in the United States depended significantly on the clinical and educational orientation of the leadership at various institutions. Those facilities with a psychodynamic orientation advocated one type of approach, whereas those with descriptive and cognitive emphases used quite different styles of interviewing. With the advent of DSM-IV, the Othmers recognized that an integrated approach to interviewing was vital for the entire field. They achieved this integration in Volume 1 and have now taken the more complex step of attempting an integrated approach to more "difficult" patients.

Beyond conceptualizing the need, the Othmers have accomplished several other tasks in making Volume 2 useful to a wide group of practitioners. Taking DSM-IV as a base, they have classified "difficult" patients into a practical system, including 1) patients with disorders that are "medically inexplicable" (e.g., conversion, dissociation), 2) patients with impaired reality testing resulting from delusional and hallucinatory experiences, 3) patients with cognitive impairment, and 4) patients with self-deceptive and dissimulating behavior. Given this classification, the Othmers illustrate how to conduct an interview with patients who have each of these types of problems. The interviews are provided in great detail, along with a logical rationale for the specific choice of words, methods, and sequences.

The DSM process has provided us with a base for developing rational options for treatment of those with specific disorders. Practice guidelines will be a central feature of this evolution of the mental health field. Clinical interviewing is a transitional process between diagnosis and treatment. The interviewing, of course, is a vital part of making the diagnosis. To recognize that variations in styles of interviewing may be necessary is very important, especially in difficult clinical encounters. The Othmers have helped to teach us that the successful diagnostic interview may also be a useful key for successful treatment.

I am particularly pleased that the Othmers have transcended old ideological schools (they call this "Old Think") and have come up with a "New Think" approach. In a practical way, they have shown that "difficult" patients with different clusters of symptoms may be best interviewed by specific combinations of methods. They have also once again organized their book and their chapters into clearly understandable interviewing segments. This superb organization will be most helpful for students, but also will help their teachers to integrate the clinical phenomena more rationally.

As a long-time advocate of integration rather than ideological segmentation of our field, I am delighted that the Othmers have provided us with a thoroughly practical clinical approach to the interviewing of patients with problems that could easily puzzle the beginner. Their integrated approach is also a good model for us to utilize in many other clinical contexts. This book, like Volume 1, will become recognized as a fundamental text for our education and continuing learning.

Melvin Sabshin, M.D.
Medical Director, American Psychiatric Association

PREFACE

THE "OLD THINK" AND THE "NEW THINK"

In psychology and psychiatry, we encounter schools of thinking whose beliefs about the nature of psychiatric disorders and appropriate styles for interviewing patients with those disorders apparently contradict each other. From a *psychodynamic standpoint,* psychiatric disorders are seen as the result of unconscious, infantile conflicts that are kept out of one's awareness by defense mechanisms. An open-ended, unstructured, indirect interviewing style that focuses on introspection allows these conflicts to emerge and defenses to manifest themselves. From a *behavioral standpoint,* psychiatric disorders are viewed as results of maladaptive conditioned responses to noxious stimuli, which can be explored directly in the interview. From a *descriptive standpoint,* psychiatric disorders are conceptualized like medical disorders—in terms of symptoms and signs—even though their pathology and etiology are elusive. The descriptive interview assesses the diagnostic criteria for these disorders.

Each school in its orthodox form holds that its approach applies equally well to all psychiatric disorders. Yet present clinical and research data indicate that this claim has become an "Old Think."

In the "New Think," it is proposed that each of these different approaches is well applied to one group of disorders but not as well to some others. For example, cognitive disorders—similar to medical disorders—often show measurable and identifiable tissue pathology and can be well described in terms of symptoms, signs, and laboratory values. A descriptive approach appears to be appropriate here. In contrast, disorders that are associated with psychological factors, such as somatoform, dissociative, conversion, or posttraumatic stress disorders, can be best explored if the assessment of their symptoms and signs is augmented by a probing for their psychological factors. Thus, unstructured, indirect assessment techniques—hypnosis and other uncovering techniques—enrich the results obtained by a symptom- and sign-oriented, descriptive approach.

Furthermore, disorders that involve deceptive or self-deceptive behaviors, such as substance abuse, oppositional defiant disorder, conduct disorder, factitious disorder, malingering, and some of the personality disorders—antisocial and borderline—are difficult to explore by interviewing for symptoms and signs alone. The motivational component has to be elucidated to fully understand the patient's pathology.

The "New Think" strives to overcome generalization by providing a differential approach to interviewing. It favors multiple approaches that individualize and explore in depth each disorder and all contributing factors to prepare the patient for optimal therapeutic intervention. This "New Think" approach is followed in this book.

ACKNOWLEDGMENTS

◆ ◆ ◆ ◆ ◆

I feel about editors the way I feel about directors: they know their jobs. . . . Editors know their business and, honestly, I've never once thought, "Well, if they'd left that moment in the film, I'd have got an Oscar."

◆ ◆ ◆ ◆ ◆

Michael Caine
Acting in Film, 1990

Our colleagues donated thought and time to this project: Man Anand, M.D.; Julie Applegate, Ph.D.; Sharon Cain, M.D.; Sue Croskell; Tim Dellenbaugh, M.D.; Cherilyn Desouza, M.D.; Linda Glimcher, R.N., M.S.; Kenneth Hines, Ph.D.; Ronald R. Holt II, D.O.; Mark M. Hood; Linda L. Kalivas, M.D.; Lee Ann Kelling, M.D.; Elizabeth C. Penick, Ph.D.; Barbara J. Powell, Ph.D.; Nora Quiason, M.D.; Sandy Radom, Ph.D.; Peggy Ragland; Eric Schmidt; Ron Schaumburg; Carol Smith, M.D.; Glenn Townes; Daniel F. Ward, M.D.; and Cindy Wood, M.D. Many thanks to all of you.

We thank our panel of reviewers from both coasts and in between who volunteered much-needed critique: Robert P. Granacher, M.D., in Lexington, Kentucky; William V. McKnelly, M.D., in Kansas City, Kansas; Robert L. Spitzer, M.D., in New York City; and Gary J. Tucker, M.D., in Seattle, Washington. These busy people seemed to have the most time. And what a joy it was when they told us that they liked this book. We extend special thanks to Ronald L. Martin, M.D., in Wichita, Kansas, who as a participant of our review panel contributed many detailed suggestions on an early draft and on the final draft of the manuscript. Thank you, Donald R. Royall, M.D., and your group for your speedy response to our request to include a copy of your assessment tools in this volume. We thank Diane Buckingham, M.D., who, as an African-American psychiatrist and colleague, gave us valuable advice on issues of race.

We thank Lawrence F. Berkland, investigator, with Berkland and Associates in Kansas City, Missouri, for his valuable input and suggestions. We thank Kevin Passer, M.D., for conducting some voice-stress interviews.

We thank our family—our son Konstantin, systems engineer and director with Apple Computers, who recreated voice-stress analysis on the Macintosh computer; our son Philipp, medical student, who helped with editing; and our daughter Julia who in many counted (!) hours typed the manuscript while in middle and high school. We thank Charlotte Gierth, S. C. Othmer's mother, for her support—spiritual and practical.

Jane Carver and the staff at Dykes Library of the University of Kansas Medical Center in Kansas City, Kansas, found the most elusive authors. Thank you, Jane, for your detective work. Many thanks also to Susan Case at the Clendening History of Medicine Library and Museum of the University of Kansas Medical Center.

We thank our editor Kitty Moore for her straightforward thinking and her ever good spirits in developing this book—and us, really.

Special thanks to the American Psychiatric Press—to Carol Nadelson, M.D., who, caught in the Boston ice storm, read through this manuscript in one weekend with her red pen and smoothed out the wrinkles; to Claire Reinburg, who always kept us in the clear and on schedule; to Pam Harley, who improved the text with her preciseness; and to Ron McMillen who put up with us once again.

INTRODUCTION

FRAMEWORK

◆ ◆ ◆ ◆ ◆

What sorrow has come to your heart now? Tell me, do not hide it in your mind, and thus we shall both know.

Homer
The Iliad (eighth century B.C.)

◆ ◆ ◆ ◆ ◆

This book is about patients who are difficult to interview; those who, in Homer's phrase, hide in their mind the sorrow of their heart. The difficulties originate in the patient's symptoms, signs, and behaviors that interfere with the interviewing process.

In DSM-IV (American Psychiatric Association 1994), these difficulties are addressed in the forms of diagnostic criteria, associated features to Axes I and II disorders, and frequently observed behaviors that relate to the diagnostic criteria or associated features. Such difficult patients express their distress in some way other than straightforward complaints. One patient manifests his distress through pseudoneurological, unexplained, somatic or psychological symptoms. Another patient may withdraw into a world of her own and shut you out, or behave as if her internal world is reality. Some patients with failing brain function may hide their deteriorating cognition from you. Finally, a patient may signal suffering by deceiving you.

Such a patient does not accept the interviewer as a supportive person. He does not share his symptoms and, at times, misleads the interviewer.

For these difficult patients, we have used interviewing techniques that differ from both descriptive, criteria-oriented interviewing and open-ended, psychodynamic interviewing. We have collected the histories of those difficult patients for whom these not-so-common interviewing techniques were helpful. This inductive process led us to four groups of difficulties and their matching interviewing techniques.

The first type of difficulty is the displaying of signs and symptoms of illness that are in fact medically inexplicable; these signs and symptoms involve a patient's consciousness, identity, memory, sensory and motor nervous systems, and bodily functions (Part I of this volume). Patients in this group show conversion, dissociative, avoidance, or somatic symptoms; frequently, patients experience these symptoms simultaneously. The DSM-IV disorders characterized by these symptoms are conversion disorder; dissociative disorders; posttraumatic stress disorder; and somatoform disorders, especially somatization disorder. All these disorders are judged to be associated with psychological factors—factors that may represent a history of physical and sexual abuse, life-threatening traumatic events, or stressors often associated with the onset, maintenance, and exacerbation of the symptoms. Clinical experience indicates that a group of uncovering techniques may help to explore these psychological factors: hypnosis, free association, active listening, and symptom validation.

The second type of difficulty is a patient's impaired reality testing, resulting from delusional and hallucinatory experiences (Part II). With such patients, it is difficult to establish and maintain rapport. They act on hallucinations and delusional thoughts as if they were real. They may encapsulate themselves in mute stupor while attending to their internal world, or attack the interviewer as an enemy. All DSM-IV disorders that are associated with psychotic symptoms belong in this category. We describe several techniques useful for such patients: amobarbital and lorazepam interviewing, tranquilization with retrospective interviewing for delusional and hallucinatory experiences, and empathizing with patients' acceptable goals while diffusing their socially destructive behaviors.

The third type of difficulty is cognitive impairment, which causes patients to provide incomplete information or inappropriate feedback about their problems (Part III). Such cognitive impairment may be overlooked and misinterpreted as symptoms of major depression, schizophrenia, or an anxiety disorder. The three major categories of DSM-IV cognitive disorders—dementia, amnestic disorders, and delirium—belong to this group. However, some disorders, usually first diagnosed in infancy, childhood, or adolescence, complement this group—namely, mental retardation, learning disorders, and attention-deficit disorders. We discuss methods to alert the interviewer to the presence of a cognitive disorder and present specific examination techniques that can quickly identify the impairment.

The fourth type of difficulty is deception and self-deception (Part IV). In DSM-IV, deception is recognized in conduct disorder and antisocial personality disorder within the criteria of lying and using aliases. It is seen in the self-deceptive, dissimulating behavior that is an associated feature of substance use and eating disorders. Deceptive behavior is also addressed as a characteristic of borderline personality disorder and pedophilia. False information received from a patient can lead to misdiagnosis. Interviewers may be fooled because they may not notice deceptive behavior. In this book we present techniques to help the interviewer detect deceptive behavior and enable the patient to replace that behavior with the openness necessary for a successful therapeutic alliance. These techniques include cross-examination, voice-stress analysis, and cognitive techniques.

The Clinical Interview Using DSM-IV, Volume 2: The Difficult Patient builds on our first interview book, *The Clinical Interview Using DSM-IV, Volume 1: Fundamentals* (Othmer and Othmer 1994). The four-dimensional interviewing approach outlined in Volume 1 is now applied to the difficult patient. This approach focuses on the interviewer's rapport with the patient, on the techniques that elicit information, on the patient's mental status during the interview, and on the diagnostic decision process. However, this four-prong approach is not sufficient for interviewing the difficult patient successfully. The interviewing strategies presented here enhance the symptom- and sign-oriented interviewing style by employing specialized techniques that address the difficulties encountered by clinicians.

Volume 2: The Difficult Patient draws from many sources. It integrates interviewing techniques developed by different schools of thinking in psychiatry and psychology, such as psychodynamic, cognitive, and neuropsychiatric approaches, as well as the legal system's methods of cross-examination and voice-stress analysis. It shows how these different approaches help the interviewer elicit reliable information from patients normally tough to interview and solve their diagnostic puzzles. We discuss the effectiveness of these methods and, in those instances where they could be improved on, point this out too.

The organization of each chapter shows the following outline: First, we describe the nature of a specific difficulty in interviewing and its appearance in patients' mental status. Then we discuss interviewing techniques that might be most helpful with patients showing that difficulty, and how a given technique can best be integrated into the interview. We recommend a progression in five steps:

Step 1: Listen.   This step allows the interviewer to recognize the patient's mental status and identify his exact type of difficulty.

Step 2: Tag.   In this step, the patient is made aware that the interviewer is noticing a difficulty.

Step 3: Confront.   During this step, the interviewer signals to the patient that there is a difficulty that needs to be discussed.

Step 4: Solve.   During this step, the interviewer implements a technique thought to be the most effective for resolving the patient's difficulty.

Step 5: Approve.   In this step, the interviewer makes the patient realize the advantage of having overcome his difficulty.

We demonstrate each technique in patient interviews. We highlight the interviewing strategy and not the authenticity of the individual case. Our cases are prototypes of psychiatric pathology.

We have found that gender influences the course of interviews; thus, because the cases that appear in this book are to some extent real cases, and the dialogue, actual dialogue, we have been careful about retaining the original gender of the interviewer. Most of the interviews were conducted by E. Othmer; in these cases we therefore have kept the male gender for the interviewer. However, we have taught and observed female interviewers in situations that resemble some of our own cases; therefore, in those cases in which we have drawn on these interviews, we have used the female gender for the interviewer. For the patients, the gender of the patient in the original interview has been retained. However, to ensure the noninterview portion of the text reads smoothly, we have chosen to switch genders as each new topic is introduced in the text.

We hope this introduction gives you a framework from which to consider the interviews with various types of difficult patients.

PART I

SYMPTOM LANGUAGE

INTRODUCTION TO PART I

SYMPTOM LANGUAGE

Patients who show the use of symptom language verbalize somatic symptoms and display signs that are medically unexplained, such as pain in different body sites, and gastrointestinal, sexual or reproductive, and pseudoneurological symptoms. In the absence of any physical evidence of a cognitive disorder, they report amnesia, derealization, depersonalization, and disruption of their identity. They show avoidance behavior toward situations that others judge to be relatively safe, and emotional detachment from people close to them without evidence that these people ever insulted or hurt them. In other words, they show symptoms that are not the result of a currently identifiable general medical condition or of a psychological noxious stimulus. The disorders that are characterized by such symptoms are somatoform disorders, dissociative disorders, and posttraumatic stress disorder (classified as an anxiety disorder in DSM-IV [American Psychiatric Association 1994]).

In the case of somatoform and dissociative disorders, a general medical condition that could account for the reported symptoms is absent. In the case of posttraumatic stress disorder, a current threat that could explain avoidance of situations and people cannot be identified. According to DSM-IV (American Psychiatric Association 1994), the onset or exacerbation of the reported symptoms appears to be associated with psychological factors and conflicts that show their impact by medical symptoms, including neurological ones, and often by profound avoidance behavior. Thus, these patients express themselves in the form of symptoms rather than in descriptions of their conflicts. Therefore, the use of a symptom language is the unifying feature of the disorders discussed in Part I.

This common feature is illustrated by the comorbidity of these disorders.

3

For instance, the symptomatology of two somatoform disorders (e.g., somatization disorder and conversion disorder) and one of the dissociative disorders (e.g., dissociative identity disorder) overlap (Martin 1994, in press). For example, 40%–70% of patients with dissociative identity disorder show conversion symptoms (Coons et al. 1988; Putnam et al. 1986; Ross 1990), and 35% of patients with dissociative identity disorder have symptoms that fulfill criteria for somatization disorder (Ross et al. 1989). Conversion symptoms are part of the diagnostic criteria for somatization disorder. In Guze et al.'s (1971) study, which used criteria that did not require the presence of conversion symptoms, over 90% of patients with "definite" hysteria (i.e., somatization disorder) had at least one conversion symptom, and almost 80% had several conversion symptoms. At least two dissociative symptoms that are part of the diagnostic criteria for posttraumatic stress disorder link this disorder with the dissociative disorders—that is, dissociative flashbacks of the traumatic episode (criterion B3 of posttraumatic stress disorder) and dissociative amnesia for important aspects of the trauma (criterion C3 of posttraumatic stress disorder). Family and twin studies have indicated that the tendency to report conversion symptoms, to have dissociative identity symptoms, to experience posttraumatic stress, and to somatize is at least partially inherited (American Psychiatric Association 1994).

Manifestations of somatoform and dissociative disorders—in contrast to those of factitious disorders and malingering—are not under the patient's voluntary control (Martin and Yutzy 1994). Clinicians accept the symptoms of posttraumatic avoidance also as not being under voluntary control but as being an expression of pathological anxiety that may be associated with dissociative flashbacks.

For conversion disorder, pain disorder, dissociative identity disorder, somatization disorder, and posttraumatic stress disorder, a reciprocal relationship between the physical symptoms experienced and the psychogenic factors is considered. In DSM-IV, it is required that these disorders significantly impair social or occupational functioning. Conversely, the DSM-IV diagnostic criteria for conversion disorder, pain disorder, and posttraumatic stress disorder include psychological factors; these factors are judged to be associated with the initiation or exacerbation of these disorders. Furthermore, 85% of patients with dissociative identity disorder and 50% of patients with somatization disorder reported childhood sexual abuse; these occurrence rates are significantly higher than the 15% incidence of sexual abuse reported by patients with mood disorders (Martin, in press). Thus DSM-IV diagnostic criteria and research show an association between psychological factors previously occurring in patients with somatoform and dissociative disorders as well as posttraumatic stress disorder. Yet patients who have these disorders tend to emphasize their present somatic, conversion, and dissociative symptoms, or their avoidance behavior in posttraumatic stress disorder, but are unable or unwilling to recognize and explore the associated psychological factors. For somatoform and dissociative disorders, these patients consider their symptoms as evidence of a general medical condition rather than as symptoms associated with psychological factors.

Thus, patients who have somatization disorder emphasize the somatic nature of their disorder and often angrily refute psychological factors as responsible for their symptoms. For example, patients who have conversion disorder do not seem aware that their pseudoneurological disability is related to a demand they cannot meet. Patients with dissociative disorder frequently report amnesia for any precipitating events. They do not report an association of a current stressor with their dissociative state. The same is true for many patients with posttraumatic stress disorder who may experience elements of a trauma in recurrent, involuntary flashbacks, nightmares, and memories. They point to a past trauma to explain their current avoidances and anxieties rather than focusing on difficulties in their current life situation—yet they are unable or unwilling to review that trauma in detail. All these patients express their distress with somatic symptoms rather than with psychological complaints.

Patients' anxiety in or their inability or resistance to evaluating all aspects of their psychiatric disorder, especially the psychological factors, is the difficulty that you experience in the interview with such patients. A correct diagnosis of the patient's coping deficit is hampered by two obstacles. First, the symptoms conceal rather than elucidate the psychological coping deficit. Second, the symptom language expresses the patient's inability or unwillingness to discuss his problem with a mental health professional. The patient may prefer to speak with an internist (e.g., in the case of somatization disorder) or with a neurologist (e.g., in the case of conversion disorder and dissociative disorder). The patient with dissociative identity disorder—unless currently experiencing disabling symptoms—may not feel the need for any help at all. The patient with posttraumatic stress disorder may avoid talking to anyone about the trauma. However, a patient's inability or reluctance to discuss psychological aspects of his disorder does not validate Stekel's (1943) concept of somatization as a bodily disorder that expresses a deep-seated neurosis. Such a causal relationship has so far not been established.

It is the interviewer's task to recognize the patient's symptoms as an expression of her problems with coping and to help her directly discuss those anxieties and problems. Validating the patient's symptoms, hypnotizing the patient to bring out interpersonal conflicts, probing the patient's suppressed memory with free association, and helping the patient recall trauma by imaging and emotional pacing are strategies you may use. These interviewing techniques allow you to examine for psychological factors and traumatic events that may be associated with the patient's disorder, independent of the question of whether or not those factors are psychogenically contributing to the occurrence, onset, or course of the disorder.

The term *uncovering techniques* has been used for some of these techniques, such as free association, hypnosis, and the amobarbital or lorazepam interview. When we use the word *uncover*, we do not imply that the technique reveals etiologic, psychological factors, but that it merely reveals thought contents that the patient previously could not or would not report to the interviewer.

CHAPTER 1

CONVERSION

Summary

Patients with conversion disorder present with a deficit of the motor system (e.g., limb paralysis) or sensory system (e.g., blindness). These symptoms cannot be explained by a neurological or general medical condition. They reflect the patient's understanding of the nervous system (i.e., they differ from signs indicating physical injury to the nervous system).

Standard interviewing techniques are not effective in disclosing the underlying purpose of the conversion symptom. Hypnosis may help to uncover precipitating events and sometimes the purpose of the conversion and may reverse it.

◆ ◆ ◆ ◆ ◆

The point meriting special attention is the condition of the mind at different stages as results . . . from hypnotism. At one stage it gives an extraordinary power of concentration of thought . . . whereas, at another stage, the discursive, or imaginative faculties are excited into full play, and thus the most expanded, bright, and glowing scenes and images are presented to the fervid imagination.

James Braid
Neurypnology (1843)

◆ ◆ ◆ ◆ ◆

1. What Is Conversion?

According to DSM-IV (American Psychiatric Association 1994), *conversion* is a pseudoneurological phenomenon; *conversion disorder* occurs at a rate of 11–300 cases per 100,000 in the general population and in 1%–3% of outpatient referrals to mental health clinics. Conversion represents a medically unexplainable apparent malfunction of the voluntary neuromuscular system (e.g., as in paralysis) or the sensory system (e.g., as in loss of pain perception). Such deficiencies do not correspond to anatomic pathways but reflect the patient's understanding of body functioning. For example, a patient claims loss of pain perception in his right hand although his temperature perception is intact. Anatomically, both modalities are transmitted by the same peripheral nerves; one cannot lose the ability to experience pain yet retain the ability to perceive temperature variation.

During a patient interview, negative and positive conversion signs may emerge. Negative signs signify a loss of function (e.g., paralysis, urinary retention, deafness, anesthesia); positive signs signify pathological productions (e.g., pseudoseizures, tremors, bizarre movements, hallucinations, paresthesias).

Following the 1837 concept of the surgeon Sir Benjamin Brodie, Freud (1924) reintroduced the term *conversion* in 1894 to describe the process by which a patient transforms an emotion into a physical manifestation (Ziegler et al. 1960). In DSM-IV, the occurrence of clinically significant conversion symptoms in the absence of a superseding somatization disorder is considered a disorder.

Recent research provides three findings relevant for conversion. First, patients with a conversion symptom may show neurological disorders involving the same body part affected by the symptom. This finding is compatible with the patient's exploitation of the deficit to avoid a task or duty. The patient may simply have exaggerated a legitimate but clinically occult neurological disorder to serve her need to escape that task (Willerman and Cohen 1990). Alternatively, the neurological deficit may result from disuse atrophy. In a follow-up study (Spierings et al. 1990), 52 of 84 (62%) hospitalized children who had been diagnosed as having a conversion disorder showed a history of a general medical condition (apart from normal childhood diseases). Therefore, when you face a patient with conversion disorder, you should explore whether a neurological or other general medical disorder may be facilitating the conversion (Gatfield and Guze 1962; Stefánsson et al. 1976). Furthermore, 45% of the family members of the 84 children showed organic disorder; 44%, psychosomatic diseases; and 26%, psychiatric disorders (Spierings et al. 1990). Therefore, you should assess the presence of both stress and family dysfunction, as these have been reported in the families of children with conversion disorder (Siegel and Barthel 1986).

Second, historically, psychological factors have been intertwined with the concept of conversion (Martin 1992). They were included as diagnostic criteria in DSM-III (American Psychiatric Association 1980) and DSM-III-R (American Psychiatric Association 1987) for conversion disorder. Yet the empirically established power of these factors to distinguish a conversion disorder from a physical disorder is weak (Cloninger 1987). Raskin et al. (1966) successfully distinguished 32 patients with conversion symptoms from 7 patients with physical disorders, all referred from a neurological service because of a suspected conversion reaction, "by judgments about whether or not the symptoms were being used to solve a conflict brought about by a precipitating stress" (Cloninger 1987, p. 248). Yet those judgments were confounded by the researchers' observations that the patients had histories of medically unexplained somatic symptoms in 26 of 32 cases. Therefore, it is questionable whether the interviewer's criterion—namely, that a neurological symptom precipitated by stress and without apparent somatic findings and serving conflict resolution—would help to identify that symptom as a conversion symptom. Regardless of this argument, as interviewer you may use an uncovering technique for the suspected conversion symptom because this technique can have two positive effects: 1) it can resolve the symptom, and 2) it can lead you to a conflict the patient has, whether or not that conflict is etiologically solely responsible for the development of the conversion symptom.

Third, Breuer and Freud (1957), Charcot (Guillain 1959), and others (Janet 1907, 1911; Babinski [Gauld 1992]) observed that patients with conversion disorder can be easily hypnotized. Thus, some theoreticians believe that the psychogenetic mechanism of the conversion dysfunction is autosuggestion or autohypnosis. However, not all subjects who can be easily hypnotized develop conversion symptoms; therefore, suggestibility is a necessary but not a sufficient condition for the development of conversion symptoms. It is advisable to test a conversion disorder patient's trance capacity or hypnotizability (see below) whether you plan to use the hypnotic interview or not. Even if you do not use the hypnotic interview, the test can be used as confirmation of the presence of one necessary condition for conversion—suggestibility.

Interviewing patients with conversion disorder poses unique difficulties. According to the DSM-IV criterion B for conversion disorder, to make the diagnosis the interviewer must establish that psychological factors, conflicts, or other stressors are associated with the conversion symptoms.

When encountering conversion disorder in a patient, you are thus faced with two problems. First, you must elucidate the precipitating event, if any, that may be associated with the conversion in order to diagnose the disorder with some certainty. Second, you must exclude patients with neurological disorders, patients with other general medical conditions, patients under the direct influence of a substance, or patients acting according to culturally sanctioned behavior or experience (criterion D). Such patients may be suggestible and develop additional conversion symptoms.

In children and some patients with low intelligence, you can often reconstruct the purpose of the conversion by eliciting an account of the precipitating event. In most adults, however, such an approach will not work. Patients are not conscious of a conflict. They believe in the medical nature of their symptom or sign. They do not feign it (criterion C). Patients may act vague, anxious, and hostile toward you. Therefore, you have to use disorder-specific methods to detect the preceding, associated psychological factors.

2. Conversion in the Mental Status

Patients who have conversion disorder may show four characteristics:

1. An exaggerated emotion converted into an impairment in response to a specific demand
2. *La belle indifference* to the resulting impairment
3. A lack of psychological understanding of the impairment
4. A lack of assertiveness in synchronizing other people's demands with their own needs so that a conversion reaction becomes necessary

None of these characteristics may discriminate the conversion disorder from a general medical condition.

> Mrs. X. brings her 5-year-old son, Peter, to the outpatient clinic because at night he can only walk on his knees because he experiences paralysis in his legs. This sign is not explainable by any neurological defect; it represents Peter's understanding of a neurological disability.

In children and adolescents, paralysis is a predominant conversion symptom, as are gait problems and seizures (Lehmkuhl et al. 1989). For children under age 10 years, conversion is seen equally in boys and girls. At later ages, it is seen predominantly in females (Spierings et al. 1990).

Let us now explore how the four characteristics of conversion apply in this example.

Exaggerated response

> Peter shares a bedroom with his 8-year-old sister, Sara. Every night, after Sara has finished reading, she asks Peter to climb out of his bed (even after he has fallen asleep), walk to the light switch, and turn off the ceiling light. Peter does not like to be awakened, nor does he want to leave his warm bed to comply with his sister's demand. He is so annoyed over this chore that he develops the conversion symptom of walking on his knees. Both his anger and his knee walking are an exaggerated response to his dominating sister's request.

Spierings et al. (1990) found that 88% of hospitalized children with conversion disorder show a psychogenic etiology similar to the one in this case.

La belle indifference

> When asked whether he felt very sick or scared by the weakness in his legs, Peter smiles and says, "Oh, I feel fine." He does not appear to be concerned when told that he might not be able to play soccer or baseball or any other sports any more if his paralysis spreads. He lacks depth of emotion. He tolerates his disability with nonchalance.

The theatrical presentation of such a disability, combined with *indifference,* was first described by Pierre Janet (1859–1947; Janet 1911). However, a patient with a general medical condition may also show a stoic attitude, or if a patient has lesions of the nondominant, parietal cortical hemisphere, he may develop *anosognosia*—the inability to recognize that he has a disease or bodily defect.

Lack of psychological insight.   When walking on his knees, Peter could not oblige his sister's demand because he was unable to reach the light switch. He did not feel that he had voluntary control over his paralysis or that he was malingering. He believed in his paralysis and did not see that its purpose appeared obvious to the professional.

When patients have conversion disorder, they usually deny any connection to a stressor, even though they themselves have reported the sequence of stressor and conversion. They do not connect what the professional bystander clearly recognizes as cause and effect. These patients' introspective ability—their insight—is poor. In our example, the 5-year-old boy could claim to be disabled because he was able to overlook the purpose of the conversion.

Nonassertiveness. The boy's paralysis allowed him to refuse his sister's demand without having to oppose her directly or to complain to his mother about her. The paralysis allowed him to pretend that he wanted to oblige his sister's wishes but that he was just not able to do so. Rather than asserting himself, he expressed his wishes through conversion. Such a reaction helped him to avoid confrontation. The solution of his conflict by conversion was in keeping with his lack of assertiveness.

In this particular case, Peter regained the capability to walk on his feet after the interviewer made him understand the purpose behind his knee walking and after the mother arranged for Sara to have a bedside table lamp.

Hypnotizability

Scales have been developed to measure hypnotizability, such as the Stanford Scales of Hypnotic Susceptibility and the Harvard Group Scale of Hypnotic Susceptibility (Orne and Dinges 1989). These scales contain four classes of suggestions: ideomotor tasks, challenges, cognitive tasks, and memory tasks.

The *ideomotor tasks* are usually the easiest way to determine a patient's hypnotizability. We use three ideomotor tasks:

- *Sway test.* Have the patient stand up and close his eyes. Ask him to imagine that he is standing at the end of a board and that another person begins lifting the other end of the board causing him to fall backward. You stand behind the patient and catch him. A successful test tells you how much the patient trusts you. If he falls backward immediately, you probably have a hypnotizable patient who is willing to work with you.
- *Pendulum test* (using the Chevreul pendulum; Wright and Wright 1987). Give the patient a foot-long string with a ring or weight attached to it. Then ask the patient to hold the string up with a nonsupported arm while sitting on a chair with her legs slightly apart. Ask her to imagine that the ring starts to swing in a circle that becomes larger and larger. First you give the patient this suggestion; later ask her to give herself the

suggestion. This test measures the patient's autosuggestibility with minimum influence by you.

- *Eye test.* Ask the patient to look at your index finger, which you hold a foot away from the patient and a foot above the patient's eye level. Ask the patient to focus on your index finger without raising his head. Ask him not to blink but to imagine how tired his eyelids are becoming, that they are becoming heavier and heavier, so heavy that they close. If you can only see the half-moon of white sclera slowly disappearing under the eyelids (in other words, if the patient's eyes roll up), the patient is hypnotizable. The eye test shows good correlation with a more elaborate test for hypnotizability, Spiegel's Extensive Hypnotic Induction Profile (Spiegel 1975).

As a *challenge task,* we use the finger lock test. This complements the sway test because it measures the degree of the patient's cooperativeness. A patient who feels she has to oppose your authority will most likely fail the finger lock test because you challenge her willpower. To pass the test, the patient must submit her will to the power of your suggestion. The patient folds her hands and is asked to imagine two forces that laterally press the fingers together so that they cannot be pulled apart. Then, the patient is challenged to separate them. If she has difficulty doing this, the patient is suggestible.

A *cognitive task* that measures hypnotizability is to suggest to the patient that he close both eyes and then see and relive a suggested scene, such as sitting on a balcony experiencing a beautiful sunset. The patient who can fully visualize the scene and describe details can be considered suggestible.

A *memory task* involves giving a patient several items to recall, then telling her that her memory will be blocked and she will not be able to remember all of the items. If she cannot recall the items, you have established a high degree of suggestibility.

In summary, the faster the patient can follow the suggestion (i.e., the shorter the assimilation time to realize your suggestion), the more hypnotizable the patient is and the more appropriate it is for you to attempt a hypnotic interview in one 50-minute session.

3. Technique: Hypnosis

Hypnosis works in detecting the conflict behind a conversion symptom because it uses the same mechanism for resolving the conversion symptom that produced the conversion symptom in the first place. Under hypnosis the patient will report the conflict that previously proved elusive while the patient was conscious.

The hypnotic interview is most useful in patients with conversion, dissociation, posttraumatic flashbacks, and somatization. It may help patients with panic disorder and eating disorders. However, there is no evidence that patients who have problems with alcohol or drug abuse, major depression, mania, schizophrenia, or delusional disorder will benefit from a hypnotic interview.

When you use the hypnotic interviewing technique, proceed in two acts: first, induce hypnosis and bring the patient to a certain depth; second, interview the patient under hypnosis to detect the patient's intentions for the conversion.

Introducing Hypnosis

Before using hypnosis, you have to know what it is and what it is not. *Hypnosis* is a technique for inducing a special state of consciousness. In that state, the patient's concentration is increasingly focused on suggested images, ideomotor performances, and sensory perceptions. Memory and awareness are curtailed or enlarged to allow a journey into the past or future. This state is called a *trance*. Hypnosis may lead to *hypermnesia* (increased memory), but this memory may not be accurate even though the patient is confident about the accuracy of his recall (Sheehan 1988). Hypnosis is not a technique to induce sleep, even though the name hypnosis comes from the Greek word *hypnos* meaning "sleep." During hypnosis, the patient displays alpha waves on the electroencephalogram characteristic of wakefulness, not theta waves, delta waves, K-complexes, or sleep spindles that indicate sleep (Dynes 1947).

When considering the use of hypnosis, ask yourself these three questions: 1) How hypnotizable is the patient? 2) How should the hypnosis be induced? 3) How deep should the hypnosis be?

1. How hypnotizable is the patient? With typically 50 minutes available to complete a hypnotic interview, you do not want to fail with a patient who is difficult to hypnotize. As we have pointed out, most patients who have a conversion or dissociative dysfunction are easy to hypnotize, but they may experience an authority conflict with you and resist your hypnotic skills. Therefore, it is advisable to test the patient's hypnotizability or trance capacity beforehand. Testing hypnotizability is also a good way to tune the patient in to the hypnotic process.

2. How should hypnosis be induced? After you have determined that the patient is hypnotizable, select the method that best suits the comfort level of both you and the patient. Hypnotists have described a number of induction techniques, including progressive relaxation, number progression, eye fixation, arm levitation, guided imagery, sleep to hypnotic trance (Wright and Wright 1987), and autogenic training (Schultz 1969). A brief description of these seven methods follows.

Progressive relaxation teaches the patient to focus on the muscles of each body part, progressing from foot to scalp, by suggesting that the patient tighten and relax each part.

Number progression combines an image (e.g., the patient sitting in a comfortable chair on a moving sidewalk such as those seen in airports) with posts numbered from 20 to 1. The chair moving past the decreasing numbers represents the patient's progression toward increasing relaxation, preparing the patient for the task to come (Wright and Wright 1987).

In *eye fixation,* hypnosis is induced by asking the patient to fixate her eyes on some defined point, such as a light or the hypnotherapist's finger. The hypnotherapist then suggests relieving this eye tension by lowering the eyelids and by general body and mind relaxation (Wright and Wright 1987).

Arm levitation impresses on the patient the idea that he can experience hypnosis through unintentional arm raising as the result of some thought or image suggested by the therapist (Wright and Wright 1987).

Guided imagery is used to induce trance in patients who can imagine well. The hypnotherapist suggests that the patient imagine a setting where she feels most secure and peaceful (e.g., at home) (Wright and Wright 1987).

Sleep to hypnotic trance is used in children in combination with a therapeutic daytime program. The therapist (or parent trained as a therapist) whispers suggestions regarding a desirable daytime behavior into the child's ear during the time of transition between sleep and wakening (Wright and Wright 1987).

We have modified the autogenic training method developed by Schultz (1969) to induce hypnosis and autohypnosis (see detailed description below in Step 4a, "Induction of Trance"). This method parallels physiological changes during relaxation and sleep onset. You and the patient can monitor the degree to which he assimilates the suggestions. The responsibility of carrying out the suggestion lies with the patient, using his concentration and imagination. You direct the action away from your authority. For the novice interviewer this method is easy. Because it uses simple suggestions (e.g., experiencing the weight of the limbs), it bears little resemblance to fairground hypnotic shows and thus minimizes the risk that it is mistaken as a magic trick. The patient can practice the method successfully at home. The progressive steps allow the patient or hypnotherapist to gauge the completeness of relaxation and depth of hypnosis. A demonstration of this technique follows.

Ask the patient to sit comfortably. Then approach the patient with two-part directives. The first part steers the patient's attention to a specific body part (e.g., head, arm, leg) and body sensation (e.g., weight, temperature, breathing, heartbeat). The second part suggests a direction toward which the sensation will develop:

weight	→	heavy
temperature	→	warm
breathing	→	slow, regular
heartbeat	→	strong, slow, regular

The patient needs to be given a method by which to provide feedback. Ask the patient to raise his right index finger when he becomes aware of a specific sensation, and then ask him to raise the finger again when the sensations develop in the suggested direction.

Start with the head. First, let the patient notice that his head has weight. You might say,

Let your head hang down. Notice a pull of your muscles on your neck. Feel that your head has weight. Only when your neck muscles are really relaxed can you feel the weight of your head. If you feel the weight, raise your right index finger.

If the patient raises his finger, continue by suggesting heaviness:

You will notice that your head gets heavier and heavier. The more relaxed your neck muscles are, the heavier your head feels. Do you feel how your head gets heavier and heavier? If you do, raise your right index finger.

Tell the patient to continue thinking,

My head is heavy.

Use the same two-part directive for the patient's shoulders, arms, hands, and legs:

Your shoulders, arms, hands, and head have a weight. If you feel the weight, raise your finger.
As you relax your legs they will feel heavier and heavier. If you feel the weight, raise your finger.

Then ask the patient to keep thinking,

My shoulders, arms, hands, and legs are heavy.

Patients with dissociation or conversion reactions usually have no difficulty carrying out these suggestions. If they do, work on one part of one extremity at a time.

The next directive focuses on body temperature. Say to the patient,

Your body has a temperature. If you can feel the temperature in any part of your body, raise your finger. Now, feel the temperature at your belly area. If you feel the temperature at your belly area, raise your finger.
Notice that your belly area feels warm. Raise your finger if you feel it. Let the warmth spread. If you feel it spreading, raise your finger.
Now you feel the temperature in your arms and hands. If you feel the temperature, raise your finger.
Let the warmth spread in your arms and fingers. When you feel that your arms and hands get warmer and warmer, raise your finger. Keep thinking, "My hands and arms are warm."

Then, repeat the same directive for the legs. Summarize the command by saying,

Now your whole body feels heavy and warm. Raise your finger if you feel that your body is heavy and warm.

At this level of relaxation you can usually direct the patient to tell you in clear sequence how his conversion first developed (see Step 4b, "The Hypnotic Interview," below).

Some patients need a deeper level of relaxation to reconstruct the "purpose" of their conversion symptoms. Patients who experience anxiety and panic attacks, in particular, benefit from focusing on breathing. Tell the patient to listen to and feel his breathing,

Notice how you breathe. Your body "breathes" you. It breathes you. Recognize how it breathes you. Let it breathe you. If you have the feeling that it breathes you, raise your finger.

At this point you may notice that the patient starts to breathe more deeply and regularly even though you have not suggested it. Tie into this observation:

> Notice how your body breathes you deeply and regularly. It breathes you slower and slower, deeper and deeper, and more evenly and smoothly. Keep thinking it breathes you deeply and regularly. Slow, deep, and regular. If you get that feeling, raise your right index finger.

After the patient has been breathing deeply and regularly for 1–2 minutes, direct his attention to his heartbeat:

> Feel your heartbeat. Somewhere in your body you will be able to feel your heartbeat. You may feel your pulse in your arms and hands. You may feel your pulse in your neck, or you may feel your heartbeat directly in your chest. If you have found your pulse or heartbeat, raise your right index finger.
> Can you feel your heartbeat directly? If you feel your heart directly, raise your finger.
> Now notice how your heart starts to beat strongly, slowly, and regularly. Your heart beats strongly, slowly, and regularly. If you can feel how your heart beats slowly, strongly, and regularly, raise your finger.

At this point, summarize the relaxation state to the patient:

> Now you feel heavy and warm. Your body is breathing you slowly. Your breathing is deep and regular and your heart beat is slow, strong, and regular. If you have all these feelings, raise your right finger.

If a patient can visualize and realize all these suggestions, he has reached a state of trance. Now the patient can realize posthypnotic suggestions such as

> When our session is over, I will ask you the question, "What time is it?" In response, you will ask me for my white coat. You will not be able to know why you ask me that question.

If the patient carries out the posthypnotic suggestion, you know he has fully cooperated with you. Posthypnotic suggestions are easily carried out by patients who have dissociation or conversion disorders.

3. How deep should the hypnosis be? Hypnotherapists measure the depth of hypnotic trance by the degree of suggestibility the patient demonstrates. There are three levels: light, middle, or deep.

A *light trance* is recognized by the completion of ideomotor changes, such as the patient's arm floating up or getting heavy. This stage of relaxation is often sufficient to allow the patient to revisualize the circumstances that activated the conversion dysfunction. The *middle level* has, in addition, sensory changes (e.g., paresthesias, analgesias, anesthesias), partial amnesias, and simple posthypnotic compliance. The *deep level* shows posthypnotic compliance; visual, auditory, and tactile hallucinations; time distortions; age regression; hypermnesia or selective amnesia; profound anesthesia; and open-eye trance (Spiegel 1975).

The Hypnotic Interview

In the hypnotic interview, we follow the 10 principles emphasized by hypnotherapists (Wright and Wright 1987):

1. Use appropriate language. Use the same words as the patient does to describe her disability, her feelings related to it, and the details of the precipitating event.
2. Step back into the concrete situation. Have the patient recall in a very concrete way the scene and the situation under which she first experienced the conversion sign. The patient has to relive the very situation, not just talk vaguely about faded memories. The patient needs to see the situation—the physical surroundings, the people involved; she must hear them talk, experience their smell, and feel the temperature of the situation. Only when the patient is in sensory touch with the situation can you ask her to move on.
3. Accentuate the positive. Express your suggestions and guidance in a positive way. For example, tell the patient that her mind is fully absorbed with what happened shortly before the conversion started. Avoid double negative statements like "You will not be distraught," because the patient may hone in on the negative elements and become distracted. Instead, stress the positive: "You will be calm." Be firm and assuring about what you want the patient to do. Use the term "try" only when you in fact want the patient to fail. For example, if the patient recalls a scene clearly in detail, you may firmly anchor this "stepping back into the scene" by telling the patient, "Try to wipe the images out of your mind. You notice you can't do it. To the contrary, they become stronger."
4. Link suggestion to recall. Connect the patient's realized suggestions (such as the heavy feeling that was part of the autogenic training induction

technique) with the scenes that you want the patient to recall: "As you feel heavier and heavier, you sink back into the past."

5. Offer a reward of positive feelings. As the patient remembers past problems and conflicts, tell her that the clarity of her recall makes her feel good, gives her control, and lets her see things in a new light. This makes her want to reexperience in depth the pain, insult, or ridicule that caused the conversion symptoms. Now the patient will understand what happened; she can follow through at her own pace, with you at her side, in the safety of your office.

6. Offer reassurance. Use direct and indirect reassurances.

   Direct reassurance: "As you remember past problems and past insults, you will be safe. You will be able to control the pain and the embarrassment."

   Indirect reassurance: "Some patients may feel thirsty after going through the trauma again. I will get you something that you may need. Would you like coffee, tea, milk, or juice afterward? Let me help you with that." Indirect reassurance distracts the patient from the anger or pain of the embarrassment that she may have felt when the conversion first developed. She will reexperience the trauma with a tangible, oral reward.

7. Establish anchors for recall. These serve as reference points to which you can return later. As the past event comes back, such anchors become stronger: "The heavier and warmer you feel now, the heavier and closer the past sinks down in you and you can really see and feel what happened."

8. Repeat suggestions frequently. Reconfirm to the patient the hypnotic suggestions of the autogenic training (as outlined above), such as breathing slowly and regularly, having a slow heartbeat, and being able to visualize more clearly and in more detail what happened when the patient developed the conversion.

9. Use the patient as a guide. Help the patient "own" the hypnotic process and recall: "Because you want to understand what happened when your paralysis first occurred, you are more and more able to follow the strength of your memory. You are more and more able to recall what happened."

10. Put the patient in charge. Use the patient's authority, not yours, to assimilate all suggestions. For example, say, "The better you can imagine, the more you are able to recall." Thus, it is the patient's success, and not yours, when she realizes a suggestion. Similarly, it is the patient's failure, not yours, if it does not work.

Limitations of the Hypnotic Interview

Like any psychotherapeutic or somatic intervention, the hypnotic interview technique has its limitations and contraindications. We agree with some of the limitations identified by Spiegel (1975) and Orne and Dinges (1989).

First, the hypnotic technique affects the patient differently than a standard interview. He may suspend his critical judgment and consequently develop deep dependency feelings for the interviewer. He may display intense emotions and may be more vulnerable to the actions of the interviewer. Thus, use the hypnotic interview only when you are prepared to work with the patient outside of hypnosis at least on an intermediate basis.

Second, if you use the hypnotic interview, monitor your own fantasies of power and control and eliminate those feelings from your interaction with your patient. Avoid hypnotizing patients who indicate they may engage in a power struggle with you. For example, if a patient does not comply with the finger lock test, or cannot unlock the fingers after you have removed the suggestion, you should not induce hypnosis because he may refuse to leave the trance state or may uncontrollably fall into a spontaneous trance. He may incorporate your interaction with him as another part of his conversion or dissociative dysfunction. Hypnotize the patient only after you have established appropriate rapport with him outside of the hypnotic process.

Third, conduct all hypnotic interviews in the spirit of voluntary cooperation. Initiate a hypnotic interview only if during the prehypnotic interview the patient showed that he would be able to appreciate the benefits. Recognize any coercion, explicit or implied, and eliminate it.

No controlled studies are available that show whether hypnosis and continuous free association that give the patient temporary insight into the conversion process actually cure the dysfunction. Case reports do show that assertiveness training may help to replace conversion with more effective coping styles (Willerman and Cohen 1990). However, we do not know how durable the results of such assertiveness training are and to what extent they can be generalized.

4. Five Steps to Reverse Conversion

We interview a patient with conversion symptoms in five steps:

Step 1: Listen. Allow the patient to describe her symptoms in her own words, thus giving her ample opportunity to demonstrate the disability.

Step 2: Tag. Summarize the patient's description of the problem and explore the history of its onset. Elicit situations that seem to worsen or improve it. Doing so may give you some idea about the purpose of the conversion symptom for the patient.

If you use free association and your patient becomes evasive, avoid pushing for a clear, logical history about the development of the patient's dysfunction. Instead, approach indirectly. Without interrupting, let the patient talk about her friends, family members, and employer who were around when the conversion first started. Encourage her to talk about her likes and dislikes. In short, use free association to gather the puzzle pieces. In our experience, autosuggestive and relaxation techniques invariably help the patient report the conflict that precipitated the conversion. (For more details on the use of this method see Chapter 2, "Dissociation.")

Step 3: Confront. Tell the patient that her disability is not based on any true nerve damage but is brought on by a self-hypnotic process triggered by stress. The patient may act very surprised or become anxious or angry. At this point, introduce the idea that a special technique called "hypnosis" is available to explore and reverse the conversion.

Step 4: Solve. Use the same mechanism that produces the symptom—in this case the autohypnotic mechanism—to resolve the conversion. Resolving occurs in two parts: preparing the patient by inducing a trance (Step 4a) and conducting the hypnotic interview (Step 4b).

Step 4a: Trance induction. Describe the hypnotic technique to the patient. Tell her that patients with her type of problem are often very talented at relaxation exercises that help them attain a trancelike, hypnotic state. Explain that this trance often sharpens the memory so that she will recall scenes and events otherwise hidden from her. Tell her that she can only be hypnotized if she is gifted enough to imagine the things you suggest and if she wants to be hypnotized. Tell her that you are interested in a cooperative venture, not in a contest of wills. This strategy places the success of the hypnotic procedure into the patient's hands.

Once the patient agrees to try hypnosis, slow down the process. "Not so fast," you may say. "We first want to find out whether you have a good ability to imagine things. Let's test it." Then introduce the sway test, the pendulum test, the eye test, and the finger lock test. These tests prepare the patient for hypnotic induction. If the patient passes the tests, start with the hypnotic process.

Step 4b: The hypnotic interview. During the trance, ask the patient to visualize when her conversion symptom first occurred. From your prehypnotic interview you will usually have some clue about the onset and the purpose of the symptoms. Direct her to visualize that scene.

Tell me what you saw when you first lost the feeling in both of your legs.

Usually the patient can give a good description of that situation.

Let the story go on frame by frame, like a movie. Tell me your feelings and thoughts. Tell me what you feel, see, and hear. Tell me what you think.

After the patient has given you a clear description of how the symptom came about, tell her she will keep this understanding in mind when she emerges from the state of relaxation. Then let the patient know that the hypnotic interview is nearly over.

You have accomplished what you wanted to do. You know how you developed your disturbance. Now you want to leave the state of trance. If you want to wake up, take a deep breath, and feel how the breath refreshes you. Take another, deeper breath and hold it in. Now you feel fresh and relaxed. Take your third and even deeper breath; hold it and, as you release the air, shake your body and open your eyes. Now sense how fresh and relaxed your mind and body feel.

After the patient opens her eyes, ask her how she is feeling. You expect the cooperative patient to describe a state of freshness and relaxation as you have suggested.

Step 5: Approve. Consider that some resentment of having lost the secret to her symptom could negatively influence the patient's rapport with you. If so, reassure her during this step that she has won an insight and has overcome an ineffective method of coping. Regardless of whether the patient expresses resentment or satisfaction about her newly gained knowledge, reassure her that the new insight helps with diagnosis and therapy. Compliment her on her ability to imagine the sensations that you had evoked for her and express your satisfaction that she was able to follow your hypnotic suggestions:

You were able to relax yourself, which allowed you to open your mind and remember what happened to you when you lost the feeling in your legs. We've had a good session. I'm looking forward to our next meeting.

5. Interview: Identifying the Psychological Factors Under Hypnosis

The time: 8:00 A.M. *The setting:* Grand rounds in a neurology department at a southern university.

The resident presents the case of Mr. M., a 27-year-old, single, white male who is paralyzed on the right side of his body. The paralysis began 3 weeks earlier when the patient was bowling with his father, brothers, and sister. The patient had picked up the bowling ball but when he tried to throw it, his right arm went stiff, his right leg collapsed at the knee, and he fell down. The family tried to help him up, but he fell down again. He did not lose consciousness or report pain. On the contrary, he expressed surprise about what had happened to him. The family tried to help the patient walk with assistance, but his right knee locked and he dragged his leg. When standing unassisted, his knee would buckle and he would fall down.

The family brought him home and put him to bed. Several days later, he was able to leave the bed but he still dragged his stiffened right leg behind him. Also, his right arm hung flaccidly at his side. The patient claimed that he could not stay up for a long time because he would feel weak and tired. He had full control over excretory functions and his breathing was regular.

His neurological history showed a hospitalization for seizures; however, the electroencephalogram findings at the time were negative. A neurologist who had witnessed a seizure had diagnosed it as a pseudoseizure.

Mr. M. was a slow learner who had required special education. He had never had any behavioral problems nor any history of alcohol abuse or tobacco use. Before the onset of the paralysis, he helped his father and brothers on the farm.

Mr. M.'s physical examination was unremarkable. The neurological examination showed symmetrical reflexes in both upper extremities, even though the patient claimed that he could not move his right arm and that it felt weak. The reflexes in his right leg were difficult to evaluate because the knee joint and Achilles tendon were tense. The patient claimed only a slightly decreased sensitivity to pinprick on his right side, excluding the face, but the right-sided cremasteric and abdominal reflexes were present.

At this point in his presentation, the resident asked the nurse's aide to bring the patient in on the stretcher. To his surprise, the nurse's aide indicated that the patient could walk. The aide brought a normally walking patient into the room. (R = resident; I = interviewer; P = patient)

R: [With astonishment on his face] What has happened, Mr. M.? You are walking?
P: [Obediently] Yes, sir. I am.
R: How come?
P: [With surprise] Don't you know? The psychologist came last night. He made me walk again.
R: How did he do that?
P: [With nonchalance] Well, he hypnotized me and when I came out of it, I was walking.

Here is what had happened the previous evening at the hospital.

Step 1: Listen

1. I: Hi, I'm Dr. T. What seems to be your problem?
   P: I can't walk very well.
2. I: Can you get out of bed and show me how you walk?
   P: [Sits up in his high-legged hospital bed, his right leg sticking away from his body sideways in a 45° angle. He swings his left leg over the edge of the bed and slides out from under the covers. The interviewer notices that Mr. M.'s longjohns have a yellow stain in the crotch area and his right gray sock has a hole over the big toe. His right arm is hanging down flaccidly. He swings his stiff right leg around in a semicircle, stands on it for a moment, then makes a step with his left leg and, dragging his stiff right leg behind him, moves toward the interviewer. Then he swings it forward again and lunges toward the interviewer who catches him before he lands on his chest. A rancid odor permeates the air. The interviewer puts the patient back on his feet and asks him to walk across the room toward the wall. The patient reaches the wall, gives himself a push, turns around, and smiles, showing a missing incisor] Isn't it strange what has happened to my leg and my arm?
3. I: [Also smiling] Yes, it's strange indeed. Tell me exactly what happened.
   P: [The patient rubs his 3-day-old beard and describes how he had suddenly fallen over in the bowling alley. He answers questions about person, time, and place correctly. He recalls three out of three words (pencil, car, watch) immediately, but after 10 minutes can recall only two out of three. With prodding he produces "clock," insisting, "I know it wasn't 'watch'."]

The interviewer and patient so far have good rapport. The interviewer began the interview with one open-ended question and, as the patient related his story, used techniques that encourage continuation, such as asking, "What happened then?" and, "Tell me more!" This was sufficient to make the patient tell his version of the story.

As to mental status, the interviewer noted Mr. M.'s poor hygiene and a nonphysiological, impaired movement of the right leg. The patient's affect reflected amazement rather than concern about the disability. His smile indicated *la belle indifference*. The patient was oriented; his recall and recent memory led the interviewer to suspect that the patient might be simulating a recent memory disturbance by claiming forgetfulness about the third object but coming up with a reply close to the correct answer. (This reminded the interviewer of Ganser's syndrome, in which an individual, such as a prison or jail inmate, tries to fake mental illness by answering questions with approximation [e.g., $2 \times 3 = 5$].)

As to his diagnosis, the interviewer noted that the displayed paralysis was incompatible with any paralysis based on damage to the peripheral or central nervous system. The patient's paralysis appeared to be a product of conversion.

Step 2: Tag

4. I: Tell me what your father and brothers and sister did just before you grabbed the bowling ball.
   P: [Burps, then swallows while thinking. Then he shakes his head and shrugs his shoulders.] Nothing really. [Rolling his eyes backward] I just fell down. [He denies being able to remember what he was thinking or feeling at that moment. He further describes how he just lost his strength, his leg buckled, and from then on he could not walk any more. The patient grimaces, chews his lower lip, and looks at the interviewer. Then he pulls up his right shoulder with the dangling arm, shakes his head, and scratches his crotch.] I really can't remember.
5. I: So you draw a blank when you try to remember what thoughts you had at the moment you fell down?
   P: Yeah, I guess so.

The rapport between the patient and the interviewer remained good. The patient was in good spirits and tried to be cooperative. However, when attempting to learn details, the interviewer ran into a wall of amnesia. Therefore, the interviewer could not reconstruct a possible purpose of the conversion. He realized he would have to use free association or hypnosis to break through the amnestic block.

The patient remained friendly, smiling, and seemingly cooperative in his demeanor. However, his expressive movements gave the impression that he was only acting cooperatively. He did not offer any clues as to a possible conflict. The nonchalant way in which the patient presented his disability, his low IQ as evidenced by his past need for special education, and the demonstrated pseudoneurological deficit are compatible with conversion disorder.

Step 3: Confront

6. I: The neurologist and I both think that you don't have a nerve disorder, but that something in your life brought on your trouble with walking.

P: [With surprise] You mean there's nothing wrong with my nerves? But there must be. You can see I can't walk. [He pushes his tongue through the incisor cavity, releasing a sucking click.]

7. I: Oh, indeed, you have a problem. And we can find out what that problem is all about.

P: Oh yeah?

8. I: Yes. But I will have to put you under hypnosis.

P: Really? Is that dangerous?

9. I: No, it's not dangerous. But you have to have a special gift.

P: What do you mean?

10. I: The gift to be able to imagine what I tell you to imagine. I can't do that imagining for you. You are the one who has to do that. If you can put your mind to it, you can do it.

P: Oh, I was never any good in school. I was never good at doing things right. The teacher always yelled at me. If it's hard, I can't do it.

11. I: This is not schoolwork. It's something between you and me, and you really have been great in showing me your walking problem. I know you'll do a great job.

P: All right . . . okay.

The interviewer introduced himself as an expert who agreed with another expert that the patient did not have a nerve disorder. He offered him a diagnostic impression and a plan of action—a hypnotic interview. The patient accepted this expertise. He showed his trust by following the interviewer's plan without asking for details. His behavior demonstrated that he was assuming an obedient role. His dependency suggested that he was probably easy to hypnotize.

Mr. M.'s responses showed the low self-esteem and low self-confidence of a person who has failed repeatedly and consistently as a student (A. 10). He seemed to equate any demand on him with a school task. The patient's history and mental status were compatible with a diagnosis of borderline intelligence or mental retardation and conversion disorder.

Step 4: Solve

Step 4a: Induction of Hypnosis

12. I: I want you to be aware that, if I hypnotize you, it's not really me who's doing it. You do it yourself. I just help you to hypnotize yourself.

P: [With a soft, hesitant voice and a questioning look on his face] But I've never done that before.

13. I: [Putting his hand on the patient's shoulder and with a slow, calming voice] Well, maybe not on purpose. You just may not have known that you did it. Now, I can help you to hypnotize yourself. But first we have to find out how well you are able to imagine what I tell you. Please sit down in this chair over here.

P: Okay. [He sits down, his right leg stretched far to the side. To conduct the pendulum test, the interviewer hands the patient a short string with a ring tied to one end. The patient grabs the string with his left hand.]

14. I: No, I want you to hold it in your right hand.

P: [Pointing to his limp arm] But I can't.

15. I: Well, I will help you. Let me put the string between your fingers. [Puts the string between the patient's limp right thumb and index finger] Now, I will press your fingers together for you—okay?

P: I'll try.

16. I: [Pressing the patient's fingers together] Now, let the string hang down freely. Put your right elbow on your stiff leg. Let me help you.

P: [Ends up in an awkward, leaning-over position, but the string with the ring is hanging down]

17. I: Now imagine . . . the ring starts to swing . . . in a circle . . . [ring starts to swing] . . . the circle will become bigger . . . and bigger.

P: [After less than a minute the ring is flying around in circles.] Isn't it funny? I'm not doing it. You know, I have no strength in my arm and hand.

18. I: I know, but you passed the test. Now, feel how the string slips out of your fingers. [And indeed, the ring falls on the floor.] You really have strong mental power—you can be hypnotized. Let's try another test.

P: All right, sir.

19. I: Now, let me help you fold your fingers. Press your healthy fingers in between your weak fingers on your right hand and fold them! Very good, you are doing it. Now, imagine that a force on both sides of your hand is squeezing your fingers very hard. They stick together. Feel the force that presses your fingers against each other! Feel that force! Try to pull them apart! Try! Try to pull your fingers apart! Try harder! You can't do it! Try harder! Try harder!

P: [The patient's knuckles turn white, his fingers become red. So does his face when he tries to pull.] I can't. [He exhales loudly, shakes his head.]

20. I: Now, the force stops pressing. The force is gone. Now, take your fingers apart.

P: [Unlocks his fingers and exhales noisily]

21. I: Now you have some idea about what hypnosis is like. Let's start.

P: What do I have to do?

22. I: Nothing really. Just follow through with whatever I suggest. Put your hands in your lap . . . good. Let your eyes close [patient's eyes close] and let your head hang down [patient's chin falls on his chest]. Feel the weight of your head, feel the weight of your head. When you feel the weight of your head and feel how your head pulls on your neck, your index finger will rise. [The

patient's left index finger pops up.] Your head gets heavier and heavier. It really pulls on your neck. It pulls more . . . and more. Again, let your finger rise when you feel it.

P: [Raises his left finger. His mouth opens and saliva runs over the lower lip.]

23. I: Fine . . . you can really feel it. Now feel the weight of your shoulders and arms and hands. If you feel the weight, your left index finger rises.

P: [Raises his left index finger]

24. I: Let me put your weak arm on your stiff leg. Your shoulders and arms and hands get really heavy, really heavy. You feel the heaviness.

P: [The patient's left index finger rises by itself.]

25. I: Very good. Your finger is telling me. Now feel the weight of your legs. When you feel the weight of your legs, your finger will rise.

P: [No response]

26. I: Let your left knee fall to the outside. Let it fall to the outside and relax. Do you start to feel the weight of your left leg? [The patient's left index finger rises.] Your leg starts to feel heavy. Raise your finger, when you feel its weight.

P: [Raises finger]

27. I: Now both legs feel heavier and heavier.

P: [Raises finger]

28. I: Now your head and shoulders and arms and hands feel heavy. Your limbs feel heavy. If you feel the heaviness all over, let your finger rise again.

P: [Raises finger]

29. I: Now feel the temperature in your belly. You become aware of the temperature in your belly. If you feel the temperature in your belly, raise your finger.

P: [Raises finger]

30. I: You will notice that your belly feels warm. It feels warmer and warmer . . . and now your belly feels really warm. Feel the warmth of your belly.

P: [Finger pops up again]

31. I: Now feel the temperature in your arms, and hands, and legs. Let your finger rise! [Patient raises it.] The warmth from your belly spreads all over. Your arms and legs get warm, get warmer . . . and warmer. If you feel it getting warmer and warmer, your finger will rise again.

P: [Raises finger]

For diagnostic purposes, the interviewer asked the patient to perform the pendulum test with his "paralyzed" hand to confirm that ideomotor transmission of the hypnotic command could take place. The ideomotor response of the patient's paralyzed hand supported the diagnosis of a conversion paralysis rather than of a neurogenic paralysis. The patient quickly assimilated the interviewer's suggestions (A. 17, 19, 20). He crisply raised his finger, even before he was asked to do so (A. 22). The prompt completion of the challenge task and the effort the patient demonstrated in trying to pull his fingers apart underscored the patient's willingness to surrender his own will to the interviewer's suggestions. Thus, the patient put both his trust and the responsibility for himself into the interviewer's hands.

The interviewer formulated all suggestions as "happenings" to the patient. For example, rather than saying, "If you feel the weight of your shoulders, arms, and hands, raise your left index finger," he said, "Your left index finger rises" (Q. 23).

Mr. M. was easy to hypnotize. He was cooperative to the degree of subservience. He showed a high degree of suggestibility and rapid ideomotor assimilation. As soon as he acknowledged feelings of heaviness and warmth, the therapist began the hypnotic interview.

Step 4b: The Hypnotic Interview

32. I: As you feel the heaviness in your body, you sink back into the past. You are back in the bowling alley, and you are bowling with your family. You hear the noise of the rolling balls and the clatter of the falling pins. You see it all again. If you can see it, your finger rises.
    P: [Finger pops up]
33. I: That's good. You feel more relaxed and heavy and warm as you are back in the bowling alley. Tell me what you feel and what you see and what you hear.
    P: My brothers have high scores. My father has a high score. They grin and laugh. And Frank says, "Even Ann bowls better than you. Even your baby sister outscores you." And I'm really behind. They're all laughing when I pick up the ball. They're grinning.
34. I: Yes? What do you feel?
    P: I'm angry. They tease me. They always tease me. They say, "You dummy! You can't do anything right." I hate bowling. I always lose. [Biting his lips] I'm just not good with the ball. I'm not good with anything.
35. I: Go on! Do you feel what is coming next?
    P: [No answer. Shrugs both shoulders]
36. I: As your head is heavy and your shoulders are heavy and your arms are heavy, all your thoughts come back. . . .
    P: [No answer]
37. I: Now you feel your body. Tell me how your body feels.
    P: The ball is so heavy. My arm feels weak. I drop the ball. My leg feels weak. My leg gives in. My leg buckles and the ball rolls away. I fall down. I lay on the floor. I can't move my leg. I can't move my arm. John picks me up. "Are you all right?" he asks. "I guess," I say, "but I'm so weak."
38. I: What do you feel? Tell me what you feel!
    P: I feel good, but I'm weak. They don't tease me any more. Even John cares for me. He's always making fun of me. They still care.
39. I: Now you feel weak. Now you know they still love you. Now, when you are weak, you don't have to bowl and they won't tease you. Let me talk to your folks. If you don't want to go bowling, you won't have to do it.
    P: [Breathing heavily]

40. I: Now, feel how your strength comes back into your right hand and arm. Your right arm feels light. It rises. It slowly rises. Imagine that a balloon is attached to it; it lifts your arm.

    P: [Right arm rises]

41. I: And now imagine the string is cut, your arm falls down.

    P: [Arm drops down in patient's lap]

42. I: Your fingers move. Feel how your fingers stretch. Now, they bend to a fist.

    P: [Right fingers form a fist]

43. I: I will tell your brothers and your dad that you cannot bowl with them, because it will make you weak. Now, Mr. M., as you feel heavy and warm, your strength comes back fully into your right hand and arm. You can bend your fingers. Your fingers bend again and stretch. Now your hand moves up and down, and your arm lifts up and moves down. Feel how your hand and arm start moving.

    P: [Moves hand and arm]

44. I: Now your right knee bends. It bends and it stretches. Now you can bend it.

    P: [Right leg starts shaking]

45. I: Now your right knee bends. Now you can bend it.

    P: [With jerky movements, patient bends knee]

46. I: Now it stretches and it bends. Now you can stretch it and bend it, stretch it and bend it! You are getting your full strength back.

    P: [Patient indeed bends his right knee and stretches the leg.]

47. I: Now you have the strength back in your entire right side. You can walk and move again. You feel that you can walk and move again. Nod your head if you feel it.

    P: [Nods head]

48. I: When the hypnosis is over, you can walk and move again. [Interviewer ends the hypnosis by suggesting to the patient that he take three deep breaths as described above. After the patient opens his eyes, the interviewer asks him to walk around in the hospital room. He walks back and forth, then stops in the middle of the room.]

    P: [In a flat voice] I feel all right.

Mr. M. assimilated the interviewer's suggestion that his weakness was disappearing. He showed full cooperation when he followed the interviewer's suggestion, who told him his strength had returned. Under hypnosis, the patient could reconstruct the onset of the paralysis. His leg started to move first with jerky movements, as if it wanted to express the conflict over whether to bend or not (A. 45). The firm suggestions (Q. 43–47) finally persuaded him to give up the paralysis.

Immediately, the purpose of the conversion became clear: Mr. M. wished to escape the ridicule of his family. He felt inferior to his siblings and felt ostracized by them. These findings would be consistent with Mr. M.'s history of slow learning. He may have mental retardation with some psychomotor clumsiness. Rather than being the butt of family jokes, when he was paralyzed, Mr. M. became the center of concern for his family.

The interviewer became Mr. M.'s ally when he promised to protect him from teasing by his family members. He said he would attempt to make the family become more sensitive to Mr. M.'s poor ability to bowl (e.g., by giving him a handicap in his bowling score). Such support would solve the patient's conflict with his family and restore the patient's muscular strength in his right arm and leg. Thus, the interviewer's planned intervention served the same purpose as the patient's conversion symptom: reduction of embarrassment. Mr. M. appeared very dependent on the opinion of his clan. Future family sessions might be necessary to prevent further similar conflicts and further conversion signs and symptoms.

Step 5: Approve

49. I: Mr. M., I'm glad that you have the gift to be hypnotized. It allowed us to find out how you became weak.

P: [With an insecure smile] Hmmm.

50. I: What I would like to do is to explain to your folks that bowling is not for you. If they don't want you to become weak again, they have to quit teasing you and understand that you can't do some things as well as they can. What do you think?

P: I don't know. I'm scared. They'll make fun of me, I think.

51. I: Why do you think they'll make fun of you?

P: Because . . . I don't know. . . . They always do.

52. I: They have to understand. . . . Your weakness will show when they pressure you too much.

P: [Smirking] Do you think they understand that?

53. I: Well, we will meet with them and make them understand what the problem is.

P: [Nodding his head] They may listen to you.

The interviewer assumed the leadership role in reducing family pressure on the patient. He did not educate Mr. M. about the psychological origin of his paralysis because Mr. M. considered himself physically ill. It is a therapeutic "blind alley" to convince patients of the psychological nature of their symptoms (Krull and Schifferdecker 1990). Because the duration of Mr. M.'s symptoms was short, the treatment was beneficial. Helping the patient become more assertive and independent and helping him to stand on his own rather than resort to conversion are long-term goals that cannot be accomplished in a 1-hour interview.

The patient did not behave as if he had been cured from a crippling disability. On the contrary, he was insecure and anxious about how his cure—the reversal of his conversion—would affect his family who might not understand (A. 50–53).

Diagnosis

Axis I. Conversion disorder with motor symptoms or deficit.

1. Patient fulfills all DSM-IV criteria for conversion disorder:

   A. One or more symptoms or deficits affecting voluntary motor or sensory function that suggest a neurological or other general medical condition, i.e., acute paralysis and pseudoseizure by history.
   B. Psychological factors are judged to be associated with the symptom or deficit because the initiation or exacerbation of the symptom or deficit is preceded by conflicts or other stressors.
   C. The symptom or deficit is not intentionally produced or feigned (as in Factitious Disorder or Malingering).
   D. The symptom or deficit cannot, after appropriate investigation, be fully explained by a general medical condition, or by the direct effects of a substance, or as a culturally sanctioned behavior or experience.
   E. The symptom or deficit causes clinically significant distress or impairment in social, occupational, or other important areas of functioning or warrants medical evaluation.
   F. The symptom or deficit is not limited to pain or sexual dysfunction, does not occur exclusively during the course of Somatization Disorder, and is not better accounted for by another mental disorder.

2. Rule out related disorders of the same group of somatoform disorders (e.g., somatization disorder).
3. Rule out dissociative disorder or establish its coexistence.

Axis II

1. Possible dependent personality disorder; whether the patient meets the criteria for this disorder will have to be examined in further sessions.
2. Possible mental retardation; testing would include the Kent Test (Kent 1946), the Rapid Approximate Intelligence Test (Wilson 1967), the Shipley Institute of Living Scale (Zachary 1986), and the Wechsler Adult Intelligence Scale—Revised (Wechsler 1981).

Axis III

1. Rule out mild cerebral palsy.
2. Rule out the beginning of multiple sclerosis or another neurological disorder that may facilitate the development of or mimic a conversion sign or symptom.

Axis IV. Problem with primary support group, adult.

Axis V. Global Assessment of Functioning (GAF) Scale score = 40. Patient shows severe impairment in family relations. He has symptoms and signs that prevent him from working or participating in family life.

6. Conversion and Hypnosis in Psychiatric Disorders

In DSM-IV, the dysfunction of conversion is recognized in the following Axis I and II disorders:

- Conversion disorder.
- Somatization disorder—Conversion or dissociative symptoms have to be present to fulfill the criteria.
- Posttraumatic stress disorder—Flashback phenomena may be associated with conversion and dissociative symptoms.
- Histrionic personality disorder—Although conversion symptoms are not listed as part of the diagnostic criteria for this disorder in DSM-IV, histrionic personality disorder is often associated with such symptoms. The DSM-II (American Psychiatric Association 1968) description of "hysterical neurosis," the antecedent of histrionic personality disorder, contained two subtypes of the disorder: conversion and dissociative.

Ford, working in conjunction with other researchers (Ford and Folks 1985; Ford and Parker 1991), thought of conversion as a symptom rather than a disorder because conversion occurs in many psychiatric and neurological disorders. Autosuggestive or autohypnotic suggestions are present in conversion, dissociation, somatization, posttraumatic stress, anxiety, panic, and eating disorders. They may also play a significant role in self-deception, as reflected in patients' attempts to conceal from the interviewer the negative life influences of drug and alcohol abuse; justify secretiveness about certain symptoms, such as suicidal ideas, obsessions, or compulsions; or hide vulnerability from self-recognition, as occurs in narcissistic personality disorder.

A review of the available literature shows the lack of knowledge concerning the incidence and prevalence of conversion. Incidence ranges from a high of 25%–33% lifetime isolated symptoms in women to a low of 0.01%–0.02% conversion disorder in patients seen by psychiatrists. In our view, conversion seems to be underrecognized. Conversion can emerge at any age; according to Siegel and Barthel (1986), 27 of 563 (4.8%) psychiatric consultations in a children's hospital showed conversion. Conversion is more common in women than in men and can appear with more or less sophistication at any educational level (Barsky 1989). Total paralysis seems to be rare. Except for pseudoseizures, the emphasis in presentation seems to have shifted to less obvious pseudoneurological symptoms (such as weakness and difficulty walking).

Conversion symptoms often occur alongside dissociative symptoms (Nemiah 1991) because the mechanisms of conversion and dissociation—that is, autohypnosis—are identical for both. However, these mechanisms are divergent with respect to the function affected: conversion affects the afferent and efferent peripheral nervous and sensory systems, whereas dissociation affects the patient's identity, memory, and sense of reality.

To address conversion phenomena, a hypnotic interview appears to be preferable over other techniques if hypnosis shows an economic advantage (i.e., in saving time and sparing suffering). Clinical experience shows that conflicts that can be brought to awareness by a hypnotic interview can also be brought to awareness with other techniques, especially free association (see Chapter 2, "Dissociation").

In this chapter we discussed how to apply hypnosis to the special problem of conversion. However, hypnosis applies to all psychiatric symptoms that involve suppression and repression of experiences, memories, and thought contents. Thus, hypnosis is useful in dealing with dissociative reactions, dissociative identity disorder, somatization, and posttraumatic stress reaction.

Hypnosis is not limited to the uncovering of suppressed thought contents. It also can be used to shape and condition behavior. Examples are inclusion of hypnosis in biofeedback, acupuncture, and relaxation of the anxious patient.

Hypnotic principles have an even wider application. Hypnosis as a ritualized, specialized form of suggestion is an affirmative statement made to others with an air of truth and certainty meant to be accepted by the recipient without scrutiny. As the interviewer, you make these suggestions knowingly or unknowingly all the time. Here are typical examples:

> If you open up to me, I can help you.
> If you reveal your problems to me, you will feel much better.

Thus, all supportive, reassuring, and confirming statements are somewhat suggestive in nature. They are designed to reduce patients' anxiety, increase their comfort, deepen their trust, and modify their behaviors. Suggestion is part of most if not all diagnostic interviews. The suggestive technique follows the 10 guidelines of hypnotherapists (see "The Hypnotic Interview," above). Its judicious use enhances your effectiveness in interviewing.

What if hypnosis fails? The psychodynamic methods of focusing on defenses and transference patterns (developed by Freud) together with free association are helpful. Freud's method was developed for handling conversion and can be quite effective for that purpose.

The placebo method for handling conversion symptoms is waiting them out. Alternatively, you can approach the patient with behavior modification methods. Praise her whenever her conversion sign or symptom improves. Give her attention mainly for improved functioning and ignore with your own *belle indifference* the persistence or worsening of conversion sign or symptom. In chronic conversion, amobarbital and methylphenidate have been used (Hurwitz 1988).

DISSOCIATION

Summary

Dissociation insulates a patient from the impact of painful memories or current stressors (the latter of which can even include psychiatric treatment). There are interviewing techniques that are helpful in revealing the conflicts that underlie a patient's dissociation and in diagnosing the specific dissociative phenomenon present. *Free association* unmasks depersonalization and trance; *hypnotic switching* elucidates dissociative identity disorder (called multiple personality disorder in DSM-III-R [American Psychiatric Association 1987]).

◆ ◆ ◆ ◆ ◆

Tarde, quae credita laedunt, credimus.
Where belief is painful, we are slow to believe.

Ovid (43 B.C.–A.D. 18)
Heroides, Epistle II, Line 9

◆ ◆ ◆ ◆ ◆

1. What Is Dissociation?

As defined in DSM-IV (American Psychiatric Association 1994, p. 477), the essential feature of the dissociative disorders is "a disruption in the usually integrated functions of consciousness, memory, identity, or perception of the environment." This disruption manifests in symptoms such as amnesia, fugue states, flashbacks, derealization, depersonalization, out-of-body experiences, trance, and "splitting" of personality. Dissociation may present as a rage attack, a self-mutilating behavior, or a problem with impulse control.

Dissociation may occur more often than is currently recognized (Ross 1991). One severe form of dissociation—dissociative identity disorder (called multiple personality disorder in DSM-III-R)—has been considered to be relatively rare, although there are indications that it is diagnosed and treated with increasing frequency (Boor 1982; Kluft 1987).

Dissociative phenomena pose difficulties for the interviewer. First, dissociation may be difficult to spot. Patients cannot tell you about it because they may not be aware of it. Many clinicians have no training in recognizing dissociation or have never (to their knowledge) dealt with a dissociating patient and often are ill prepared to suspect and identify the condition. It can take as long as 5–7 years and repeated hospitalizations for a person with dissociative identity disorder to be accurately diagnosed (Curtin 1993).

Behavior that appears dramatic or uncooperative may prevent you from obtaining descriptive information about the dissociative symptoms. Thus, underlying conflicts or stressors (including severe physical and sexual abuse) may remain obscure. For example, in a patient with dissociative identity disorder, dissociation may emerge as a form of hostility that disrupts the interview but that may not be recognized as an actual sign of this disorder. Dissociative amnesia and fugue occur sporadically, whereas dissociative identity disorder and depersonalization disorder are more chronic in nature. Recognition of the symptoms of dissociation is a problem for psychiatrists mainly trained in a descriptive model.

Followers of modern descriptive psychiatry, as developed by Kraepelin (1968), are more impressed by the familial occurrence and natural history of different psychiatric disorders and less by unconscious conflicts that may play a role in conversion and dissociative disorders, the assumption made by Breuer and Freud (1895) and his followers. According to the latter group, the different clinical pictures of that illness presented by a patient are determined by the patient's developmental stage when the conflict occurred and by the defense mechanisms the patient unconsciously employed.

Second, when you identify dissociation, you may mistake it for a neurological symptom or vice versa. It is necessary to differentiate dissociation from organic conditions (Mesulam 1981). For example, the differential diagnosis of dissociative amnesia would include the following:

- Neurological amnestic states (e.g., Korsakoff's psychosis)
- Transient, reversible, drug-induced amnestic states (e.g., an alcoholic blackout)
- Transient ischemic amnestic attacks
- Seizure disorders

You may misinterpret a dissociative symptom as being intentionally designed to mislead, annoy, or distract you. You may miss the patient's lack of control over both the switch into the dissociative trance and the altered behavior displayed during the trance. Even if electroencephalograms and repeated drug screens are negative and you accept the altered state as involuntary, you may discount it as unexplained, thus omitting a dissociative reaction from your differential diagnosis.

Third, dissociation or conversion may appear as a pseudoseizure. These seizures can be manifested as motor phenomena showing characteristics of a conversion symptom with voluntary neuromuscular activity (e.g., arm and leg thrashing, eye closing, teeth chattering) or as symptoms of altered consciousness with depersonalization and derealization. The patient may report that either he was cognizant of his surroundings during the seizure and can reconstruct the conversation that transpired during it, or that he was in a different world, unable to respond to you. If conscious, the patient may claim that he was unable to control the thrashing. A patient with pseudoseizures may report that he cannot recall what happened during the seizure. This amnestic type of pseudoseizure is both a dissociative and a conversion symptom.

Dissociation and conversion may reflect the same psychogenic mechanism—namely, autosuggestion or autohypnosis. Breuer and Freud (1895), Charcot (in Guillain 1959), and others (Janet 1907, 1911; Babinski [in Gauld 1992]) observed that a patient with dissociative and conversion symptoms is easily hypnotized. However, suggestibility is a necessary, but not a sufficient, condition for the development of these symptoms.

Fourth, after you show that a symptom is indeed pseudoneurological, you have to detect the precipitating conflict and the stressors that preceded it.

According to DSM-IV, a trance is not dissociative if it occurs exclusively during a psychotic disorder, a mood disorder with psychotic features, or a brief reactive psychosis. Such exclusions may be risky. Some severe, near-miss suicide attempts seem to occur during a dissociative trance in the course of an affective disorder with delusional pessimism, guilt, and low self-esteem.

Dissociative trance appears to be distinct from general suicidal rumina-tions and planning in that it is triggered by an outside stressor, such as an imagined insult, or by a real or imagined threat of desertion. Usually the patient can remember the stressor, but not his suicidal reaction to it. In trance, the patient may be obsessed with the sudden urge to carry out a self-injurious act without being able to tell why. All energy is funneled into that act, and the patient does not question its purpose.

2. Dissociation in the Mental Status

The mental status of the dissociating patient is characterized by two states of consciousness. One is the patient's interactive awareness and responsive-ness, a state that is easy to access; the patient's responses are predictable and continuous in time. In the other state, the patient suddenly shows one of five phenomena: amnesia, trance, flashback, personality switch, or mood change.

Amnesia.   The amnestic state usually occurs when you talk and expect the patient to listen. The patient's gestures disappear. She shows no symbolic or goal-directed movements. She just stares at you or into space. There is no dramatic occurrence of any autonomic response. The patient has a blank facial expression. No grooming movements occur. She appears absent-minded and disconnected. She seems unaware of what she just told you minutes ago, or she ceases responding at all and needs to be addressed several times. And then, suddenly, a startle response may occur and the patient may ask you to repeat your question, or she may explain that she was absentminded.

Trance.   The patient slips into an intense emotional state. His attention is focused exclusively on stimuli of particular interest to him while he filters out other environmental stimuli. He starts to discharge his emotional reac-tion like a fusillade, such as in the form of uninhibited crying or screaming, a prolonged angry tirade, or fanatical speech. In a clinical setting, the patient may fall into this trance state showing acute suicidal, homicidal, aggressive, or self-accusatory behavior. At the end of the state, he may claim amnesia for what he just told you.

His facial expressions may freeze into an expression of puzzlement. His reactive movements may stop. He may automatically repeat a grooming movement, such as stroking his left forearm with his right hand. He may stare at one particular spot while talking with a monotonous voice. Then he may tell you that all of a sudden it felt as though you and the room became unreal (derealization), as if he had left his body, and as if he was watching the scene from outer space (depersonalization).

Flashback. This state occurs most often when the patient relives and enacts a trauma. She begins to report the traumatic event but becomes more and more emotional, relives and enacts the event, and ignores outside stimuli and your interventions.

Personality switch. Like an actor, the patient slips into a different role, talking with a different tone of voice, showing an unfamiliar affect and psychomotor movements. He may be disoriented to the environment, ask you who you are, and introduce himself with a new name, a new profession, and a new place of living.

Mood change. Certain personalities may represent an extreme emotional state, such as childlike trust, dependency, fear, or hostility. The latter is most disruptive to the interview.

Hostility is easy to spot but difficult to deal with. Hostility blocks rapport with the interviewer and overshadows other traits that might otherwise be evident in the patient's mental status (compare the differential diagnosis of hostility in Chapter 5, "Psychotic Acting Out").

Hostility in the dissociative personality emerges in response to a threat from within. The patient may be reexperiencing a childhood trauma, such as severe physical or sexual abuse (Braun 1990; Putnam et al. 1986; Ross et al. 1991; Whitman and Munkel 1991). As a protective response, she splits off this intolerable memory from her consciousness and embeds it in a specific personality. She wants to kill in herself both the victim and the witness of that abuse. She transfers this hatred onto anybody whom she experiences as forcing her to face up to her memories.

In your effort to understand the patient, you may become the target of her aggression. You may unintentionally evoke dissociative hostility whenever you explore the patient's traumatic memories. She may become anxious because you are invading her private space, trespassing on her territory. Feeling threatened, she wants you out. If you push ahead with your exploration and confront her too pointedly with her hostility, she may feel cornered and attack you.

Verbal Strategies

Patients differ in reporting dissociative phenomena. You have to address this topic and assess the frequency, duration, and intensity of these signs. You need to explore with the patient whether he has experienced

Amnesia
- Do you lose time?
- Do you lose memory when you drive? When you try to pay attention?
- Have you lost memory for certain key events or time periods in your life?
- Have you ever ended up in certain locations, found yourself dressed in certain clothes, or found yourself in possession of certain objects and had no recollection of how all this came about?

Depersonalization
- Have you ever had the feeling the person in the mirror is not you? That you are not really in your own body?
- Have you ever experienced pain and other sensations as if they were coming from a distance?
- Have your thoughts ever sounded like voices inside your head who make comments about you?

Derealization
- Did you ever have the feeling that familiar places and people seem unfamiliar and unreal, far away, or behind glass or fog?

Trance
- Do you become absorbed in movies, in your own daydreams, or even in daily activities and either don't respond to the world around you or forget it altogether?

Personality switch
- Have you ever felt or been told that you switch into another personality?
- Have you ever been able to do things at certain times that you could not do at others?

The Dissociative Experiences Scale (Bernstein and Putnam 1986) quantifies these phenomena (Frischholz et al. 1990; Ross et al. 1988).

3. Techniques: Free Association and Hypnotic Switching

Two methods for exploring dissociative trance are *free association* and *hypnotic switching*.

Free Association

Free association was first used by Breuer in treating the patient Anna O., who experienced dissociative symptoms (Breuer and Freud 1957). Breuer and Freud showed that free association could take the place of hypnosis in overcoming dissociative amnesia. Practitioners who use hypnosis agree that many tasks accomplished with hypnosis can also be accomplished without it (Wright and Wright 1987).

Free association helps ease the patient into remembering painful events, feelings, and thoughts. As it relieves pressure, free association enlarges the frame of reference and encourages the spontaneity necessary to reveal the patient's innermost thoughts. It puts the patient in touch with her thoughts and helps her to openly express her flow of thinking.

When using the technique of free association, you need to make an effort to achieve an atmosphere of relaxation and safety. Unlike in traditional psychoanalytic free association, in which the practitioner attempts to detect, over many sessions, the unconscious conflicts that may contribute to the patient's character structure and psychiatric disorders, the interviewer of a dissociative patient needs to direct the free flow of ideas toward specific topics. What are the steps to take?

- Create a rapport so that the patient feels safe, supported, emotionally understood, and empathized with.
- Encourage the patient to report whatever comes to mind. Explicitly introduce free association as a technique that will unravel the mystery of the dissociative or conversion symptom.
- Use the dissociative or conversion symptom as your target. Try to uncover the specific conflict underlying the specific symptom.

The advantage of free association is that it is less disruptive than hypnosis because it does not require an induction technique. Free association attaches thoughts to dissociative behaviors and symptoms, enabling you to understand them psychologically. It may induce the patient to reexperience a conflict, express it, and share it with you. Free association does not feed into the patient's tendency of autosuggestion. It may lead to a better integration of the amnestic material, and it may prevent future amnestic splitting. The disadvantage of free association is that it is time consuming.

Why does free association work for autosuggestive phenomena? Clinical experience shows that a goal-directed inquiry into a patient's conversion and dissociative symptoms often fails to reveal their purpose. The patient simply does not remember. Neuropsychologically, one can argue that logical functions involve the dominant (usually the left) hemisphere of the brain, whereas autohypnotic suggestions work via images processed in the nondominant (usually the right) hemisphere. Therapeutic hypnosis uses images and therefore involves right-brain functions. Similarly, free-floating associations are also more suitable for evoking spontaneous right-brain images than are logical questions.

Hypnotic Switching

Standard clinical interviewing is ineffective in patients with dissociative identity disorder and, in most cases, free association is too time consuming. Hypnosis works best with cooperative patients. The sudden and unexpected emergence of a personality with an extreme mood, such as hostility, will not allow you the luxury of inducing hypnosis. In this situation, hypnotic switching can work. *Hypnotic switching* is the positive response to the request to produce or give up a dissociative state on an announced signal, such as counting to 3.

Virtually all patients with dissociative disorders are hypnotizable. This feature is most prominent in patients with dissociative identity disorder "because they experience spontaneous hypnosis and autohypnosis on an ongoing basis" (Kluft 1992, p. 162). If you know that a patient has dissociative identity disorder, you can call on a different personality to come forth. This switching technique uses such patients' capability to change quickly from one discrete personality to the other. Hypnotic switching is therefore useful in working with these patients.

Prepare to use hypnotic switching from the moment you suspect the presence of dissociative identity disorder. If you can activate in the patient the identity feeling of another personality, the switch follows predictably. Because the patient is pathologically susceptible to suggestion, tell him that you are ready to listen to another personality. Thus, you can induce a dissociative state without formal hypnotic induction. This switching technique is simple. Avoid pressuring the patient to perform. Instead, declare your readiness to receive. Tell the patient,

> I'm ready to listen and talk to [give the name of the alter if you know it].
> I'll count to three; then let [name] come forth.

Address the patient by the name of this other personality if you know it. If you do not know the alters' names, address them by their characteristics (e.g., the friendly one, the promiscuous one, the boisterous one) or simply "the other one." If you do not know name or characteristic, simply say,

> Maybe another personality within you looks differently at this topic and wants to come out and tell me about it.

The hypnotic switching technique has four advantages:

1. It turns off the hostile and dangerous personality.
2. It confirms that the patient indeed has dissociative identity disorder rather than is experiencing a dissociative amnestic state.
3. It allows you to explore the patient's host personality through the eyes of a secondary personality.
4. It allows you to detect some of the childhood experiences that precipitated the first dissociative splitting into separate personalities.

4. Five Steps to Reconnect

Step 1: Listen.   The patient may describe a dissociative symptom, such as amnesia, derealization, depersonalization, or flashback, or you may directly observe a sign of dissociation, such as a trance or a flashback when the patient reports an emotionally charged event or when it occurs.

Step 2: Tag.   Tag the symptom or sign by pointing out to the patient that one of the problems that she mentioned is of particular importance, such as her memory disturbance, as manifested in her inability to recall certain things, her finding of some objects in her possession that she does not know how she acquired, or her apparent intense reliving of a past event during the interview.

Tag a dissociative symptom or sign in an indirect way. Tell the patient that she just seems to be more absorbed, like in a daydream, or seems to be reliving a certain event, but that you are not sure. Tell her that you would like her to tell you what just happened in her mind. Now she may describe an amnestic event, a flashback, derealization, or depersonalization. Her report will help you to classify the event. Then ask her for similar occurrences in the past. Assess in detail what she remembers of these events and what preceded and followed them without asking her for a causal interpretation.

Step 3: Confront. Hone in on the most intense, most recent, or most frequent event and highlight its importance. Focus in detail on precipitating factors and on feelings and events that followed the dissociation.

Step 4: Solve. Pick the interviewing technique that most likely will help you to elucidate the dissociation: free association, hypnosis, or hypnotic switching. Familiarize the patient with whatever method you have chosen. Then, depending on the method, ask her to tell you whatever comes to her mind about her dissociative experience, trace her through that experience under hypnosis, or switch her identity if she gives evidence of the presence of a dissociative identity disorder.

Step 5: Approve. Show understanding for the patient's dissociation and explain the psychological meaning of the symptom or sign. Express empathy for the trauma that led to the dissociation and for the discomfort that the patient may experience from the dissociation. Make sure that your remarks lead to an integrative rather than another traumatic experience.

5. Interview A:
Free Association and Dissociative Amnesia

The following is an example of the interviewer exploring a dissociative, suicidal urge with free association. The patient, Ms. C., is a 34-year-old, white, twice-married mother of three girls. At the emergency room of a university hospital, she requests admission because of recurring depression and a sudden urge to commit suicide. (I = interviewer; P = patient)

Step 1: Listen

1. I: Hello, Ms. C. What seems to be the problem?
   P: Call me Marleen, please! Ms. C. sounds so stiff. I cannot stand it. Everybody calls me Marleen.

2. I: Okay. Now, Ms. C., please tell me what I can do for you.
   P: Don't you like me? Or don't you listen? I feel more comfortable if you call me Marleen. [Patient then reports symptoms of depression of moderate severity without agitation or psychomotor retardation. She seems able to talk about her suicidal urges and exhibits no crying or shame. She displays her feelings dramatically; genuine despair is missing. This disparity between drama and lack of depth gives her presentation a histrionic flavor, suggesting the possibility of a diagnosis other than depression.]

Step 2: Tag

3. I: [Interviewer tags the patient's suicidal behavior and asks her to elaborate on the circumstances that seemed to trigger it.]
   P: [Patient describes a sudden switch.] "I daydream a lot. I doze off with my eyes open. I've done that since childhood. All of a sudden I'm in the bathroom holding a razor blade or swallowing a lot of pills. And then somebody finds me, or I have a sudden awakening and call my husband or the hospital. I know it must sound crazy. [Patient reports neither precipitating events, repetitive thoughts, nor feelings of despair.]

Step 3: Confront

4. I: You are telling me you get the urge to kill yourself and that it hits you out of the blue.
   P: It seems that way.
5. I: Does anything happen before you feel the sudden urge to kill yourself?
   P: [Frowns and looks up to the ceiling] Nothing in particular.
6. I: Do you feel that anything causes your urge?
   P: [Shakes her head] No, not that I know of.
7. I: Do you have any thoughts that keep coming back when you are depressed?
   P: I feel lousy. I think it will never end. What's the use of living if I feel like that?
8. I: I see. These are common thoughts that occupy a person's mind during a depression. But is there any specific topic that you seem to worry about?
   P: No . . . [then, with a frown] I don't understand what you mean.
9. I: You're right. I'm putting you on the spot.
   P: [With a sudden flirtatious smile] You are?

The patient was well groomed and alert. She comprehended questions and answered them without circumstantiality or tangentiality. She showed no psychomotor retardation or agitation. Her affect was bright and appropriate to her thought content.

The interviewer initially screened her with closed-ended questions for precipitating thoughts or events that could explain her suicidal urges

(Q. 4–8). Her feelings that life was useless appeared unrelated to her sudden urge to kill herself. The interviewer could not explain the suicidal urge as a symptom of depression, as a response to a rejection, or as anger directed against the self. Because the goal of this interview was to explore one symptom in depth (i.e., the patient's sudden suicidal urge), the interviewer did not assess diagnostic criteria for major depression, bipolar disorder, or for a personality disorder.

Step 4: Solve

Step 4a: Free Association

10. I: [Ignoring the patient's flirtatious quip, in the same tone of voice] Maybe I can make it somewhat simpler for you. I'd like you to tell me whatever pops up in your mind. Don't worry whether it answers my questions or not. Just say what comes up.

  P: You mean just anything?

11. I: Yes, just anything. Even if it seems embarrassing or unimportant or doesn't answer my question. We call this free association.

  P: Sounds like rambling to me.

12. I: That's just what it is. But there may be a message behind that rambling— a message that we often miss.

  P: Hmmm . . .

13. I: Can you try to do that? Just answer without worrying whether it's right or wrong, or whether it's the answer I'm looking for.

  P: [Smiling] Let my mouth do the talking?

14. I: Yes. Instead of your brain, you mean?

  P: Yeah. [Laughing] That should be simple.

15. I: [Laughing too] Let's try it—okay?

  P: [Shrugs her shoulders without saying anything]

16. I: Think about your urge to kill yourself. What kinds of thoughts cross your mind?

  P: [Closing her eyes] All kinds of thoughts, but nothing's clear, nothing sticks out.

17. I: When you think about killing yourself . . . how would you do it?

  P: Right now? I don't feel like it right now.

18. I: Imagine you felt like it right now.

  P: [Slowly with a soft voice and eyes closed] Hmmm, slashing my wrist . . . throwing myself under a car . . . [opens her eyes] or just trying to jump out of these windows up here [from the fourth floor of the medical school building].

19. I: What comes to mind right now when you think about killing yourself?

  P: [Looks puzzled]

20. I: Tell me what you are thinking.

  P: It makes no sense. [Wrinkles her nose as if smelling a stench]

21. I: That's what free association is all about. Say anything, whether it makes sense or not.
    P: [After a pause] My husband. . . . [Shakes her head] That's nonsense.
22. I: Your husband?
    P: Yeah. It makes no sense. [Laughing sarcastically] I don't want to kill myself because of my husband. [Sits up in her chair] Let's just stop that free association stuff.
23. I: Let's not worry right now about whether it makes sense or not.
    P: [Slumping back in her seat] Okay.
24. I: [With vigor] As you said, we just want to let the mouth do the talking. You mentioned your husband. What else pops up?
    P: What he says about my father. [Pressing her lips together, grimacing] Oh, that's stupid . . . I don't want that.
25. I: [Urgently] Just keep talking, Marleen.
    P: Do I really have to? [Pausing] Okay. I saw my father about 3 months ago . . . and I called him 2 months ago. I don't see him that often. We're not very close. I stay away from him. My husband doesn't want him around. He doesn't trust him. I call him only when I need something, like money. He never says no.
26. I: Your husband does not trust him?
    P: Nope. It's my fault because once when I was depressed, I told him what my father did. It was kind of stupid to tell him.
27. I: [Surprised] What your father did?
    P: [Looking down in her lap, whipping one foot, biting her lower lip] What he did to me.
28. I: What he did to you?
    P: [Biting her nails, looking down] Yes . . . [pause].
29. I: Marleen, you seem to have a hard time talking about it.
    P: [Leaning her head to the side, smiling, suddenly flirtatious again] I do?
30. I: Well, you started to whip your foot, to bite your lip, and you looked away from me.
    P: [Puzzled] I did?
31. I: Did you notice that?
    P: Kind of. I guess.
32. I: You seem to feel uncomfortable.
    P: Yeah. [Squirms and scoots around in her chair]
33. I: You seem to have difficulties talking about it.
    P: [Reluctantly] Yeah.
34. I: Can you tell me how you feel?
    P: [Blushes] Ashamed.
35. I: You feel ashamed when you think about your father?
    P: No . . . only when I'm depressed.
36. I: When did you get depressed?
    P: About 5 or 6 weeks ago. I was so stupid to tell my husband.
37. I: What did you tell your husband that was so stupid?
    P: Just stuff. I'm stupid to talk about it. . . . I told him that my father had molested me.

38. I: That he had molested you? And did you say how he had molested you?
    P: Oh, I didn't do that. I wasn't that stupid. I just told him that he had molested me. And that was enough to make him mad. Now he hates him. He doesn't want him around our daughters or me.
39. I: How did your father molest you?
    P: He . . . I don't really know. I don't remember. [Looks out the window]
40. I: Let's see what comes to mind.
    P: I just have that feeling. It's kind of fuzzy.
41. I: Just say what comes to mind.
    P: He's holding me . . . [closes her eyes with a painful expression in her face] kind of holding me . . . close . . . [shakes her head] . . . and he is touching me. . . .
42. I: [After a pause] Touching you?
    P: [Opens her eyes and looks the interviewer in the eyes]
43. I: How do you feel?
    P: [Gets a deep fold between her eyes] Just terrible. [Starts crying]
44. I: Just terrible?
    P: [Starts to whip her foot, turns her head toward the door, gets up, sits down again]
45. I: You seem to want to run away. Do you?
    P: [Looks up to the ceiling, then whips her crossed-over leg, and looks at the door] I feel restless.

Because Marleen's suicidal impulse represented a specific thought content that was not hallucinatory or delusional yet appeared unconnected to any conscious or logical stressor, the interviewer felt that the patient unknowingly had suppressed some memories that were triggering her suicidal urges. In other words, the suicidal urge was dissociative in nature, especially as her suicide attempts had an amnestic quality (see Step 2). Therefore, he was trying to access these triggering thoughts through an indirect interviewing technique—free association.

To introduce free association, the interviewer became a teacher (Q. 10–15). The patient showed initial resistance by degrading free association as rambling (A. 11) and nonproductive in that it evoked no clear response (A. 16). However, her apparently illogical thoughts (A. 16–19) evoked her resistance (A. 20, 22). The interviewer's encouragement (Q. 23–25) kept her compliant. Continuation techniques (Q. 20, 21, 24, 25) enhanced the flow of thoughts, but the patient's anxiety (e.g., nail biting [A. 28]) brought that to a halt. The interviewer identified the patient's emotions and interpreted them as discomfort. The interviewer pointed out her gestures, which were an indication of her anxiety (Q. 30).

Rather than pressing for details when blocking occurred (A. 39), the interviewer invited free association and the patient followed through (A. 40,

41). Instead of verbalizing, the patient acted out her resistance in a desire to escape (A. 44, 45). However, when the patient expressed her painful feelings (A. 41–43), the interviewer failed to accept them with empathy, and continued with exploration instead (Q. 34–45).

Step 4b: Interpreting a Suicidal Trance

46. I: You are looking at the door.
    P: I wish I could forget it, just forget it.
47. I: [Softly and encouraging] Let it come to mind. What comes to mind?
    P: [Closes her eyes. Suddenly she jumps up, hits her thighs with her fists, runs to the door and out of the office. She dashes down the stairs and into the street. Car brakes squeal; she misses being hit by just a few feet. She tears along the street toward a nearby park and falls down on the grass, breathing heavily.]
48. I: [Catching up] What happened?
    P: [With glazed-over eyes looking through the interviewer into distant space] Go away. Leave me alone. I want to die. I just want to die. [Hitting her thighs with her fists again]
49. I: You want to die?
    P: [Crying, without listening to the interviewer, rocking back and forth, talking in a low voice] I want to be dead.
50. I: Dead?
    P: [Crying and shaking, holding her hands in front of her face, rocking again; long pause]
51. I: Marleen, you want to be dead?
    P: [Silent, looking through the interviewer, shaking her head, puzzled]
52. I: Marleen, what do you want to kill?
    P: [Staring at him longer, then looking into space]
53. I: What do you want to kill in you?
    P: [Silent, with glassy eyes, not answering the interviewer] I can't take it, I can't take my feeling.
54. I: What feeling?
    P: [Talking to herself] I can't take it. I don't want to remember this.
55. I: You can't bear your memory?
    P: [Mumbling] Myself.
56. I: You want to kill your feeling? What feeling?
    P: [Looks down, blushes; no answer]
57. I: Your feeling?
    P: [Talking to herself, pounding her thighs again] No, no, no! [Jumping up and trying to run further]
58. I: [Blocking her way] You want to run away again. Rather than running away, let's talk about your need to run away. Calm down. [Patient stares into space] Let's go back to the office. [Patient hesitates, sits down, rocks, then stops; she looks away, then into her lap] Okay, tell me when you are ready.

P: [After several minutes, she gets up without looking at the interviewer, and walks toward the medical school building, muttering to herself, looking puzzled and perplexed] What happened?

59. I: You ran away from the interview. You said you wanted to kill yourself.

P: I did? I don't remember. I must have had a blackout.

60. I: A blackout. . . . What do you feel now?

P: I'm awful. I hate myself. I can't stand it but I have to ask you anyway. [Stares the interviewer in the eye without blinking]

61. I: [Walking with her] Ask me what?

P: [Stepping close to the interviewer and pushing her breasts against him] But I have no chance, do I?

62. I: [Stepping to the side] What do you mean?

P: [Begging intensely] Would you go on a date with me?

63. I: [Looking her in the eyes] I'm your doctor, Marleen. It would not help you. It would hurt you if I met with you.

P: I knew you'd say that. I was afraid of that.

64. I: What made you ask that question?

P: My feeling of wanting to have sex all of a sudden.

65. I: [They reach the medical school building, enter, and cross the lobby.] Let's take the elevator back to the office.

P: Can't we take the stairs?

66. I: Why?

P: [Walks close to the interviewer] Can I touch your hand?

67. I: Let's take the elevator to the office. [They reach the office. He lets the patient enter and sit down. He discreetly asks the receptionist to check in on them every 10 minutes as the patient is in distress. He then enters his office, leaving the door ajar. He sits down behind his desk at an angle to the patient.]

P: [Whips her leg, trying to hit the examiner's foot] Can't you close the door?

68. I: Marleen, you say you get a sudden urge?

P: Yes, yes. [Shaking her head, blinking fast, wiping her eyes]

69. I: You talked about sex after the blackout.

P: I'm so sorry. I say things . . . I feel things. . . .

70. I: You ran away from this interview. You told me you wanted to kill yourself, and you told me you wanted to kill a feeling and afterward you talked about sex.

P: [Starts screaming in a high pitched voice] Ahhh! [The receptionist comes in and asks if everything is all right.]

71. I: [To the receptionist] I don't know. [To the patient] Marleen, is everything all right?

P: [Looks at him, mocking him] "Marleen, is everything all right?" I think I'd prefer that you call me Ms. C.

72. I: You're right. I prefer to call you by your last name too.

P: [Begging] Oh no, I don't mean it, please call me Marleen. Please! Please! Please!

73. I: [To the receptionist who is still standing at the door] It's fine. Just leave the door open a bit. [To the patient] Marleen, you talked about the feeling that you want to kill in yourself, then you talked about sex. What comes to mind?

P: No, no, no! Can't you stop it?

74. I: Okay, we've talked about it long enough.

P: I feel so bad.

75. I: Let's talk about it later.

P: No, no. Can I ask you a favor?

76. I: Okay.

P: Can we spend a few more minutes? I feel so bad.

77. I: Are you sure?

P: I want to get it out . . . that feeling.

78. I: Okay.

P: [Silent]

79. I: Well, Marleen, you wanted to talk?

P: [Silent again, looks down and blushes]

80. I: You are blushing.

P: Yes . . . no . . . yes . . . no.

81. I: You look so upset.

P: It's worse. It's much worse. I'm so bad. . . . [Starts crying] I feel so bad . . . I didn't fight my father. [Her crying becomes more intense] I let him have sex with me. I'm a monster.

82. I: You sound so ashamed. How old were you when he had sex with you?

P: Quite young . . . until I was 17 . . . when I met my boyfriend. When I talked to you today, it all came back to me. I remembered . . . I went along with it. [Keeps on crying]

83. I: Hmmm.

P: Yes, I'm such a slut. [Starts crying, then sniffles, grabs a tissue from the interviewer's desk, and quickly glances at him from the corners of her eyes]

84. I: And that's what you want to kill in yourself?

P: [Stops sobbing] Yes, I want to get it out of me, you see. I even asked you to have a date with me.

85. I: You try to distract yourself from your old feelings, but you can't. So you transfer them from your father onto me. And you repeat now what your father forced on you.

P: Is that what I'm doing? I do it all the time. I do it with my husband's boss. My husband found out about it . . . he forgave me.

86. I: What about your husband's boss?

P: I don't know. He's old and fat, his stomach sticks out, and he's married.

87. I: So what comes to mind?

P: I always try, I don't know why. He's disgusting.

88. I: What pops up?

P: It makes me feel better. I don't understand. And then I slash myself. It worries me. I know about sexual abuse. And I know that my father has done it with other young girls. I'm disgusted. Other girls hate it, but I . . . [cries, cries, cries] I didn't fight it.

89. I: [After a pause] Marleen . . .

P: [Stops crying, looks at the interviewer, then in an angry voice, mocking him] Get it in your head! I'm a monster! I'm such a slut!

Changes in the patient's level of consciousness and the interviewer's neglect in acknowledging the patient's distress by offering her comfort disrupted the interview (A. 47). Marleen then acted out her emotions, which interrupted the process of free association (A. 47, 57, 61–67). Surprised by the patient's impulsivity, the interviewer did not intervene when she first took to flight (A. 47). He could have said, "You look anxious, Marleen, let's take a break." Instead, he insisted on free association. His pressure precipitated a trancelike state in which the patient relived a past event. Completely focused on her inner feelings, she shut out the interviewer and denied him access to her thoughts and feelings (A. 47, 48). She dissociated from her normal self and from the interview situation.

When the interviewer allowed the patient to stare into her lap without pressuring her to talk to him, she switched back to the present—claiming amnesia for the previous few minutes (A. 58, 59). The interviewer was able to address and control her acting out when it reemerged (Q. 58, 63, 67, 70, 71). He gave her space rather than pushing for answers (Q. 58). He combined empathy with setting limits. Focusing his concern on her well-being and her state of mind (Q. 71) rather than reflecting on her behavior or her emotions helped him to control her acting-out behavior.

The patient transferred her sexual feelings onto the interviewer (A. 60–69) and, in so doing, appeared to experience a role confusion among her father, her husband's boss, and the interviewer. Her mixed-up feelings were the cause of her self-injurious and suicidal urges (A. 88). On one hand, she seemed to replay and act out the sexual abuse by her father with her husband's boss and the interviewer; on the other hand, she expressed self-condemnation (A. 69, 81, 83, 84).

Her interaction with the interviewer changed several times. First, she wanted to seduce him (A. 60–67) and became angry when he neutralized the situation (A. 71). Then she gave up her seductiveness and cooperated with the interview. The interviewer's suggestion that they terminate the interview (Q. 74, 75) motivated her to ask for more time. As soon as this request was granted, she became silent again (A. 78).

The interviewer's interpretation of her blushing as shame (A. 80, 82) allowed the patient to share with the interviewer the reason for her blushing—namely, her inability to prevent incest (A. 82). Free association helped the patient talk about her distress and gave the interviewer an understanding of its cause. He recognized that the patient was upset about her embarrassing images and feelings. He then had to motivate her to share her memories. Therefore, he asked specific questions (A. 82, 84).

To restore rapport, the interviewer interpreted the patient's behavior as a replay of the past (Q. 85). This interpretation was designed to relieve her embarrassment. She appeared to accept this view because she offered supportive examples (A. 85–87). Yet she continued to act out her self-condemnation rather than reflecting on it (A. 88, 89). She wanted to kill "the slut in her" who had asked the interviewer for a date. The interviewer interpreted this proposal as a result of her sexual abuse. Thus, he attempted to solve her guilt. Such an interpretation would require proper timing and appropriate comprehension.

The timing for pointing out a particular behavior depends on the patient's readiness to recognize that behavior. If you are unsure, ask the patient to interpret her behavior herself. If this fails, offer your interpretation. An interpretation obvious to you may not at all be obvious to the patient, making it critical that you move cautiously. Offer an interpretation only when you are reasonably sure your patient can accept it. Present small, concrete interpretations rather than global ones. Wait for the patient's affirmation before moving on. Mainly use interpretations that relieve guilt, anger, anxiety, and embarrassment rather than those that provoke such feelings. This emphasis shows an important distinction between a diagnostic and a therapeutic interview. A diagnostic interview is time limited; its task is to identify the disorder. In the therapeutic interview, patient and therapist will be working together over a longer period of time. The goal is to help the patient both become aware of her problems and overcome them.

As to Ms. C.'s mental status, she was alert, yet her level of consciousness changed. She showed stereotyped movements: thigh pounding (A. 47, 48, 57), staring (A. 48, 51–53), rocking (A. 49, 50, 58), and eye blinking (A. 68). She slipped into a dissociative state (A. 47–58) governed by intense feelings of transference (A. 58–90). She did not answer questions while dissociating (A. 47–58). When she resumed answering (A. 58), her responses were tainted by her transference feelings.

Her affect appeared labile, impulsive, dramatic, intense, and possibly exaggerated; she acted out her emotions rather than verbalizing them. Her mood was overshadowed by her feelings of disgust and self-condemnation. The suicidal impulse connected with memories of incest, which represented her attempt to punish herself, appeared to be part of a dissociative trance.

Her self-condemnation had an overlay of insincerity because of her flirtatiousness (A. 67). Even though she volunteered that she may have had a sexual relationship with her husband's boss, it remained debatable whether she had gained an emotional understanding of her behavior; she still referred to herself as a slut. The interviewer made her aware of her resistance by transforming her acting-out behavior into talking-out behavior.

Although the patient's mental status did not show any push of speech, flight of ideas, or grandiose thinking, there were other indications of mania, such as mood fluctuations from despair and suicidal ideation to flirtatiousness.

This patient's switch into a dissociative trance and the state of intensified transference are compatible with dissociative disorder and somatization disorder (although the interviewer did not assess somatic symptoms). Major depression would still be a diagnostic consideration because the patient felt guilty about the incest only when depressed.

The request to have a date with the therapist and the patient's acting out of emotions with flirtation and seductiveness (A. 61, 62, 65–67) would support the diagnosis of a personality disorder of Cluster B, histrionic and borderline personality disorder. The latter is supported by her suicidality.

Step 5: Approve

90. I: Marleen, you're right. You have this strong memory and you feel guilty about it.
    P: [Looks at him attentively]
91. I: Let me explain something to you. When a parent abuses a child, going along with the abuse is one common way of handling the situation. Doing so allows you to still love that parent, someone on whom you are dependent.
    P: You just want to make me feel good. But I know deep down I'm a slut. The worst is I keep on behaving like one.
92. I: [Looking at her] Marleen, I'm glad you spilled it out. Let's find out what is behind that feeling.
    P: I can't stand that feeling.
93. I: I know. You want to kill it in yourself. Your consciousness does not enjoy what you are doing.
    P: [Melodramatically, jumps up, stares at the interviewer, clenches her teeth]
94. I: You see, Marleen, you condemn yourself for doing what you did. That tells me that you really did not go along with the abuse by your father.
    P: [Relaxes, sits back down, holds her hands in front of her face] I'm so confused.
95. I: Why don't you stay at the hospital for a while so that we can help you to sort out your feelings. And we will treat your depression.
    P: Thank you. I couldn't stand to be at home now. I don't know what I would be doing.

The interviewer adopted a double role as the expert who recognized the reason for the patient's seductive behavior and the healer who ameliorated her guilt and self-condemnation by offering her acceptable interpretations (Q. 91, 93, 94) and providing a solution—namely, hospitalization. She responded by claiming confusion (Q. 94) but did not repeat her feelings of self-hatred or her suicidal wish. She showed insight into her need for help.

Differential Diagnosis

At this point, the interviewer does not have enough information to make a definite diagnosis. The differential diagnosis includes

Axis I

1. *Dissociative amnesia.* The patient dissociates, and afterward she is partially amnestic for her dissociative episode. Her symptoms appear to fulfill all three diagnostic criteria for this disorder; however, her dissociative amnestic episodes, both reported and observed, appeared to be relatively brief.
2. *Dissociative fugue.* The patient suddenly runs out of the interviewer's office in an apparent dissociative state; however, she does not appear to assume another identity.
3. *Dissociative disorder not otherwise specified.* The incomplete database suggests that the patient indeed has a dissociative disorder, but at this point it does not fit any of the four specific dissociative disorders listed in DSM-IV.
4. *Major depressive disorder.* The predominant mood symptoms appear to be depressive rather than manic.
5. *Bipolar disorder.* The patient describes mood swings of a rapidly changing pattern.

Axis II

1. *Borderline personality disorder.* The patient shows impulsive behavior, including sexual advances toward the interviewer. She has made frequent suicide gestures or threats. She asks for an extension of the interview and does not want to be abandoned. She shows transient dissociative symptoms.
2. *Histrionic personality disorder.* The patient appears to be attention seeking. She is inappropriately sexually seductive and provocative. She displays rapidly shifting and shallow expression of emotions. She appears theatrical.

Axes III through V. Not enough information was gathered to allow an assessment.

Epilogue

It is not always easy to determine what is truth and what is fiction in a patient's account (see Part IV [Chapters 12–15], "Self-Protective and Deceptive Behavior"). There are instances of false memory, of course, and mental health professionals have been accused of leading their patients to stories of sexual or physical abuse (Wakefield and Underwager 1992). In this case, the interviewer received Ms. C.'s permission to contact her mother, who had divorced Ms. C.'s father. The mother reported that she had caught her former husband abusing her daughter. It appeared that Ms. C. was now repeating that incestuous behavior with other fatherlike figures. Her suicidal behavior represented an attempt to resolve her conflict.

5. Interview B: Hypnotic Switching and Dissociative Personality Disorder

Robert Chris R. is a 37-year-old, muscular, 5'10", 190-pound, married Native American with a dark complexion and shiny black hair groomed in a buzz cut. He has been on the Veterans Administration psychiatric ward for over 2 weeks. On admission, his drug urine screen was negative. A sleep-deprived electroencephalogram and a magnetic resonance imaging scan were normal, and his physical examination showed no abnormal findings except a blood pressure of 135/90. He has no history of substance abuse.

While in the hospital, the patient is oriented. He can recall four out of four objects immediately and after a 10-minute delay. His Shipley Institute of Living Scale score (Zachary 1986) shows an IQ of 112. His past work record as a surgical nurse is excellent. However, on several occasions he has disappeared from home, only to be found on a highway embankment with a gun in his mouth. When asked about these episodes, he gets very irritated and explosive. One psychiatrist noted that one is "walking on eggshells" with this patient. Even open-ended, nondirective questions set him off. He denies hallucinations. Previous treatment with haloperidol (Haldol) 20 mg/day for possible persecutory delusions had no effect on the explosive behavior. However, the patient is friendly to the staff and all the other patients.

The interviewer introduces himself and explains that he has been asked to give a second opinion on his case. He talks to the patient within the view of two orderlies in a semisecluded area of the ward lounge. (I = interviewer; P = patient)

Step 1: Listen

1. I: Mr. R., what brought you here?
   P: [Smiling, with a soft voice and looking at the interviewer] The highway police. [Shrugs his shoulders] They say they found me with my gun in my mouth.
2. I: Things must be pretty bad for you to go pointing a gun at yourself.
   P: Yeah, I don't know. [Smiles, shrugs his shoulders]
3. I: Did you really want to kill yourself?
   P: [Leaning back in his chair] That's what they thought.
4. I: What did you think? What was your plan?
   P: [Closing his eyes] I'm confused.
5. I: What do you mean?
   P: [Keeping his eyes closed] Things don't make sense. [His relaxed facial expression changes to tension; he frowns.]
6. I: Can you give me an example of something that confuses you?
   P: [Stiffly pops up in his chair] What did you say?
7. I: Can you give me an example of something that does not make sense to you?
   P: [Briskly shaking his head, with a sharp tone, glaring at the interviewer without blinking] No. You'll have to do without one.
8. I: I'd like to help you, but I need to know what's wrong.
   P: [Hostile, with a tense face, narrowed eyelids, and a sharp cutting voice] Just figure it out, doc.
9. I: [Pauses] We have to do it together. You have to help me understand you.
   P: [With increased pressure in his voice] You know enough already. [Still glares at the interviewer without blinking]
10. I: Well, all I know is that you had a gun in your mouth and that you feel confused.
    P: [His neck stiffens] Just drop that. Don't dwell on "confused." I'm sorry I said that.
11. I: Okay, let's talk about the gun then. Why did you have a gun?
    P: [Sarcastic] Isn't that obvious?
12. I: The police thought you wanted to kill yourself. What did you think?
    P: I don't know. [Presses his lips together, fixates on the interviewer's eyes without blinking]
13. I: That sounds like you are not certain.
    P: [Sharply] Did I say that?
14. I: You said you don't know what it means and a while back you said that you were confused.
    P: [With a cutting voice] Don't rub it in.
15. I: I'm sorry. But, let me ask you. . . . Have you put a gun to your head before?
    P: [Relaxing] Several times.
16. I: And when you did that, did you want to kill yourself?

P: [Some tension returning] I want to kill somebody.
17. I: Do you know who?
P: [Startled, with an angry voice] What do you know about me? [With increased intensity] How come you know who I want to kill?
18. I: I don't know who you want to kill. I only know what you told me.
P: I didn't tell you anything.
19. I: That's right, but you mentioned you wanted to kill somebody and I had the feeling you didn't mean yourself.
P: Goddamnit! I told you to stay out of this!
20. I: You told me not to talk about your confusion.
P: So don't!

The patient's initial eye contact, relaxed voice, and acceptance of the interviewer's empathy (Q. 2) seemed to suggest rapport. Suddenly, this positive attitude was threatened by a change (A. 6). Mr. R. rejected the alliance (A. 8, 9) and switched into distance and hostility. However, he kept talking, even though he excluded broad topics from exploration (A. 6–20). His insight appeared poor (A. 4, 17). The relationship between patient and interviewer soon became adversarial (A. 8–11, 13, 14, 17–20).

The interviewer's effort to clarify the patient's suicidal gesture, a topic that the patient brought up himself, failed (Q. 6–14, 17–20). At Q. 8 and 9, the interviewer should have switched from gathering information to discussing the patient's anger. Instead, he tried to handle the patient's anger indirectly by changing the topic (Q. 11). The patient's anger increased even though the interviewer permitted him to avoid a sensitive topic (Q. 11, 12). Distraction did not work. The patient grew even more furious when the interviewer confronted him with two of his statements (Q. 14). At Q. 15 the patient relaxed temporarily but then returned to a tense, angry stance while the interviewer tried to find a less offensive approach. The interviewer failed to find a topic that the patient could answer without anger (Q. 17–20). An alternative technique, switching from exploring the patient's problems to discussing his sudden onset of hostility (A. 6), might have been a better way to handle the patient's anger and explore his psychiatric diagnosis indirectly.

As to mental status, the patient's muscular appearance would suggest that he was involved in body building. He showed no abnormalities in his psychomotor behavior, except for an increase in expressive movements throughout the interview. He appeared to understand the interviewer's questions clearly and answered them to the point, except once when he showed a lack of concentration in not registering the question (Q. 6).

Most remarkable was Mr. R.'s sudden change of affect from friendly (A. 1–5) to hostile, angry, and suspicious (A. 6). The patient remained hostile after his outburst in A. 6. He adopted a different affective mode, which he maintained (A. 6–20). The hostile outburst (A. 6) might have indicated a form of spontaneous abreaction to an internal problem. Such a hostile abreaction could become unresponsive to the interviewer's intervention.

The patient depersonalized his suicidal gesture (A. 1, 3, 16) and reported confusion about some of his experiences (A. 4, 5). There was some concreteness in his thinking (A. 1). The patient's thought content about the interviewer's ability to read his mind appeared to be delusional (A. 9, 17). Mr. R.'s ability to recall a recent event (A. 1) indicated that his recent memory was most likely intact. Orientation and intelligence were not tested during Step 1, but the patient was oriented throughout his hospital stay. He also showed good recent memory at admission. By admitting that he had pointed a gun at himself and was confused (A. 2–5), the patient showed at least the partial insight that he had a problem. The history of suicidal gestures and the irrational responses to the interviewer's questions would suggest impaired judgment.

Differential Diagnosis

Mr. R.'s rapid changes in affect, and his suicidal preoccupation reported with depersonalization, hostility, suspiciousness, poor concentration, and confused thinking, are all features of the following diagnoses.

Axis I

1. *Bipolar disorder, mixed.*
2. *Major depression.* Affective disorder is often associated with deficits in registration, concentration, and retrieval, as well as with slow thinking. Therefore, patients may feel that they are losing their memory and may report feeling confused. However, such mental slowing would probably emerge during the interview in the form of increased latency of response and slow speech. The interviewer did not observe these signs.
3. *Mood disorder due to complex partial seizures with mixed features.* A mental disorder due to brain tissue damage often manifests itself as a memory storage problem. Patients with complex partial seizures may experience derealization and depersonalization. Mr. R. seemed to experience his suicidal attempts as alien to him (A. 1–5), but he was not willing to talk about this experience. Such angry resistance is rarely seen in patients with complex partial seizures—unless they want to conceal having seizures at all.

A mental disorder due to chronic alcohol abuse, stimulant abuse, phencyclidine abuse, and cocaine abuse would be excluded because the patient and his wife gave a history negative for drug and alcohol abuse. The patient had a negative drug screen at admission and had been in the hospital for 3 weeks without access to substances of abuse.

4. *Beginning dementia* is unlikely because the patient has good recent memory and an above-average IQ.

5. *Amnestic state.* This diagnosis would not explain the patient's hostility and his specific thought content (i.e., the suicidal thinking) associated with his confused state.

6. *Delusional (paranoid) disorder.* Delusional disorder often involves a feeling that thoughts are being stolen from the patient's brain and that alien ones have been inserted. The patient's difficult-to-understand hostility would be compatible with persecutory delusional thinking. However, Mr. R.'s course of intermittent states of suicidal behavior surrounded by amnesia could not be easily explained.

7. *Dissociative disorder.* Amnesia, depersonalization, and rapid switch in affect are all compatible with dissociative disorder. Dissociation may involve blocking personal experiences of the host personality and alters. This patient's rigid responses could indicate the emergence of a personality who lacked a broad range of emotions. Indeed, some alters frequently represent a one-dimensional emotional state that the host splits off as unacceptable.

Axis II

1. *Borderline personality disorder.* Rapid switches in an interpersonal relationship—in this case with the interviewer—and suicidal tendencies are both compatible with borderline personality disorder. However, the patient's intense hostility was difficult to explain on the basis of this diagnosis alone.

2. *Paranoid personality disorder.* Unprovoked hostility can be a feature of this personality disorder. However, the patient's confusion and suicidal behavior would be insufficiently explained with this diagnosis.

3. *Schizotypal personality disorder.*

Step 2: Tag

21. I: I feel if we want to understand why you had a gun in your mouth, it would be helpful to learn more about your confusion.

P: You can't get off that subject, can you?

22. I: We can talk about something else . . . but I want to help you and [pausing and observing the patient] I feel I can help you best if we talk about things that sound important.

P: Important to you!

23. I: Is there any reason why you don't want to talk about your confusion?

P: I don't owe you a reason.

24. I: You're right, you don't. But, if we can share your feelings about the confusion, we may prevent you from sticking a gun in your mouth.

P: Let's skip it.

25. I: Maybe we can talk about it in a different way.

P: How's that?

26. I: Like talking about your memory. For example, can you repeat four words now—such as eyedropper, yellow, honesty, and tulip—and remember them later on?

P: Yellow, honesty, tulip . . . what was the first word? Okay, eyedropper. Hmmm, that psychiatric crap, I don't see what that can tell you. I could do it before.

The patient remained in his hostile state (A. 21–24). Yet, at the same time, he listened attentively and was interested when the interviewer shifted to a new topic (Q. 25, 26). Because the patient's refusal to explore his confusion appeared to be central to his problems, the interviewer tagged that problem (Q. 21–25), but the patient remained hostile. Therefore, the interviewer backed off (Q. 25, 26), but at the same time kept the subject in focus.

The patient's hostile affect together with his vigilant suspiciousness dominated. He responded with rigid hostility even when the interviewer changed his approach. However, he agreed to the memory test, repeating four out of four words successfully.

Differential Diagnosis

This step does not add any new disorders to the list of possible Axis I or Axis II disorders, nor does it exclude any.

Step 3: Confront

Step 3a: Backing Off

27. I: Recalling four words is easy. But I wonder whether you have some other memory disturbances. Ever have any gaps in your memory? Just can't remember what you did?

P: [Patient crouches down into his seat like a cat ready to jump at the interviewer's throat, his eyes narrowing to a slit. He inhales and holds his breath, then bites his lower lip, curls his hands into fists, white knuckles popping out. The air in the area seems to stop circulating.]

28. I: [Leaning back, relaxing, looking at the ceiling, shaking his head] Oh, Mr. R., don't answer that one. When I think about it, it's really not that important.

P: [Relaxes, releases his breath, and stares at the interviewer] Not important? What do you mean?

29. I: Well, I mean that we can talk about something else first. I want you to feel relaxed when you talk to me.

P: [Stares at the interviewer; then, sitting up straight in his chair] You thought it was important a minute ago, didn't you?

30. I: Maybe later. But not right now.

P: I don't like what you are doing. I don't trust you. You are playing some kind of game with me.

31. I: You're right. I feel that you don't trust me. What I ask you seems to make you angry. I apologize to you that I asked about your memory. I want to help you and not upset you.

P: What makes you think I got upset?

32. I: I don't know for sure, but all of a sudden you made fists, and your eyes became narrowed. I want you to feel comfortable. It's really not so important that you talk to me about your memory now. You don't have to if you don't want to.

P: So, what do you want to talk to me about?

The rapport between patient and interviewer remained strained. The patient became angry and hostile when the interviewer explored his memory gaps. The patient's hostility and anger kept the interviewer on edge. He felt uncomfortable, as if he was circling an area protected by an electric fence. Whenever he came too close, he received a shock (Q. 27, 32). He feared the patient would attack him physically or break off the interview. He wanted to avoid any form of abreaction, yet if he stayed away from the patient's inner sanctum the interview might not yield a diagnosis. However, backing off alleviated the patient's hostility and showed he was at least somewhat responsive to the interviewer. This interactive responsiveness allowed the interviewer to continue with his task rather than break off the interview and sedate the patient medically.[1]

---

[1] As illustrated in this interview, as long as the patient responds to your strategies in the expected direction, you may continue interviewing. If you cannot reach the patient with your strategies, you are at the limits of verbal intervention. You may have to resort to pharmacological intervention or physical restraints if you are attacked physically.

When the interviewer confronted the patient with his confusion and interpreted it as a memory disturbance (Q. 27), he provoked violent anger (A. 27). Backing off (Q. 28, 30, 31) released the patient's tension, but the patient's hostility remained (A. 28, 30, 31). The interviewer kept the topic of memory disturbance in focus by repeatedly de-emphasizing it (Q. 28, 32). The interviewer's soothing statements in suggestive form (Q. 29, 31, 32) kept the patient's hostility below the boiling point.[2]

Mr. R. responded to the technique of confronting, backing off, and then soothing by displaying intense affect. He was not frozen in an autistic, hostile stance but was reactive to the interviewer's intervention. Such a response would indicate that verbal interventions with this patient could still possibly be effective. It should be noted that this patient was being treated with haloperidol 20 mg/day, which had not eliminated the patient's hostility or suspiciousness.

Differential Diagnosis

The patient's hostile response to the interviewer's interpretation of memory lapse (Q. and A. 27) was most compatible with delusional thinking. Such thinking may occur in bipolar disorder, schizoaffective disorder, delusional (paranoid) disorder, or even dissociative disorder. It is unlikely in non-psychotic major depression, during which memory problems become exaggerated, and even less likely in complex partial seizure disorder, during which patients are concerned about their memory gaps rather than hiding them. Hostile remarks are seldom a feature of early uncomplicated dementia of the Alzheimer's type, in which patients usually do not recognize the memory disturbance and deny it without hostility.

The nature of the memory disturbance is important for the diagnosis, yet the patient becomes hostile when confronted with memory gaps. Therefore, the interviewer gives the patient space without losing sight of the diagnostic problem of the memory disturbance. In other words, he looks at the memory disturbance from a distance. He explores the patient's fear of anybody getting too close to him. He follows the patient's thought process while keeping distance from the memory impairment. We call this technique of pursuing a subject without using direct confrontation "trailing" the problem.

---

[2] In the nonhostile patient, continuous and repeated confronting is usually effective. However, the hostile patient does not tolerate such perseverance. Therefore, you should back off when the patient's anger increases, as this interviewer did.

Step 3b: Trailing

33. I: Well, we may talk about things that go really well for you.
    P: Things that go well for me?
34. I: Yes.
    P: That sounds phony. You make me angry.
35. I: How can I help you, Mr. R.?
    P: You can't. I have to figure it out myself.
36. I: You're right. And I feel you can do it because of your background in the health field. You have seen a lot of problems.
    P: Bullshit! I don't see how that can help me.
37. I: You understand suffering. You know what it takes to cope with it.
    P: [Hostile] What do you know?
38. I: I know that it is a tough job to be a surgical nurse.
    P: [With a sarcastic voice] But you're a shrink. What would you know about medicine?
39. I: I rotated through surgery in a small hospital. Often during a procedure there was just me and the nurse. It was the nurse who helped me through. I was scared and didn't know what to do.
    P: [Suddenly leans back in his chair, closes his eyes, and with a friendly soft voice] Psychiatry isn't that easy either. I worked in a psych ward too.
40. I: Hmmm.
    P: I do some agency work and pick up some hours in psychiatry.
41. I: So you know what psychiatric problems are like. How do you think your own problem fits in with what you've seen?
    P: You know I didn't want to be here. It was the police who brought me here, when they found me on the highway. They said I was sitting in the car with a gun in my mouth.
42. I: But then you signed yourself in.
    P: Yes, because of my wife. She wanted me to.
43. I: What made you so desperate that you wanted to put a bullet in your head?
    P: It's a useless life.
44. I: Can you help me understand?
    P: I wish I was never born. I don't want to take care of that body of mine and that person of mine.
45. I: It sounds like you don't want to be you.
    P: [As if struck by a bullet, stands up and points his finger at the interviewer] You sneak up on me. [With a sharp voice and narrowed eyelids] Get off my back! Leave me alone! You're coming too close.
46. I: Then tell me what we can talk about without my coming too close.
    P: [With a sharp voice, stepping toward the interviewer] Just stay away, you hear? You can't ever understand! You're a white man. You can't understand the Indian way.
47. I: You are right. Is there anyone who can understand you?
    P: [Stares at interviewer] After death, maybe somebody on the other side. . . .
48. I: Please sit down! Can you understand yourself?
    P: [Patient sits down and closes his eyes; with an angry voice seemingly to

himself] I'm going around in a daze. [With a very low but angry voice] Maybe my wife. Sometime she's right, gets very close. . . .

49. I: Does that help if she gets close?

P: [Opens his eyes, looks bewildered and then hostile] Just shut up. You make me angry. I want to kill you.

50. I: How would that help you? If I'm dead in front of you, how would that solve what you are going through?

P: You wouldn't push me anymore.

51. I: You're right. I'm sorry. But you say your wife is coming close, too. Should she be dead, too?

P: Sometimes . . . but she really cares for me.

52. I: I understand. I don't envy you.

P: Why do you say that?

53. I: I think you understand better than I do.

P: [Looks at interviewer without saying anything]

54. I: You want to kill me because you think I'll get too close; you sometimes want to kill your wife because she's coming too close. And then, you put the gun on your own head because you are coming too close to yourself.

P: [Screams out and jumps up, stretching out his hands toward the interviewer's throat. The two attendants come over.]

55. I: [Stares the patient in the eyes] I'm not close, but you are.

P: [Stops his screaming and his motion]

56. I: Let's talk it out, Mr. R. You scare me. I'm afraid; I can't help you when I'm scared of you. Please sit down!

P: [Sits down]

57. I: [To the attendants] Mr. R. is fine, but I'd like you to stay around in case I upset Mr. R. again. [Turning to the patient] Mr. R., earlier I gave you a list of four words. Do you remember what they were?

P: Call me by my first name! Now wait . . . you said eyedropper and yellow . . . honesty, yes, that's what it was, I wondered why you asked me to remember that. And there was another one, yellow tulip.

58. I: You remember them all. That's great, Mr. R. Oh, excuse me . . . you wanted me to call you by your first name—Robert? Is that what you want me to call you?

P: My name is Pete.

Up to this point in the interview, the level of rapport between interviewer and patient had been determined by an alternating pattern switching between empathy (Q. 1–5), hostility (Q. 6–38), back to empathy (Q. 39–44), and then back to hostility (Q. 45–58). Hostility emerged at Q. 6. The switch to empathy was then induced (Q. 39) when the interviewer admitted to experiencing anxiety when he was a fledgling surgery intern. This triggered a role reversal: the patient adopted a therapeutic stance toward the interviewer (Q. 39–44). When the interviewer tried a third time to interpret the patient's desire to be somebody else (Q. 45), the patient's hostility returned

(Q. 19, 27, 45). The hostility intensified when the interviewer put forth a key interpretation (Q. 54).

So far throughout the interview, the patient displayed two contrasting attitudes: warmth, empathy, and receptiveness on the one hand (Q. 1–5, 39–44), and hostility and opposition on the other (Q. 6–38, 45–58).

In his countertransference, the interviewer experienced tension until he finally admitted to the patient that he was scared. This made the patient turn off the current, so to speak, and temporarily allowed the interviewer to enter the "wired area." The interviewer tried to create a safe space that would allow him to probe for information without evoking the patient's anger and hostility. Distraction from the topic of memory gaps (Q. 33) failed. Therefore, he backed off and turned to the patient for help (Q. 35). The attempt to establish common ground (working in the health field) and expressing empathy for the patient's tough work situation (Q. 38) eventually failed too. The third technique, backing off by admitting weakness (Q. 39), succeeded in triggering a switch in the patient from hostility to empathy. The interviewer used this switch to probe the patient for more information (Q. 41, 43–45) and confronted him with his signing in (Q. 42) as evidence that he was aware of a problem. But when the interviewer honed in on the patient's feeling of depersonalization with an interpretation (Q. 45), a topic that the patient had introduced on his own (A. 44), the patient switched back to hostility. The interviewer again backed off by turning to the patient for help (Q. 46–48), yet he continued probing the patient's fear of somebody getting too close to his problem (Q. 47–51). He combined this probing with an expression of his wish to help the patient (Q. 49–50).

The interviewer's working toward a central interpretation (Q. 52–54) provoked the patient to attack. At this point, *trailing* to pursue a topic while maintaining safe distance temporarily failed. The patient abreacted his problem again by turning the aggression he felt against himself toward the interviewer. Yet, the interviewer concluded his interpretation (Q. 55) and then backed off, following a strategy that had helped before: admission of his own vulnerability (Q. 39, 56). Again, the patient responded positively, and the interviewer once again found himself in the safety zone.

In summary, the interviewer's backing off and soothing contained the patient and prevented him from becoming physically aggressive, but it did not convert the patient's hostile attitude into a cooperative one. The only technique that worked so far in this case was the interviewer's revealing of his own vulnerability.

Alternative approaches that the interviewer could have tried include higher doses of neuroleptic medication for a longer time and a long-term, client-centered approach. However, the patient stayed with the interview, although in a predominantly hostile attitude. It thus seemed clear that his need to get his problem out in the open overrode his need to scare off intruders who were becoming too close to his problem. The patient's displayed aggression against himself (i.e., threatening to shoot himself) and against the interviewer became a protective shield that the interviewer tried to remove.

As to mental status, so far in the interview the patient showed two attitudes: a hostile and a friendly one. The patient's hostile attitude was associated with the name of Pete and presented with hypervigilance; increased psychomotor activity; a cutting, sharp, cold voice; a hostile, angry, and labile affect (Q. 6–39, 45–58); and suicidal and even homicidal tendencies (Q. 49–54).[3] The patient's friendly attitude was visible for a brief time at the beginning of the interview (Q. 1–6) and again later (Q. 39–44). The mental status associated with the friendly attitude was characterized by good eye contact with blinking, psychomotor movements with normal rate, a relaxed muscle tone, and a soft voice. The affect associated with this attitude, however, appeared somewhat discouraged and depressed. Up to this point, the interviewer had not explored whether the patient associated a name other than Pete with this friendly mental status.

Differential Diagnosis

The patient stated that he felt confused (A. 4, 5). He showed perplexity (A. 6) and signs of depersonalization (A. 1–3, 12, 16, 17, 41, 44). Furthermore, he presented with two distinct forms of mental status, one of which was identified with the name Pete. These observations provided sufficient evidence for the interviewer to believe that the patient was switching back and forth between two states of identity and consciousness associated with the dissociative dysfunction, thus suggesting the diagnosis of dissociative identity disorder. Therefore, the interviewer's next step was to prepare the patient for hypnotic switching.

Step 4: Solve by Hypnotic Switching

59. I: Your record shows the name Robert Chris, not Robert Pete.
    P: I hate Chris. The people who adopted me called me that.
60. I: You hate Chris?

---

[3] It should be noted that suicide attempts are a common feature of dissociative identity disorder (Ross and Norton 1989).

P: Because it sounds like a female name.

61. I: It does?

P: To me it does.

62. I: Several American names are used for males and females alike, like Kay or Pat, yes, and Chris.

P: That's not for me. [Folds his arms in front of his chest as if holding on to himself]

63. I: It's not for Pete. Pete sounds angry. What about Chris? I'm ready to talk to Chris. I want to meet Chris. I will count to three and then I'm ready to meet Chris. One, two, three. Chris?

P: [Suddenly, the patient shows a soft smile on his face but looks puzzled; he crosses his legs] What did you say? Who are you?

64. I: I'm Dr. O. And who are you?

P: [With a change in voice to a higher pitch] I'm Chris. You can call me Chris.

65. I: Are you a nurse?

P: Oh no, Pete is a nurse. I'm a beautician. I do haircuts for my friends at home in the evening. [Giggling] It's kind of moonlighting. [Giggles again]

66. I: Does Pete know you?

P: I know him.

67. I: Does Pete like you?

P: He does not know much of me but he hates me. He would kill me if he knew more of me. He wants me dead. He hates Chris. He only likes Pete. Pete is macho. [Giggling some more]

68. I: Why is Pete so angry about Chris?

P: Because she's a woman.

69. I: He was adopted and they called him Chris.

P: He hates it. He hates it. He hates it. [Giggles]

70. I: He hates it?

P: His stepbrother made him do things.

71. I: Made him do things?

P: Made him suck him. He raped him [giggles] and teased him and always called him "Chris, my little sweet darling." [Giggles, then starts crying in a child's voice] Don't! John, don't hurt me! Please, please, it hurts when you do that to me . . . no . . . no . . . don't hurt Bobby.

72. I: I'm going to count to three and I want Mr. R. back. One, two, three . . . Mr. R.?

P: [Looks bewildered and speaking with a soft voice] What happened?

73. I: Do you remember?

P: No.

74. I: Mr. R., do you know Chris?

P: Yes. I'm Robert C.

75. I: Robert C.?

P: I'm friendly. Pete is angry. You can talk to me, you can talk to Robert C.

76. I: I think I can help Pete better if you talk about Pete's anger. Pete gets angry when we talk about him losing his memory. I think his anger comes up about Chris. And he gets angry when he comes too close or his wife come too close.

P: [Looks at interviewer and frowns]

77. I: Pete tells me I don't understand Indians and he may be right. But I understand a person who turns into somebody else and cannot remember it.

P: But I can remember Chris.

78. I: You can?

P: I can.

79. I: Pete hates the fact that one of his personalities is a woman?

P: He doesn't really know that. It would be awful for him, but he does not really know.

80. I: Awful? I can feel his pain. Chris is not a nurse.

P: No, she has a feminine occupation. She is a beautician.

81. I: But a nurse can be a feminine profession, too.

P: [Screams, with a sharp voice] What are you doing to me? I'm not a queer. I'm a Shawnee.

For the first time in the interview, the patient's hostile alter, Pete, cooperated with the interviewer by describing his hatred for his middle name. A second personality, Chris, has a submissive and flirtatious attitude toward the interviewer (A. 63–71). This personality did not emerge prior to the induced switch (Q. 63).

A third personality emerged, identified as Robert C. (A. 74). This alter showed a cooperative, friendly attitude, not at all flirtatious or submissive toward the interviewer. He dominated the interview from A. 72 to A. 80 and had insight into the workings of the alters.

The interviewer was having difficulty exploring the personality of Pete without provoking the patient's anger. Therefore, he searched for a more cooperative personality that would allow him to explore the structure of the multiple personalities. One way to spot a personality is to have the patient give his full name and ask if he has any other names, or whether he is aware of personality characteristics different from the one that he is currently showing. This patient facilitated the first approach by introducing himself as Pete (A. 58). This statement allowed the interviewer to connect with Robert Chris and then switch the patient by addressing a simple suggestion (Q. 63) to the character of Chris. With open-ended (Q. 64, 68, 71) and closed-ended (Q. 65–67, 70) questions, the interviewer could explore the relationship between Chris and Pete and uncover why Pete is so hateful and defensive toward the emergence of the Chris personality.

The mental status of the Chris personality was effeminate and flirtatious; she had a high-pitched voice, comprehended questions fully, and answered them to the point. Her affect appeared to be silly and seemed to ridicule the personality of Pete. She displayed histrionic giggling (A. 65, 67, 69, 71).

All personalities could be easily switched by the interviewer. This was not surprising. A patient with a dissociative disorder is highly suggestible and easy to hypnotize.

Differential Diagnosis

The interviewer set the stage for the patient's admission that he hated his female name. This admission, coupled with the induced personality switch, confirmed the suspected diagnosis of dissociative identity disorder. The patient showed two common features of dissociative identity, according to descriptions in DSM-IV: suicide attempts and the classic predisposing factor of sexual abuse in childhood.

Step 5: Approve

82. I: Robert!
    P: I hate you. I'm Pete. I hate you.
83. I: I'm sorry. I understand why you don't want to talk about it. I promise, I will stay out of it. Let me talk to Robert C. Robert C.!
    P: [Looks down at his knees, relaxes] Yes?
84. I: I see it must hurt for Pete to talk about it. I understand why Pete got angry.
    P: You do?
85. I: I understand that Pete wants to keep me away. Let me map out what I've learned about your personalities. [The interviewer takes a piece of paper and maps the personalities. At the end of the interview, the interviewer switches the patient to Robert R., the host personality, and thanks him for helping him understand the different personalities.]

The patient had described five personalities. Looking back at the interview, the interviewer, with the patient's help, determined when each personality had surfaced. He obtained such a map by asking a given personality which other personalities he or she knew and whether that personality had surfaced during the interview. This endeavor resulted in the following list:

1. Robert R., the dominant personality, was host to all the other personalities (A. 1–5, 72–80, 83–85). Robert R. appeared to be the even-tempered personality with the best access to the other four personalities. He could neither integrate Pete's macho needs nor Chris's female need for submissiveness. Of all the personalities, Robert R. was most aware of his identity but was the weakest in preventing a switch into the other personalities. Robert R. and Chris both knew of each other and both knew Pete.

2. Pete was a Shawnee who showed much hostility, a macho surgical nurse (A. 6–38, 45–62, 81, 82) who wanted to eliminate Chris, whose personality threatened to break through into Pete's consciousness. Pete knew Robert R. but not Chris.
3. Robert C. was a friendly psychiatric nurse. He surfaced in A. 39–44.
4. Chris was a flirtatious beautician (A. 63–70). She identified with the sexual abuse and accepted the female role. She was seductive and flirtatious and undermined Pete's need for machismo.
5. Bobby was a frightened, crying child. He surfaced in A. 71.

After the interviewer induced a switch from Pete to Robert C., good rapport void of suspicion and hostility and a therapeutic alliance were established. In terms of transactional analysis, the adult interviewer was then talking to the adult patient. This personality had comprehensive knowledge and was most tolerant of the other alters, except for Bobby. Robert C. was not the dominant personality. That role belonged to Robert R., who was responsible for most activities but did not know the other personalities.

The interviewer initiated this integrative step of approval by expressing to Pete his understanding about Pete's self-protective behavior (Q. 83). The switch to Robert C. was made to approach the most interactive personality and to identify the alter who knew the most about the others and was willing to share this knowledge. The interviewer mapped the personalities to obtain the most comprehensive picture (Ross and Gahan 1988). Pete felt suicidal or, more correctly, homicidal toward Chris (A. 67). This answer explained why the patient, when asked earlier about his suicide wishes, responded that he (as Pete) wanted to kill somebody (presumably Chris; A. 16, 17). However, it was possible to diminish the patient's hostility, suspiciousness, and suicidality by backing off, and to abolish these behaviors by switching personalities.

The exploration of the patient's thought content revealed a pattern of interrelationship among five personalities. Of all personalities, Robert C. had the best insight into the patient's psychiatric problem, but he had no access to Bobby, the personality who represented the one who had experienced the sexual abuse.

The interviewer examined Robert R.'s short-term memory across personality boundaries (Q. 57). The memory test was given to Pete in Q. 26; the interviewer could not dismantle the amnesia barrier. He did not focus on the failure to remember because he did not intend to demonstrate perceptual dissonance to the patient at this point (Ross and Gahan 1988). In the personality of Robert C., the patient had insight.

Diagnosis

Axis I. *Dissociative identity disorder.* Several personalities have been identified and can be switched by hypnotic suggestion.

Delusional disorder should be ruled out because of the high degree of suspiciousness shown by the Pete personality.

Axes II through V.   Not assessed.

As noted in DSM-IV, studies have shown that adult females with dissociative identity disorder outnumber males by a factor of 3 to 9. Furthermore, females tend to have more alters ($\geq$15) than do males (mean of 8). Patients of either sex can harbor destructive, hostile, suicidal, and homicidal personalities, but such alters are generally more threatening in a male than in a female patient. Inducing a switch in personalities can be a powerful technique to master the interview.

6. Dissociation, Hypnotic Switching, Hypnosis, and Free Association in Psychiatric Disorders

In DSM-IV, five dissociative disorders are listed:

- Dissociative amnesia
- Dissociative fugue
- Dissociative identity disorder
- Depersonalization disorder
- Dissociative disorder not otherwise specified (including derealization, brainwashing, dissociative trance disorder, loss of consciousness, stupor, coma, and Ganser syndrome)

In *dissociative amnesia,* memory but not identity is disturbed. During the amnestic state, the patient is in a trancelike, depersonalized state. After the amnestic period, he cannot access thoughts, feelings, sensory impressions, or actions that occurred during this period.

In *dissociative fugue,* both memory for the past and identity are lost. However, skills acquired prior to the onset of the fugue may be preserved. Also, the patient is oriented to time, place, and her new person. She also can learn new things but is cut off from her remote memory.

In *dissociative identity disorder,* several identities with their respective memories become inhabitants of a host. The host and the individual personalities may have familiarity with some but not all of the personalities.

Dissociative identity disorder splits the patient's identity into two or more distinct personalities, each with a unique perception of himself or herself, of others, and of the environment (Thigpen and Cleckley 1957). Each has his or her individual expression of affect, tone of voice, choice of vocabulary, and physiological responses (Putnam et al. 1990). A female patient may have one or more male personalities, and a male patient may have one or more female personalities.

The identity that is most often present or that has the most control is called the *dominant* (or *primary* or *host*) personality. This personality often describes his dissociative experiences as "lost time," periods too extensive to be dismissed as ordinary forgetfulness. Often the primary personality cannot describe the characteristics of the secondary personalities (also called *alters*), but these alters are frequently aware of the primary personality's strengths and shortcomings. Once considered to be rare, dissociative identity disorder is now thought to affect as many as 1 in 100 individuals, virtually all of whom have a history of severe sexual abuse, physical abuse, or both (Halleck 1990; Ross and Gahan 1988; Ross et al. 1991).

In many cases, dissociative identity disorder goes unrecognized or is misdiagnosed for years (Kluft 1987). To diagnose a dissociative personality change, you must first rule out substance intoxication, dissociative amnesia or fugue states, complex partial seizures, and other mental disorders due to a general medical condition (including neurological disorders), such as brain tumors. A diagnosis of dissociative identity disorder is confirmed by the ability to call up at least one secondary personality.

In *depersonalization disorder,* identity but not memory is disturbed. The patient, however, does not assume a new identity but experiences herself at some physical or internal distance. She feels like an onlooker of her own behaviors.

Autosuggestive and autohypnotic phenomena appear to be essential to conversion and dissociation. According to DSM-IV, individuals with dissociative amnesia and dissociative identity disorder achieve high scores on measures of hypnotizability. Patients with dissociative disorders, especially dissociative identity disorder, report childhood trauma such as severe sexual and physical abuse. As noted in DSM-IV, however, the accuracy of these reports remains controversial.

Both dissociative and conversion symptoms occur in somatization disorder. However, they are rarely the center of the disorder. They seem to be called on when the patient is in acute distress but, unlike some other somatization symptoms such as abdominal pain, they are rarely chronic. Thus, patients with somatization disorder show at times conversion and dissociative symptoms. Conversely, 35% of patients with dissociative identity disorder fulfill diagnostic criteria for somatization disorder (Ross et al. 1989).

In addition, acute stress disorder or posttraumatic stress disorder (acute or chronic, immediate or delayed onset) may be associated with dissociative symptoms. Patients with a history of somatoform, conversion, histrionic, or borderline personality disorder are highly susceptible to falling into a trance state.

Dissociation as a psychiatric symptom and sign remains a topic of discussion. There are two views: One (Halleck 1990; Kluft 1991; Ross 1991; Ross et al. 1991; Whitman and Munkel 1991) claims that dissociation plays a major role in many psychiatric disorders but is presently underdiagnosed. The other (Coons 1991; Kluft 1989b; Mersky 1992) debates that dissociation could be a thinly veiled face-saving device often introduced iatrogenically to excuse patients from taking responsibility for some of their actions. In this view, dissociation is not seen as a legitimate, discrete category of psychiatric signs and symptoms but as a form of lying and deception. Those who accept the concept of dissociation recognize the distinct phenomena of fugue state, dissociative amnesia, and dissociative identity disorder as real. Those who reject the concept consider such phenomena to be errors of clinical judgment on the part of the diagnosing therapist. Researchers in the United States (Braun 1989; Kluft and Fine 1993), Canada (Bowers 1991; Ross et al. 1991a), and Netherlands (Boon and Draijer 1993; van der Hart and Boon 1990) are more likely to accept dissociation as a clinical phenomenon, whereas clinicians in Japan (Takahashi 1990; also compare the discussion of Takahashi's research by van der Hart 1990) are more prone to deny it at this time.

DSM-IV supports the stance that dissociative phenomena are real. They are distinct from lying and pretense and should not be equated with malingering or factitious disorder. However, the interviewer's ability to discover the traumatic origin of patients' dissociation does not constitute therapy, nor does it sufficiently explain the nature of the disorder. The essence of these conditions is not that an individual dissociation can be reversed by free association, hypnosis, or by a switching process; instead, the critical point is that patients repeatedly dissociate even after they have learned that their dissociating is trauma induced and psychologically reversible. Thus, expect dissociative symptoms to recur even if in the past you have reversed such symptoms and believe patients have gained full insight into their psychogenic nature. In this way, relapse into dissociation is similar to relapse into delusions in psychotic patients, even after treatment with neuroleptics and psychotherapy has given the patients full insight into the morbid character of their delusions.

For the treatment of dissociative phenomena, you may try hypnosis, its acute variant hypnotic switching, and free association. Because most diagnostic interviews last less than 1 hour, you may attempt hypnotic switching because it is the least time consuming. The technique of hypnotic switching is indicated if the patient's dissociative symptoms were sudden in onset, which—in clinical experience—is frequently the case. Thus, hypnotic switching uses a mechanism of acute autohypnosis for therapeutic intervention that is similar to what was possibly operational in the acute production of the dissociative symptoms themselves. If the switching process does not work initially, you may use the lengthier hypnotic technique and then condition the patient via posthypnotic suggestion for hypnotic switching in the future. For more recurrent dissociative symptoms, we recommend free association.

Use free association to detect the trauma that precipitates the dissociation or conversion symptom. Furthermore, free association can aid in identifying the patient's vulnerability to certain traumatic events and conflicts. This relatively narrow application of the free association method goes back to its historic roots—to Freud's work on hysteric patients—and to the experience that posthypnotic amnesia can be reversed with both hypnosis and free association.

Free association has become the mainstay of all insight-oriented, psychodynamic psychotherapy. Therapists of different orientations favor open-ended questions and semistructured and unstructured interviewing styles to invite patients to reveal a wide variety of thought contents and emotionally charged materials rather than limiting them to endorse or refuse preconceived symptom lists. Non-goal-oriented, indirect questions, with a corresponding broad, associative style of answering, have become the preferred style of interviewing. In most instances, the interviewer guides the patient indirectly to free associations rather than directly, as was done in interview A, above.

Consider this technique whenever you encounter a barrier of nonremembering, curt yes and no answers, silence, or anxious censorship. Circling the subject of interest from a distance often generates the answers that a goal-directed inquiry cannot.

If free association and hypnotic switching fail, use a behavioral approach and praise the patient whenever she is able to stay with her main personality, or when she is able to give up dissociation in favor of controlled thinking and behavior. In especially complex cases of dissociative identity disorder, the amobarbital interview (see Chapter 6, "Catatonia") has been useful (deVito 1993).

CHAPTER 3

POSTTRAUMATIC STRESS

Summary

A patient who has posttraumatic stress disorder has faced a life-threatening event or severe injury or a "threat to the physical integrity of self or others" (DSM-IV [American Psychiatric Association 1994], p. 427). The traumatic event is reexperienced in intrusive images, thoughts, perceptions, dreams, flashbacks, and even hallucinations. Anxious avoidance prevents the patient from recalling the trauma contextually in thoughts, sensory impressions, and feelings. He also avoids discharging the trauma-induced fear, anger, and grief; in other words, he avoids catharsis.

In this chapter, we show how the interviewer can help patients reexperience the trauma and make a differential diagnosis that distinguishes posttraumatic stress disorder from other anxiety, dissociative, and psychotic disorders.

◆ ◆ ◆ ◆ ◆

Crux est, si metuas, vincere quod nequeas.
It is torture to fear what you cannot overcome.

Anacharsis (early sixth century B.C.)
Septem Sapientum Sententiae

◆ ◆ ◆ ◆ ◆

1. What Is Posttraumatic Stress Disorder?

Posttraumatic stress centers around a trauma. The DSM-IV criteria indicate that "(1) the person experienced, witnessed, or was confronted with an event or events that involved actual or threatened death or serious injury, or a threat to the physical integrity of self or others" (p. 427) and "(2) the person's response involved intense fear, helplessness, or horror" (p. 428).

The patient experiences splinters of sensory recollection of the event, such as smells, noises, and images of the event. Flashbacks, nightmares, dissociative states, illusions, hallucinations, and, in extreme cases, reenactments intrude on the patient. In replaying the flashbacks, the patient repeats the same segment of the event over and over again in her mind, asking herself repeatedly how she could have prevented the painful outcome. She is unable to find a satisfactory solution retrospectively or to process the event as a fate of human existence, so her wounds stay open.

Posttraumatic stress leads to active resistance to remembering thoughts, images, and memories associated with a trauma; an amnesia-like state may develop. The patient also blocks recollection of the affect experienced at the time of the trauma. This effort to avoid any recollection leads to a numbing of affective responses to current events and results in emotional detachment from significant others, including family members. Over time, this behavior worsens; activities, places, objects, or people that arouse recollection of the trauma are avoided. Instead of free-floating anxiety and fear, the patient experiences hypervigilance, distractibility, irritability, and exaggerated startle response during the day, and initial and intermittent insomnia interspersed with nightmares during the night.

Researchers have applied a number of models to understand the development of the symptoms of posttraumatic stress disorder. Peterson et al. (1991) reviewed 10 such models and attempted to integrate these models in their ecosystemic model.

1. In the *information processing model,* Horowitz (1973, 1974, 1979) postulated that a catastrophic event leads to an information overload, which cannot be matched with the person's cognitive schemata because the information lies outside the realm of his normal experience. The unprocessed information remains as an active form of memory and disturbs ego functioning.

2. In the *psychosocial model* (Green et al. 1985), the importance of the environment is emphasized. A supportive environment enhances and an adverse one hampers the working through of the traumatic experience.

3. In the *behavioral model,* Keane et al. (1985a, 1985b) posited a two-factor theory. The first factor represents classical conditioning in which a fear response is learned through association. The second factor represents instrumental learning by which patients avoid those conditioning cues that evoke anxiety.

4. In the *cognitive appraisal model* (Epstein 1991; Janoff-Bulman 1985), it is postulated that the catastrophic trauma disrupts the patient's basic assumptions of a safe world and personal invulnerability.

5. In the *psychodynamic model* (Freud 1919; Grinker and Spiegel 1945a, 1945b; Hendin et al. 1981; Kardiner 1941; Krystal 1968; Worthington 1978), the development of war neurosis or traumatic neurosis of holocaust survivors is explained as interaction between early childhood conflicts and the traumatic event.

6. The *psychosocial developmental model* (Erikson 1968) was used by Wilson (1978, 1980) to explain how a catastrophic trauma afflicts a person during a stage oriented toward the development of personal identity, disrupts this maturation process, and induces identity confusion and social isolation. This disruption also interferes with the development of generativity and integrity and leads to stagnation and despair.

7. In the *psychoformative model* (Lifton 1967, 1976, 1979), connectedness, integrity, and progress are emphasized; according to Wilson (1978), these qualities are disrupted by the traumatic event, which results in separation, disintegration, and stasis.

8. Brende (1982, 1983) used the *objects relation model* (Kernberg 1975;

Kohut 1971; Masterson 1976; Rinsley 1982) to diagnose a disorder of self in patients who respond with posttraumatic stress disorder to a catastrophic trauma. Two personality disorders—borderline and narcissistic—are seen as facilitators for posttraumatic stress disorder. (For more details see Peterson et al. 1991.)

9. The *psychophysiologic and biologic model* (de la Pena 1984; van der Kolk et al. 1984, 1985) is built on the biological model of learned helplessness developed by Maier and Seligman (1976), who observed that inescapable shock leads to a depletion of norepinephrine, dopamine, and serotonin in the brain and to an increase of acetylcholine and endogenous opioids. These biochemical changes reduce escape behavior and initiative to respond to stress. The increase of opioids leads the patient to become addicted to the trauma and to develop a tendency to seek reenactment of the trauma in order to experience the associated excitation.

10. In the *cybernetic model* (Schultz 1984), it is postulated that there are feedback loops between memories of combat and increased physiological arousal, which explain the balance between recall and suppression of the trauma.

Even though these models of posttraumatic stress disorder differ in the use of terminology and emphasis, they overlap and complement each other in content. In each, at least one of the following four factors is usually discussed:

- The trauma itself
- The patient's characteristics
- The environment
- The phases a patient passes through in the development of an adjustment reaction to the trauma

The trauma.   The magnitude of the trauma is thought to be in the range of events that involve facing death or serious injury as, for example, in man-made catastrophes (e.g., a bombing raid, combat, rape, mugging, car accident) or natural disasters (e.g., flood, fire, earthquake) or witnessing or learning about such events, especially when they affect family members or close associates. It is important that the nature of the trauma be accurately classified, such as whether it was acute or persistent, abrupt or gradual, faced alone or as a group, and actively or passively experienced (e.g., as pilot or passenger in an airplane crash) (Green et al. 1985; Wilson 1983).

The nature of the trauma may be important for two reasons: 1) the magnitude of the trauma may determine the degree of information process-ing necessary (Wilson and Krauss 1985), and 2) a complementary relation-ship may exist between the patient's pretraumatic anxiety level and the magnitude of the trauma (Trimble 1981). The greater the patient's preexist-ing, free-floating, phobic, generalized anxiety, the less serious a trauma is needed to elicit a posttraumatic stress response in that patient.

The patient's characteristics. Most authors seem to feel that each human has a breaking point (Trimble 1981) that is determined by her premorbid development; her cognitive beliefs about the safety of her world; her personal vulnerability; her emotional ability to discharge affects such as grief, anger, and fear; and her biological disposition to respond with anxiety, hyperarousal, and avoidance. The patient's developmental stage during which she is traumatized may also determine her response. For example, in adolescence or young adulthood, when the patient's identity is not yet fully developed, she may be more vulnerable to trauma than in a stage where she has reached a sense of identity (Peterson et al. 1991).

Patients with posttraumatic stress disorder frequently display two prom-inent characteristics: 1) They feel victimized. They feel they had no control over the event, yet wonder whether it could have been prevented through more efficiency, skill, or courage. 2) They feel guilty about their actions or the event. They feel that their actions contradicted their belief system and challenged the integrity of their self-image.

The environment. An important factor in the nature of the trauma is whether the environment is sympathetic toward the trauma victim (e.g., victims of accidents and natural catastrophes, veterans of honorable wars such as World War I and II) or cold, critical, and rejecting of the victim (e.g., victims of rape, veterans of the Vietnam War). A sympathetic environment allows successful processing of the traumatic event rather than forcing the patient to suppress his memories and emotions. (For further details, see Green et al. 1985.)

Phases in the development of an adjustment reaction to the trauma.
Horowitz (1974, 1986) developed a five-phase model for the general course of posttraumatic stress disorder:

- *Phase I:* Outcry
- *Phase II:* Denial, numbing, and withdrawal
- *Phase III:* Oscillation between denial and involuntary repetition of the

trauma by intrusive thoughts, feelings, images, memories, flashbacks, and nightmares

- *Phase IV:* Working through the trauma versus suppression
- *Phase V:* Completion of response to the trauma versus avoidance

Horowitz's Phases IV and V represent an adaptive response to trauma. However, a maladaptive response may occur in Phases IV and V in the course of a delayed or chronic posttraumatic stress disorder in which the main symptoms of the disorder become cemented. These symptoms include generalization of fear, anger, withdrawal, trauma, and pathological splitting off in the form of dissociation (e.g., amnesias, flashbacks, nightmares).

Because the patient avoids the topic of her trauma, you may mistake her detached and numb affect and her mood as major depression combined with a generalized anxiety or panic disorder, thereby missing her posttraumatic stress disorder. Even after you are able to elicit flashbacks, nightmares, and avoidance from the patient, she may resist in describing the trauma to you so that you are left wondering whether indeed the patient experienced a trauma—significant or minor—at all.

In the following sections, we describe in which disorders posttraumatic avoidance may occur, how you can recognize it in the mental status, and how to overcome it.

2. Posttraumatic Stress in the Mental Status

During the interview, posttraumatic stress may be evident in the patient's psychomotor behavior, affect, mood, speech and voice, and thought content.

Psychomotor Behavior

The patient's gestures are sparse. The hands often rest folded in the patient's lap. He uses them mostly when he describes how he stays away from things or shoves something away. While describing his trauma, he often remains motionless.

The use of hand and facial signals is usually diminished. When they occur, they help him to avoid talking. For example, if you tell him that he went through a lot, the patient may remain silent, slowly nodding or closing his eyes. When expressing disbelief, he may just shake his head.

Goal-directed movements are usually slow. He avoids activity or initiates it slowly. For example, when the interviewer sits down at the beginning or stands up at the end of the interview, the patient may lag 2–3 seconds behind. *Psychic numbing* (Lifton 1967), *emotional anesthesia* (used in DSM-III [American Psychiatric Association 1980]; Shatan 1973, 1978), and *diminished responsiveness* (used in DSM-IV) are terms used to describe this phenomenon.

According to DSM-IV, a patient's reactive movements are often dramatically increased: he startles when the door shuts or the telephone rings; he may report difficulties concentrating and falling and staying asleep. His grooming movements may be minimal except for a repeated stroking of a leg as a soothing mechanism or wetting of the ever-dry lips.

Affect

The patient's autonomic response during history taking is dampened. However, if you tap the avoided area and show empathy for her suffering, she may blush, become tearful, or have a quiver in her voice and become tremulous. The patient may also show irritability and sudden angry outbursts.

Some patients carry a stiff smile that changes little during verbal interaction. Their facial expression is usually flat when they finally agree to recall their trauma. If you discuss their feelings that result from the trauma, their facial features express sadness, helplessness, and, although rarely, anger. Fear, despair, pain, and helplessness may also emerge when you are able to connect these patients with their suppressed impressions and feelings, or when you pace them through their traumatic event.

Mood

The patient describes that he feels detached from others and lacks warmth, even for family members. He says he cannot enjoy his hobbies anymore, feels neither stimulated nor challenged by his work, and experiences the world through a glass wall or rubber skin. He may report loss of tenderness, intimacy, and sex drive, which may translate into family and marital problems and may diminish his ability to grieve. This experience of detachment gives his surroundings an air of unreality (derealization).

Speech and Voice

The patient communicates most fluently when she describes her job, social history, or daily routine. She stalls when it comes to the trauma. She steers away from reexperiencing the thoughts, feelings, images, and ideas of the trauma. When redirected, she becomes visibly anxious, starts to sweat, breathes harder, trembles, and shows increased reactive and grooming movements without verbalizing her anxiety. However, she may express numbness, depressed feelings, lack of interest, and lack of concentration without linking it to the trauma. The tone of her voice may show little modulation, with only falling pitch expressing sadness when she describes her trauma. If you identify the trauma, the patient may stop to answer your questions and become mute, or refuse to recall the trauma. She may say,

> I just can't do it.

or

> I'm unable to talk about it.

Speech starts only after some delay. It lacks fluency and is often limited to yes and no answers. An affective tone may be lacking. You get a sense of personal uninvolvement and distance. Some patients show sudden blocking in their stream of verbal or nonverbal interaction. They may explain,

> I sometimes lose my train of thought.

Here is an example.

> A 36-year-old Vietnam veteran who denies symptoms of posttraumatic stress disorder is reprimanded at his job as a warehouse stock manager for tardiness and an increase in error rate. He complains that he cannot get along with his oppositional teenage son. As he is discussing with the interviewer how to confront his son about breaking his curfew, the patient suddenly withdraws from the interview and stares into space. When asked what happened he apologizes and explains he was daydreaming but he does not know about what. With free association the interviewer elicits a flashback of an interrogation of a Viet Cong youth 15 years ago. When the youth resisted cooperating, he was pushed out of the flying helicopter to scare the other detainees into submission. The patient reexperienced seeing the white sclera in the prisoner's fear-widened eyes and hearing his scream as he plummeted to his death. The patient is unable to shield himself from the harassment of the past while facing another "interrogational situation," this time with his son. The Vietnam trauma has sensitized him for related stress. If such stress occurs, the memory of the old trauma breaks through as symptoms of delayed chronic posttraumatic stress disorder, which so far has gone undiagnosed. (Blank [1985] used the term *unconscious flashback* for this phenomenon.)

Thought Content

Intrusive recollection. An intrusive recollection is a recurrent, involuntary, and emotionally distressing remembering of parts or all of a traumatic event. Splinters of recollection may focus on one sensory element—an image, a sound pattern, a smell (e.g., of burnt flesh), a taste (e.g., of one's own blood in the mouth), or a vibration (e.g., that of an explosion); an emotion—fear of bodily harm and destruction, loss of control over anxiety or aggression, grief over a loss, anger against the threat, or guilt of having failed or unjustifiably survived; or a thought—of vulnerability, injustice, or helplessness—or search for an alternative outcome. These recollections occur in at least 75% (Horowitz et al. 1980; Kinzie 1986) to 85% (Wilkinson 1983) of patients who have posttraumatic stress disorder.

The patient may recall the trauma with some residual fear and psychomotor inhibition:

I can't go back to that part of town where the accident occurred.

or

I can't return to live in that empty house.

A recollection of a traumatic event may take a stereotyped, fixed form. The patient may respond to these recollections with fear, panic, violent acts (Krupnick 1980; Wilmer 1982), or incapacitating indecision. Here is an example.

A patient with posttraumatic avoidance accuses himself of a wrongdoing and ruminates about alternatives he should have taken. He relates how he lost his wife in a bombing raid. Before the bombardment, he told her to go to the public and not the private bomb shelter of her apartment building. She obliged. The public shelter was hit and all perished. The apartment building stayed intact. The patient felt that his wife would have survived if he had told her to stay home. He mentally played back her last words on the phone: "Don't worry, I'll go to the public shelter, if that's what you want."

When he returned home after the war, he had flashbacks and dreams about that conversation and about the telegram that had informed him about his wife's death. He felt that because he had loved her so much, he had cared too much and given her the wrong advice. The loss was unbearable. To prevent a recurrence of any loss in the future, he never dated again. He also neglected his four children who had survived the air raid in a school shelter. They reminded him of his trauma, and he could not bear the guilt. He was unable to come to peace with the past. Instead, he rehearsed his advice, looked back in despair, and devoted time, energy, and attention trying to rectify his past, thereby draining energy from the present.

In DSM-IV, it is recognized that traumatized patients may have a sense of a foreshortened future. The anticipation of being hurt may even lead to a paranoid adaptation in which the patient blames others and refuses to accept responsibility (Hendin et al. 1984).

Flashbacks. A *flashback* is defined as a dissociative reaction to extreme traumatization (Peterson et al. 1991). It differs from a recollection in its intensity and in the patient's response to it. A patient may experience his sensory recollection as illusion or hallucination and may enact parts of the event by reliving it as a quasi-psychotic attack and pseudohallucinatory dissociated state (Jaffe 1968), or in chronic, psychosis-like pictures (Niederland 1968). In DSM-IV, it is emphasized that such a hallucinatory experience is more common in children. In adults, these flashbacks appear to occur primarily in combat veterans and survivors of death camps (Jaffe 1968). Hendin et al. (1984) noted them more in veterans of the Vietnam conflict than of World War I and II.

Blank (1985) discussed unconscious flashbacks, which he was first to observe. We have observed such "unconscious" flashbacks in several of our patients. The following is an example.

> From ages 10 to 14 years, a boy was sexually abused by his cousin, who was 11 years older than him. The boy's school grades dropped. He restricted his social contacts to a girlfriend with whom he had no sexual relationship. He denied having nightmares or flashbacks. Suddenly, during the interview, he ignores the interviewer's questions and stops talking. When asked why, he says, "I don't know. I'm spacing out." After being invited to freely associate about what happened, he realizes, "I'm thinking about something else." He then reveals that that "something else" is a sudden memory of a scene with his abusive cousin. He does not recognize that he has been experiencing flashbacks.

Distressing dreams and nightmares. An estimated 70%–75% of posttraumatic stress disorder patients experience anxiety dreams and 40%–45% experience nightmares, as noted by Wilmer (1982; studying Vietnam veterans), Wilkinson (1983; studying witnesses of a hotel collapse), Krystal and Niederland (1968; studying concentration camp survivors), Kinzie (1986; studying Cambodian refugees), and Krupnick (1980; studying victims of violent crimes). These anxiety dreams and nightmares occur mainly in the first half of the night (van der Kolk et al. 1984). Their content is diverse, ranging from replications of the trauma to unrelated anxiety themes devoid of elements of the traumatic event (Wilmer 1982). The dreams emphasize the dreamer's lonesomeness, helplessness, and defenselessness (DeFazio 1978; Goodwin 1980). Such dreams may continue into wakefulness (Blank 1985; Hendin et al. 1984; Krystal and Niederland 1968).

Memory. The patient may complain about having a poor memory. According to DSM-IV, the source of this complaint appears to be related to the traumatic event and to the experience that his recollection of other events unrelated to the trauma may become disrupted by intrusive thoughts as well.

3. Techniques: Imaging and Active Listening

For the purpose of the interview, we make two assumptions about the patient whose posttraumatic withdrawal and avoidance interfere with the interview.

First, the patient is unable to discharge her traumatic emotions (e.g., her fear, by fleeing the traumatic situation; her aggression, by destroying the traumatizing force; her grief, by crying for the person she lost in the trauma). Reasons for this lack of abreaction may include lack of time or threat of being killed. For example, a rape victim may decide not to fight back out of fear of death. Therefore, the rape experience remains emotionally unfinished (Perls 1969).

Second, the emotion that is not discharged persists. Authors have proposed at least three different models for such bottled-up emotions (Guinagh 1987):

- In the *hydraulic container model* (Bohurt 1980; Jackins 1978; Janov 1970), memories and nondischarged emotions are visualized as filling up neurons (Breuer and Freud 1895/1957). This "primal pool of pain has to be drained so that misstored distressing experiences do not jam the ability to adapt and learn" (Guinagh 1987, pp. 8–9).
- In the *unfinished business model* (Perls 1969), it is postulated that emotions have to be transformed into motoric energy to lead to a closure. Thus, anger may be discharged by changing something, and fear by fleeing. If such transformation is missing, the emotions remain unfinished.
- In the *conflict model* (Freud 1896; Scheff 1979), the need to abreact the

emotion is balanced by a counterforce to suppress, withdraw, or avoid because the patient fears the recall may resubmerge her into a state of helplessness, or the suppressed emotion may overwhelm her with fear, rage, or grief.

Your interviewing technique has to shift the balance away from the patient's defenses expressed in her avoidance and withdrawal behavior toward the urge to recall the trauma and discharge the bottled-up, unfinished emotion. Clinicians have used two approaches to uncover a trauma: imaging and active listening.

Imaging

Imaging returns the patient to a past situation and helps him to reexperience sensations, emotions, and the progression of the event. Most uncovering techniques contain an element of imaging. For example, Horowitz (1973, 1974) used images in his dynamic approach to reduce controls and change information processing. Imaging is also used in various behavioral treatments, such as in imaginal flooding (Keane et al. 1985b), systematic desensitization (Schilder 1980), stress inoculation training (Meichenbaum and Cameron 1983), hypnotherapy (Brende 1985), and narcosynthesis (Kolb 1985).

To introduce imaging, invite the patient to focus on one or all four components of imaging:

- Time regression
- Sensual recall
- Emotional reexperiencing and expressing
- Sequencing of the situation

Time regression.   Ask the patient to go back in time to the point where the trauma occurred. If the time regression is intense, he may talk with a different voice, especially if the regression leads an adult back to early childhood.

Sensual recall.   Focus the patient by shielding him from outside stimuli. Ask the patient with a strong visual or auditory ability to achieve some sensory shielding by closing his eyes. Then ask him to let the scene of the traumatic events roll by, to capture images and to listen for the sounds that he heard during the trauma. Ask the patient to keep his eyes closed and experience whatever sensation of the trauma comes back—whether it be visual, auditory, gustatory, olfactory, or kinesthetic. Ask him to hold the sensation in his mind and to supplement it with all the other previously coexisting sensations.

After the patient seems to have the complete picture, put the still frame into action and let it reel off. Simple continuation techniques keep the story moving without interrupting it, without stimulating reflection, and without addressing the mood (Othmer and Othmer 1994). Some authors who use hypnotic techniques in their interviewing and therapy refer to the vivid recall of a past event as *time regression* (Pettinati 1988).

Emotional reexperiencing and expressing. When the patient shows an emotion during the sensual recall, ask him to stay with this emotion. Have him experience it, and encourage him to intensify it and hold it for the moment. Encourage the patient to express the emotion in words, facial expressions, gestures, and body positions.

Sequencing of the situation. The first three components enable the patient to experience a still frame of the traumatic event. Now ask him to walk through the trauma. Ask for the next frame:

What is happening next? Tell me what is next that you hear, see, smell, and feel.

You induce a reexperiencing mode in the patient when the patient fulfills the following criteria:

● He continues to show facial expressions while keeping his eyes closed.
● He describes sensations rather than gives editing remarks about the event, such as "I wish it had not happened," or "The company does not observe safety precautions."

Active Listening

Active listening is a process by which the patient is invited to bring past experiences to the here and now of the interview situation. Initially, you do not ask the patient to put herself back in time into the situation but to stay in the here and now. Although imaging can be conceptualized as a process that involves mainly right brain functions, the recall of active listening may involve initially more left brain functions. Some of the techniques of active listening (e.g., mirroring the patient's expressions, anticipating her expressions, pacing) have been developed by neurolinguists (Bandler and Grinder 1975; Haley 1986; Watzlawick 1978).

With active listening, you entice the patient to reconstruct the traumatic event. For this purpose, you try to anticipate her movements and affect and display them so that the patient may deliver the words that fit the affect and psychomotor expression anticipated and displayed by you. The patient's recall does not exclude time regression, sensory reexperiencing, or reliving of emotions, but these are not the focus of attention. Active listening links interviewer and patient emotionally and facilitates communication.

Patients who appear more kinesthetic and haptic in their mode of experience may respond to active listening better than imaging. For this purpose, use the following techniques: mirroring the patient's expressions, anticipating her emotions, pacing her verbal production, and timing the techniques properly.

Mirroring.   When *mirroring,* as interviewer you imitate the patient's body position, gestures, facial expressions, breathing pattern, and tone of voice. Mirroring indicates acceptance of the patient's thoughts, feelings, and intentions. You share the patient's personal drama and reflect her pain, anguish, and emotional despair. When you reflect the patient's verbal and nonverbal expressions, watch that none of your expressions mock her. Make sure that your expressions are in pace with the patient's—similar but not identical. Picking up and resonating the patient's demeanor intensify the patient's feelings. Work with a short time delay: trail the patient by a few seconds to be sure that you are indeed in tune with the way your patient feels. Use

- Verbal feedback of thoughts
- Verbal feedback of emotions
- Enactment of the patient's stance and emotion
- Imitation of the patient's breathing rhythm
- Mirroring of the patient's facial expression
- Copying of the patient's gestures
- Re-creation of the patient's voice in volume, tone, timbre, and cadence

Mirroring must be carried out with sensitivity so that the patient does not feel mimicked, but comforted and understood.

Anticipating.   After you feel that you have accurately read and mirrored your patient's feelings, start leading the nonverbal conversation. In your own psychomotor and affective expression, anticipate the patient's emotional discharge. For example, if you expect the patient to report a painful event, display a painful expression when the patient initiates her verbal report. This helps the patient to ventilate her trauma. Your anticipation raises her awareness about her feelings. Anticipating keeps her focused. Hopkinson et al. (1981) observed that the patient's emotional expression followed the interviewer's interpretations 44% of the time. The degree of emotion the patient displayed depended on the degree of emotion the interviewer displayed when making the interpretation: when the interviewer's response was made with emotion, the patient gave an emotional response in 75% of the cases; when the interviewer responded with no emotion, the patient gave an emotional response in only 26% of the cases. Thus, an emotional expression can be used to entice the patient to continue her story by providing an emotional bridge.

The technique of anticipating is useful for patients who let you see some of their emotions. It is less helpful for totally withdrawn patients who talk little or who have limited facial expressions and gestures.

Pacing. Align your body posture to the patient's and move at the same speed as she does. First let the patient lead; then synchronize your movements; finally, anticipate and guide her movements (Bandler and Grinder 1975; Haley 1986; Watzlawick 1978).

Timing of techniques. Time your mirroring and anticipating well. When you start to mirror the patient, adjust your body position first. You may trail the patient for seconds. Then start to move your body in unison with the patient's, reflecting a similar but not identical position and similar psychomotor movements, such as gestures. Do not mirror goal-directed or symbolic movements. A symbolic movement is used instead of words; it requires an acknowledgment, not an imitation. Therefore, respond to a symbolic movement as you would respond to a question or statement.

Next, start to mirror the patient's affective expressions. Show reactive responses, facial expressions, grooming, and tone of voice that are similar to those of the patient. Bring your psychomotor movements and affective expressions in line with those of the patient. This will help you to understand better her psychomotor and emotional response.

Use this knowledge to complement the patient's recall of sensory impressions of the trauma by magnifying and displaying the psychomotor and affective components, especially when her recall fades and she may stop talking. By anticipating her psychomotor and emotional expressions, you urge her to fill in the words about sensory impressions that she experienced during the trauma. In other words, use a nonverbal continuation technique. Rather than saying, "What came next?" or "Hmmm," express the feeling of the horror that the patient is ready to talk about; she may then tell you what it is you are experiencing horror about. Thus, you first trail the patient, then catch up with her, and finally lead her.

Enhancement Techniques

To enhance imaging and the effect of active listening, interviewers have used a number of enhancement techniques.

1. *Biochemical disinhibition:* A sedative-hypnotic, such as amobarbital or lorazepam, can be used. Kolb (1988) found that 14 out of 18 posttraumatic stress disorder patients responded with time regression and an emotional catharsis of the trauma during an amobarbital infusion called *narcosynthesis*. Similar results may be expected with lorazepam. However, use of amobarbital or lorazepam does not ensure that the account is accurate. Anxiety and wishful thinking appear to distort such catharsis (Pettinati 1988). (For a description of the amobarbital technique, see Chapter 6, "Catatonia.")

2. *Cognitive enhancer:* A stimulant drug may be used, such as 20 mg of dextroamphetamine or 30 mg of methylphenidate, as pretreatment. This will take 1–2 hours to become effective, so the interview will have to take place later. Such a drug will increase fluency of thinking and verbal production.

3. *Relaxation:* Various relaxation techniques can be used to prepare the patient for imaging and hypnosis.

4. *Hypnosis:* Clinicians frequently use a hypnotic-induction technique to place the patient in a trancelike state before they induce time regression and reimaging of the traumatic event.

5. *Free association:* This technique is used to reduce the patient's controls and allow him to access traumatic material.

6. *Analysis of defenses:* By analyzing the patient's defenses, the interviewer can focus on the patient's resistance and avoidance behavior in the hope that the patient can overcome his anxiety of recall.

7. *Change of perspective:* The patient is asked to visualize the traumatic event as a spectator rather than as the victim that he was.

8. *Recall with different outcome:* The patient is asked to fantasize a different outcome of the traumatic event to ease the pain of recall.

9. *Reframing:* The patient is asked to discuss the traumatic event from a perspective that allows him to experience the trauma as meaningful.

10. *Controlled catharsis:* The patient is asked to enact his anger, cry for the lost one, and express his anxiety. For therapy, some traumatologists postulate that, besides recall, an emotional abreaction (i.e., catharsis) is desirable. Such catharsis means that the patient vents his anger against the traumatic and life-threatening force, expresses his fear by imagining his escape from the threat, or cries out in grief by enacting his desire for reunification with the lost one.

You can facilitate catharsis verbally and nonverbally. For example, if the patient recalls his sexual abuse, you may ask him what he feels would be the just punishment for the perpetrator. You may ask him to describe how he would like to see the perpetrator hurt. Alternatively, you may express anger in your gestures and by your facial movements when the patient reports the abuse, thus providing the affect that he tends to block from his own recall. If the patient describes the loss of his child in a car accident, you may ask him to call for the child by name, or you may reflect grief in your nonverbal language. If the patient describes how he was trapped in the flood, you may ask him to describe how he could escape in a motorboat, or you may show fear followed by relaxation while you listen to his account.

Our diagnostic interviewing technique is directed toward the accurate reconstruction of the trauma with or without catharsis. You may use the patient's need for catharsis to facilitate the recollection of the trauma. However, you may want to curb the catharsis to preserve the integrity of the interview situation and prevent the patient from becoming overwhelmed by his emotions. You may curb catharsis by interrupting the recollection process and return to the here and now with statements such as,

> I see that this event still upsets you. I'm glad that it is over now and that you are here, safe and protected.

4. Five Steps to Reexperience the Trauma

Step 1: Listen. Invite the patient to talk about the trauma. Often such a report remains abstract, incomplete, edited, and void of affect. Ask for sensory impressions, for the sequence of occurrence and feelings. The severely traumatized patient usually does not comply.

Step 2: Tag. Highlight the elements of the patient's traumatic event as it emerges from Step 1. Encourage her to elaborate and magnify these impressions. The patient is often unable to recall the trauma in detail.

Step 3: Confront. Confront the patient with the discrepancy between her social disability and the faintness of the reported trauma that supposedly explain her disability. For example, tell her the trauma does not seem to affect her, yet her school grades have dropped, she has lost her job, or she has become isolated. Tell her that her faint and flat recollection of the trauma may not be the result of a fading memory but of her success in suppressing it from her consciousness. Confront her with her avoidance. Then, ask the patient to attempt to overcome her anxiety and to give you a report of the trauma that reflects the horror she experienced at the time of the event.

Step 4: Solve. The goal here is to have the patient recall the traumatic event in detail. Merely confronting the patient with her phobic defenses does not motivate her for this task. Two proposed techniques may now help—imaging and active listening.

In the first interview below, we demonstrate the technique of imaging; in the second, the technique of active listening with dextroamphetamine enhancement.

Step 5: Approve. With the help of imaging or active listening, most patients can give a detailed recall of the trauma but usually without catharsis. If the patient recalls the trauma, express empathy for her suffering. If she displays self-accusation, express understanding for her attempt to undo the past.

If the patient has a catharsis, let her reexperience the pain of the trauma. Build a bridge between the pain of the traumatic event and the present incapacity. Let her experience the connection between the past and the present. Point out the relief that she may get from integrating her past with the present. For a moment, at the end of the interview, such a patient may sense the relationship between the past stimulus and her present response. Now, the numbing influence of her avoidance that separated the trauma from the response may lift.

5. Interview A: Imaging to Visualize the Trauma

Mr. P. is a 54-year-old, white, married meat cutter. Two years previously, he lost four fingers of his right hand in an accident at a meat plant in Chicago. At a Chicago hospital, four surgeons took shifts in a 17-hour operation and were able to reattach only two fingers before the prolonged anesthesia became hazardous. The other two fingers perished on the surgical tray. Mr. P. did not regain the ability to move the joints of the attached fingers, but he did regain the sense of temperature and pressure in them. He had to wear a protective glove to avoid freezing sensations in the attached fingers, triggered at temperatures below 80°F.

Mr. P. returned to work on a rehabilitation schedule: 1 hour a day, then 2, then 4, and finally 4 hours for 3 days of the week and 6 hours the other 2 days. When he went back to work for 6 hours daily, he became unresponsive to those around him, withdrew from his family, and became monosyllabic and finally mute. He was hospitalized for major depression, severe, without psychosis.

During the hospitalization, Mr. P. was asked whether he had daytime flashbacks or had dreamed about the accident. The answer was a reluctant and delayed no, and the interviewer excluded posttraumatic stress disorder as a diagnosis. At discharge, his dexamethasone suppression test had normalized. Routine laboratory tests were negative. On 100 mg of nortriptyline and supportive and cognitive therapy, Mr. P. reported feeling 70%–80% better. Yet he froze when he considered the idea of returning to work—any kind of work, not just returning to his old job at the plant. Before the accident, Mr. P. had never had a phobic disorder, agoraphobia, a panic disorder, or depression. His mother did experience depression and nervousness.

The interviewer was asked to determine Mr. P.'s disability. Why couldn't he return to work? He had had a perfect work record for 33 years. He had not even sued the company, although the Chicago company was penalized for neglect of safety regulations. The consulted psychologist, who was experienced in worker's compensation cases, could not help.

The interviewer was not able to make a diagnosis that explained the patient's disability. Mr. P. had overcome severe depression. He was left with mild initial and intermittent insomnia, irritability, and difficulty concentrating. Neither the past depression nor the present symptoms appeared to justify his present disability. He refused to go to work despite a premorbid personality void of oppositional defiant disorder, antisocial personality disorder, malingering, or any plotting for compensation. Did his morbidity and dysfunction fit the criteria for posttraumatic avoidance?

Step 1: Listen

The patient is well groomed. He wears a checkered flannel shirt and dress pants. (I = interviewer; P = patient)

1. I: Mr. P., when did your depressive feelings start?
   P: About the time when I had my accident and lost my fingers.
2. I: How did that happen?
   P: [In a monotone voice, sitting straight] Well, the supervisor of the plant had ordered us to remove the safety guards from the meat cutters.
3. I: Why was that?
   P: So that we could work faster—the guards slowed us down.
4. I: Hmmm.
   P: [Sitting straight and still] It's illegal, and after my accident they got fined.
5. I: How do you remember the accident?
   P: Oh, it's been 2 years now.

Mr. P. did not show any signs of personal anguish. He and the interviewer did not become engaged emotionally; they did not bond against the patient's pain.

The patient responded normally to the interviewer's questions. Although his answers were goal directed, he did not elaborate. He rarely changed his body position. His gestures were sparse. His facial expression changed little, except for some eye movements. His affect was restricted, flat, and detached. He did not volunteer to talk about his mood. Missing were modulations in voice, images, feelings, sound recollections, and dramatic descriptors of the accident. He sounded more like a bureaucrat who was quoting safety violations than a trauma victim. His detached way of reporting was compatible with emotional numbing secondary to post-traumatic stress disorder and with restricted affect secondary to major depression.

Step 2: Tag

6. I: Do you remember any thoughts you had?
   P: [As if looking through the interviewer] Not really.
7. I: Any memories?
   P: [Squinting] Not really.
8. I: Any pictures?
   P: [Shakes his head] I don't really know what you mean.
9. I: What about the accident? Did it ever come back as a flashback exactly the way it happened?
   P: Not really. [Frowns] You asked me that so often. [Frowns more] The accident is a thing of the past—like many other things.
10. I: Mr. P., how do you feel about the accident?
    P: [Shrugs his shoulders] It happened 3 years ago. [Pulls down the corners of his mouth] They violated the safety regulations to make us work faster—they got penalized for that.

The interviewer probed the patient's thoughts and images regarding the accident to tag them using symptom-oriented, closed-ended questions (Q. 6–9). Mr. P. denied having nightmares, flashbacks, or intrusive memories. Tagging encouraged the patient to give more details about the accident but did not engage him in reliving it. He remained emotionally detached. He showed only a few facial expressions: squinting (A. 7), frowning (A. 9), shrugging his shoulders, and pulling down the corners of the mouth (A. 10). He did not recall any sensory impressions from the accident either. When Mr. P. mentioned that his company had violated the safety regulations for increased production (A. 10), the interviewer could have used the enhancement technique of catharsis (see discussion of controlled catharsis, #10 under "Enhancement Techniques," above) by asking the patient to express his anger about the company. However, the interviewer focused on the patient's defense, his inability to go back to work.

Step 3: Confront

11. I: You say the accident happened 3 years ago. You seem to have forgotten about it. Can you explain why you still can't go back to work after 33 years with a perfect work record?
    P: [Looks the interviewer in the eye] I don't know. I just can't. [Leans back and looks up to the ceiling] I can't figure it out myself. [Looks at the desk] I just freeze when I hear about work.
12. I: How did you feel when you first returned to work?
    P: [Eyes drifting down] I felt I didn't do my job. I was sitting around. [Pauses; looks to the right, then to the left] I had no idea what to do first. I had no idea what to do at all.
13. I: What do you feel now when you think about the accident?
    P: [With a bland expression] Nothing. Kind of empty. [Gets a deep fold between his eyebrows and closes his eyes]

Because the patient did not show any engagement, the interviewer confronted him with the discrepancy between a fading trauma and the high degree of morbidity that still resulted from it—namely, Mr. P.'s cessation of work, dissolution of social relationships, and general withdrawal. This attempt to focus the patient on his resistance and defenses is another enhancement technique for interviewing the posttraumatic patient (see #6 under "Enhancement Techniques," above). Yet, this focus classified only two of the patient's symptoms: his apparent amnesia (A. 6–8) and his emotional anesthesia (A. 13) about the accident.

The interviewer's attempts to understand the patient's refusal to return to work were blocked. To obtain access to the patient's emotional state and to find an explanation for his resistance to return to work, the interviewer decided to use imaging.

Step 4: Solve

14. I: Mr. P., please keep your eyes closed. Is that okay with you?
    P: I don't mind. [Bends his head and keeps eyes closes, hands folded in his lap]
15. I: Well, Mr. P., go back in time . . . try to see, hear, and feel the accident again, like a movie. Can you see it?
    P: Yeah, there's nothing to that. [Keeps his eyes closed]
16. I: Tell me what's happening.
    P: I'm cutting meat. I'm behind. I feel hurried. I have to catch up.
17. I: You sound hurried. Keep on talking.
    P: I know when I grab the meat closer to the cutting line, it doesn't bend away from the knives, and I can cut it faster. I'm doing real well, I have it down pat. It's real mechanical: Grab a piece of meat, hold it close, run it through the knives, run it through the knives, run it through the knives, up to the end piece and throw it away. Grab another piece, hold it close, run it through the knives, throw away the end piece. Grab another piece. . . .
18. I: You sound as if you are part of the meat-cutting machine.
    P: Yeah, that's how it feels. I really like it.
19. I: Tell me what you hear!
    P: It's like marching to a rhythm. It kind of calms me down. Zing, zang, zing, zang. Zing as it cuts the air . . . and then zang as the cutter cuts the meat. Zing, zang, zing, zang.
20. I: I hear and feel the rhythm.
    P: [Monotone, in a matter-of-fact voice] And it goes on all morning. And then . . . there is a sting. I try to grab the meat . . . I can't. My fingers are gone. My hand looks like part of the cut meat. The only thing that moves on the cutting table is my thumb. I can still move it. I can't move my fingers. They lay still on the meat table, they don't move. I shut off the machine with the other hand and grab my fingers. They are still warm. [His lips start to quiver.]
21. I: Stay with this feeling, Mr. P. Tell me what you feel.
    P: I feel as if I'm holding four cigars in my hand. They don't feel really cold. [The fold between the patient's closed eyes gets deeper and he presses his eyes tight.]
22. I: What do you see, Mr. P.?
    P: The stump, the bloody stump that is . . . that was . . . that is my hand. I see it.
23. I: Do you feel any pain?
    P: No.
24. I: Stay with that vision.
    P: Oh, I do.
25. I: Do you ever see it in your dreams?
    P: No.

26. I: Do you ever see it in a flashback?
    P: No.
27. I: Do you ever see it any time?
    P: Oh, yes. I see it all the time. I see my hand is a stump, whether I sleep, whether I walk, whether I talk. Whatever I see, part of it is that stump, right down here. [Points to the right at the height of his chest]
28. I: Zero in on this!
    P: If you look right on, it's in the right lower field, that's where I see my stump.
29. I: All the time?
    P: It never leaves me. I see the red of the meat and the white of the bones that were my fingers. I hear the zing zang of the saws and smell the freshly cut meat. It sticks with me. . . .
30. I: You see the stump all the time?
    P: Yes, I carry it with me. I see it always whether I have my eyes open or closed.
31. I: Mr. P., it must feel awful how this sticks in your face all the time.
    P: Yeah, it is part of me. Like a part of my eye, my inner eye. [Opens his eyes]
32. I: [Silent]
    P: Yes, I see the stump all the time. I don't remember a time when I didn't.
33. I: Is there any smell that stays with you?
    P: No. [After some hesitation] When they took me to the hospital, it really smelled like a hospital. Usually hospitals don't smell anymore, but this one really smelled like a hospital.
34. I: What about sounds?
    P: You know I have that high-pitched sound in my ear . . . like of locusts. I went to an ear doctor and he said that there is nothing wrong with my ears.
35. I: Does that sound remind you of anything?
    P: I haven't thought about it.
36. I: What does it sound like?
    P: [After a pause] It sounds like the meat cutters when they are empty and spinning. Yes, that's it! I never thought about it.
37. I: So, those things are with you all the time as if you are frozen in that experience?
    P: Yes.
38. I: It sounds as if the movie stopped there on the last frame.
    P: Frozen. Like frozen in time.
39. I: So, you are really going through a lot.
    P: [Starts to sob, then cries]
40. I: When you came to the hospital and you were so depressed that you didn't talk, I think you were really withdrawn into your pain.
    P: [Sobs more] I earned my living with my hands and now one of them is gone.
41. I: How painful it must be to look at your hand now.
    P: And see a fixed-up stump. I don't know what is worse: the bleeding stump or the dangling useless fingers sewn onto it.
42. I: Work crippled you. I understand how that makes you feel.
    P: It made me dependent on my wife.
43. I: You feel helpless.

P: The work that supported me, crippled me. My hand that I needed to work is gone. I couldn't stand any more of that. I'm not the same.

44. I: You feel that work will crush you?

P: It will make me a bleeding stump. Nothing will be left of me.

45. I: This sounds as if work will wipe you out. And that prevents you from going back to it.

P: I feel how little I can do now. It's making me feel helpless, dependent on my wife, and unable to protect myself. I start to shake inside if I think that I have to show up for work again. I feel lost and destroyed.

46. I: They tried to give you office work.

P: I feel useless there. I've always worked with my hands. My whole family did.

Step 5: Approve

47. I: Was there anybody in your family who had an injury like yours?

P: Yes, my grandfather. His arm got caught in a corn picker. He lost his right arm.

48. I: Oh?

P: And my father. I was there when he lost his fingers. He was working in a sawmill. He tried to clean the teeth of a saw and came too close. His hand was caught. His fingers were flying right over his shoulder. He lost the tips of three fingers.

49. I: Hmmm.

P: It's always with me. Most of my family seems to work with that kind of equipment.

50. I: Now I understand your fear of work much better.

P: I want to work but I feel so useless in what I can do. I was good with my hands, but my right hand is gone. I'm no good anymore.

The interviewer decided to use the patient's spontaneous response of eye closing (A. 13) to introduce the technique of imaging. The patient's response of eye closing seemed to call for this technique. Enhancement techniques that could have been introduced at this time are relaxation or formal hypnosis, amobarbital, or application of lorazepam.

In contrast to his previous laconic responses, Mr. P. did well with time regression and eyes-closed imaging (A. 15) even without enhancement. He reported impressions that were

● Visual (images of his fingers and the stump)
● Auditory (the noise of the cutting knives)
● Kinesthetic (the work rhythm and its relaxing effect)
● Sensory (the warm, cut-off fingers)

Yet the patient's affect remained restricted; his only emotion was the quivering of his lips (A. 20). The interviewer seized this moment to ask Mr. P. again to stay with the feeling and to describe it. Mr. P. then offered an intense perception: the sensation of holding his four warm fingers as if they were cigars.

At this time, the interviewer could have used a cathartic enhancement technique by asking the patient to call for his fingers:

I want my fingers back.

The patient's cathartic response would have been an outburst of sobbing, crying, and calling for his fingers. However, the interviewer kept the patient in the imaging mode, which so far had allowed him to review the trauma. The reason the patient denied pain, nocturnal terror and nightmares, and flashbacks of the accident (A. 23, 25, 26) was because visions of his hand were present all the time (A. 27).

The interviewer's empathy (Q. 31, 39–43) set free the patient's thought content and feelings of dependency (A. 42, 45), worthlessness (A. 46), defenselessness (A. 45), helplessness (A. 43, 45), uselessness (A. 46, 50), and expectation of being a total cripple (A. 43, 44). At first, Mr. P. could not answer the question why he could not return to work; eventually, the interviewer's tuning in to the patient's feeling of being a "cripple" brought out the emotional answer to this question: Mr. P. feared that work would cripple him further (A. 43–44). Except for his hand injury, he was physically fit to return to work. However, he did not think that his avoidance of work was silly and out of proportion—he identified with his posttraumatic avoidance rather than experiencing it as ego-alien.

Mr. P. was living with an ever-present image of the result of the accident: the image of his bleeding, fingerless stump. It had become part of his internal field of vision—not an on-off phenomenon as is implied by the term "flashback." It never occurred to him to call the vision of his cut-off fingers a flashback. With the technique of imaging, the interviewer was able to confirm that the patient was paralyzed—not by the process of the injury, but by the frozen image of its result. He confirmed the diagnosis of posttraumatic stress disorder, chronic, and that Mr. P. was reexperiencing the event in an unusual manner. Instead of retaining an image of the event itself, he retained an image of its aftermath: his crippled hand. He did not experience this memory in recurrent images or dreams but as a constant visual presence that became part of his self-image. He felt intense stress related to the workplace. In the aftermath of the accident, Mr. P. had responded by a prolonged depression with psychomotor retardation, loss of sleep, and loss of appetite. He was emotionally paralyzed, not able to formulate or express his thoughts or feelings about the accident. He had become so distanced from his emotions that he did not perceive them and, therefore, could not express them. The interviewer helped Mr. P. connect with his feelings of being a "cripple" and express them.

Diagnosis

Axis I

1. Posttraumatic stress disorder with delayed onset
2. Major depressive disorder, single episode, in remission

5. Interview B: Active Listening to Enhance Recall

Mr. G. is a 43-year-old, white, divorced male who had requested to be admitted to a Veterans Administration hospital a few days before Christmas. He felt he could not survive the holidays in his hotel room. He sits slumped over in his chair, ashen faced, bags under his eyes.

Step 1: Listen

1. I: How can I help you?
   P: I'm not sure.
2. I: You came here to get help. What was on your mind?
   P: I just knew I couldn't stay in the hotel during Christmas by myself. I didn't feel safe.
3. I: You live in a hotel?
   P: Yes. After my divorce I couldn't stay alone in our luxury home. I would wake up in cold sweats. I would hide behind a sofa. Vietnam came back to me.
4. I: After so many years? You must have gone through hell.
   P: It's been 18 years. Now, I have nightmares.
5. I: What are the nightmares about?
   P: I can't tell you. I haven't told anyone. Not even my wife. [Looks down in his lap] My wife couldn't stand my screams during the night and the brooding during the day . . . just sitting there . . . staring.

Step 2: Tag

6. I: You never talked about your nightmares?
  P: I couldn't. Something has to happen if I want to keep on living.
7. I: You must be going through a lot of pain. You even lost your wife over it. Are your nightmares always about the same things?
  P: Yes. The same two.
8. I: Can you tell me about them?
  P: Impossible. I just can't. I have no words. [Looks lost, gazes at the ceiling, shakes his head, blushes, bites his lips, raises his eyebrows, flinches as if somebody jams a knife into his body, looks pain stricken and desperate]
9. I: When did these nightmares start?
  P: Two years ago. We had just sold our business for a lot of money.
10. I: What kind of business?
  P: When I came back from Nam, I didn't know what to do. My wife had started to paint porcelain and I helped her. We were very successful. In $2\frac{1}{2}$ years we had 15 people working for us, and it continued to grow. We started wholesale and worked up to 18 hours a day. We had over 50 employees when we sold the business. We had no vacations for 7 years.
11. I: You buried your life in work.
  P: Yes. We had that expensive house, but we really lived in the back room of our office. If not for the dog, we wouldn't have gone home.
12. I: And then you sold the business?
  P: Yes. My wife and I were dreaming of a life where we would enjoy our home, visit relatives, and travel. All these dreams. . . . [Looks at the wall and shows a painful expression in his face]
13. I: [Mirrors the painful expression]
  P: And the dreams came . . . as nightmares about Nam. [Closes his eyes, opens them, and looks at the interviewer] I woke up screaming in a cold sweat. [Stares at the wall] During the day I'm in a daze.
14. I: Do you have flashbacks during the day?
  P: [Looks at the interviewer] Two. I feel I am back in Vietnam. [Eyes wide open with a fearful expression]
15. I: [Mirrors the wide-open eyes and breathes faster]
  P: My living room is the battlefield.

Step 3: Confront

16. I: Share your pain with me.
  P: [Closes eyes, presses lips together] I'm not ready for that. [Shakes his head] I'll never get that far. [Looks at the interviewer] My wife has asked me a hundred times [looks at the ceiling] but I can't.
17. I: [Looks up] You are wrapped in your past as if in a cocoon.
  P: [Sighing] That drove my wife away. [Looks into space]
18. I: [Leans back, looks at the patient]

P: I was alone in that mansion . . . I hated every minute of it . . . I wanted to feel alive . . . be with people. All I saw was furniture, glass, wood carvings, and painted porcelain. [Looks at the interviewer]

19. I: Like a mausoleum.

P: I couldn't stand it. I moved to a hotel. That's where I live, no contact with people, just TV, not even watching.

20. I: And you can't share your memories?

P: I can't be with people. I'm losing my mind. I can't sleep. I'm scared of the nightmares. During the day I sit and brood, don't shave, don't shower, don't eat.

21. I: You are depressed and caught up in your past with no escape.

P: [Buries his head in his hands]

   The interviewer began with a routine question to elicit the patient's chief complaint (Q. 1) and then followed this lead with clarification (Q. 3–14). She expressed empathy verbally (Q. 7) and nonverbally (Q. 13, 15). With Q. 13 and 15, she started to mirror the patient's expression of pain and fear and trailed him by a fraction of a second. The interviewer chose this pacing technique because the patient displayed distress in his affect and in his psychomotor movements (A. 8, 12, 13, 15–17, 21). The interviewer used these displays of expression as opportunities to mirror the patient's actions, thereby using mirroring to communicate active, attentive listening and empathy for his story. It is a nonverbal method of communicating to the patient,

   I understand. I'm interested in what you are saying.

Step 4: Solve

22. I: Let me help you. Dextroamphetamine may help you talk. It may lift your mood. [The interviewer explains the action of dextroamphetamine and its predictive value for tricyclic response (Little 1988)].

P: [Shakes his head] I'm not ready for talking but I'll try the drug. [The patient receives 20 mg of dextroamphetamine. One hour after the dose, he reports no change in mood but he is talking with other patients, whereas before he would sit in the smoking lounge by himself, brooding. Two hours after the dose, the patient is conversing with the nurses, joking with the mental health worker, and initiating conversation with two patients. He smiles, walks faster, and holds his head up and body erect as if he had grown 2 inches. He looks 5 years younger. Mr. G. smiles at the interviewer.]

23. I: I never knew you had teeth.

P: [Blanches] Why do you say that?

24. I: Because for the first time since I met you I see you smiling.

P: They are artificial.

25. I: Well, I meant that you are smiling.

    P: [Releases breath] I just feared you could read my mind.

26. I: You make me curious now. Why did you think I could read your mind?

    P: I thought you knew about my teeth. Let's forget it.

27. I: I meant that you seem to feel better.

    P: I never thought a drug could make me feel better. Nam messed me up. How can a drug make me overcome Nam?

28. I: Nam made you feel bad but you allow it to do that.

    P: I feel better now. I feel like calling my ex-wife.

29. I: The medication lifted your mood. Could you talk now about Vietnam?

    P: [Deep folds freeze his face into a bloodless mask] I'm sorry, I'm so sorry.

30. I: [Closes her eyes and mirrors the fold between the eyes] I hear you . . . [leaning back] I'm ready to hear about Nam. [Opens her eyes]

    P: [Looks at her face as if seeking to read something from it. He stares at her nearly as if unaware of her glances. His mouth opens, his eyes roll up, he looks to the ceiling, then to the left and to the right; he is breathing hard.]

31. I: [Looks at the ceiling too, breathes deep as if she has to tell the story and then releases air] It started . . . when?

    P: [Looks at her, takes a deep breath, then releases the air slowly and speaks as if talking to himself] It was in '66. Nobody at home knew about Vietnam. [Looks at the white wall opposite him] I'd been with the special forces since '63. We were all very close. We never had any contact with the regulars. There were no ranks, just first names. Closer than family. I'd not been as close to anyone before. We lived in a village with the Vietnamese, whom we could trust.

32. I: I've heard about the special forces.

    P: There were just a few thousand of us. Our mission was reconnaissance, not fighting. We stayed out of any fights even though we were trained in jungle fighting.

33. I: So you were the eyes of the army.

    P: That's pretty much it. We were looking for North Vietnamese storage places and we found a huge underground armory, four stories deep, impossible to hit from the air.

34. I: Hmmm.

    P: Some guards saw us and they fired some shots. We took out a few of 'em but didn't get 'em all. So the North Vietnamese knew that we had found it. They knew we would be back. I wired headquarters and asked for regulars [makes a sweeping hand motion] to help us wipe 'em out.

35. I: [Looking at the patient, narrows her eyelids as if to look ahead]

    P: They sent about 50 people from Fort Sells in Lawton, Oklahoma . . . with lots of explosive—enough to wipe out a storage four times as large. They had no experience in fighting, let alone jungle fighting. A bunch of healthy-looking kids, smiling, not ready to take anything on, and by no means the gooks, as they called the Vietnamese.

36. I: [Pulling the angles of her mouth down] Gee.

    P: Usually, when we got reinforcements, I stayed in charge. This time, they sent a major with them, senior to me in rank.

37. I: Did he have any jungle experience?
    P: No. He had done maneuvers in Oklahoma, not known for its jungles. [Biting his lips]
38. I: [Biting her lips too]
    P: He insisted that he was in charge. [Louder] I told him what we had to do: fight our way through the jungle and wipe out that camp. It could take up to 5 days. "That's too much time. They'll get too much reinforcement. We'll go right up the road and hit them fast," he said. [Clearing his throat] I told him that's exactly what they'd expect us to do. It'd get us killed in an ambush. "Nonsense," he said. "They won't be ready. We'll start right now and hit them before they know what's hitting them." [Sighing]
39. I: [Sighing too and slowly shaking her head] Could you change his plan?
    P: [Shaking his head] He pulled rank on me.
40. I: [Sighing and nodding her head]
    P: [Nodding his head] He ordered me to do what he said because he was in command. [Sighing, angry] I told him we would all get killed. [Louder] We had been fighting the Vietnamese for 2 years, we knew what they are like. But nothing could stop him. So we started marching up the road . . . [Closing his eyes, shaking his head, silent]
41. I: [Looking at the patient, after the patient opens his eyes, she closes hers and very slightly shakes her head as if thinking to herself]
    P: [Wrinkles his forehead] We hadn't been on the road for more than a day.
42. I: [Wrinkles her forehead too]
    P: And there the T mines went off from the jungle trees all around us . . . and fire decked us from the left. We jumped off the road into the jungle on the other side. We had run into a horseshoe ambush. With me, 3 of my men survived and 13 of the regulars. Our men were moaning in the street. Among them the major. He was going to get us all killed. I called back to headquarters. I gave them our position, told them to hit the road and the jungle west of us. They told me that they'd be there in 5 minutes with white phosphorous. [Rolling lips in, bending his head back, looking at the ceiling]
43. I: [Mirroring the patient's movements slightly]
    P: [Digs his head into the elbow of his left arm, breathing heavily, after several seconds lifts his head with a frozen facial expression] I can't do it.
44. I: [With a fearful expression stares at the patient, as though frozen in fear]
    P: [Looking at her]
45. I: [Starts to breathe faster and shakes her head very slowly]
    P: [Shakes his head slowly too, breathes faster, and then takes a deep breath]
46. I: [Looks through him with a painful, determined look on her face, pressing her lips together]
    P: [Face relaxes, his mouth opens]
47. I: [Takes a deep breath and raises her clenched fists into the patient's eyesight]
    P: [Clenches his fists too while his face becomes tense, eyes wide open] I've seen what phosphorous does. [Shakes his head] We could not get the wounded off the road. We could not let them burn. [Wrinkles his forehead]
48. I: [Wrinkles forehead too, presses lips together, narrows eyes to a small slit]

P: [Narrows eyelids too] So we started to shoot into the moaning bodies until it was silent. It was so very quiet.

49. I: [Looks up as if listening for the silence]

P: Then the sound of the planes. The engine noise hurried toward us.

50. I: [Pressing fists against her stomach and bending over as if ducking]

P: [Ducking too] You have to see what phosphorous does . . . a white flash . . . all is gone. Bodies shrink, trees vanish, and then silence. Just the wind. It blows the smoke of burnt trees and burnt bodies into our faces.

51. I: What a horror! That memory forced you into the hospital now at Christmas?

P: It's worse. It's the Tet offensive that really gets me.

The interviewer gave the patient feedback about his improved mood and used this as the reason to expect the patient to be able to talk about his trauma (Q. 23–29). The patient picked up on the positive feedback of his mood but still declined to talk (A. 29). Next the interviewer increased her nonverbal communication by mirroring the patient (Q. 30, 31) and set a verbal cue, which the patient responded to (Q. and A. 31). The patient began with the nontraumatic part of his trauma, needing only a little encouragement (Q. and A. 31–36). This introduction was abstract and void of sensory impressions and emotions. However, the patient repeated the deep breath that the interviewer induced to pace the patient (Q. and A. 31). This response showed that the patient was responding to the techniques of active listening.

The interviewer acknowledged that she was familiar with what the patient was talking about and that she understood what he was saying (Q. 32, 33). The patient expressed feelings of disdain (A. 35), which the interviewer reflected nonverbally (Q. 36) and verbally (Q. 37). She also mirrored the patient's nonverbal expression of helplessness (Q. 38). The interviewer mirrored the patient up to Q. 39, then introduced an anticipating head movement that expressed a negative outcome (Q. 39) that the patient picked up, thus showing that he could be led. The interviewer used another head movement (Q. 40), which also paced the patient. Again, the interviewer mirrored the patient's expression until Q. 43.

Despite the mirroring, the patient broke off his report (A. 43). The interviewer paced him back into the horror-inducing affective state that he had just abandoned (Q. 44, 45). The patient then restarted the story with a general statement (A. 47) and returned to a recall mode. The interviewer mirrored him and once again began to pace him (Q. and A. 48) by maintaining the facial expressions of painful determination that she could induce in the patient. The patient followed and began to visualize the traumatic situation (A. 47–50).

Up to this point, the history the patient gave of the traumatic event seemed to indicate that the patient's unfinished emotions were the source of his continued trauma. First, the patient could not discharge his anger against the higher-ranked officer. He had to follow orders instead, or risk mutiny charges. Second, he could not grieve and call for his wounded friends. To the contrary, he had to shoot them to save them from death by fire. Third, he could not act out his fear by escaping because he was trapped in a cross fire. His helplessness was augmented by the fact that he had foreseen what was to happen, but had been unable to change the course of the disaster. Thus, at this juncture, it appeared that the unfinished business model (Perls 1969; see Section 3, "Techniques," above) applied to Mr. G.'s posttraumatic stress. However, when the interviewer judged the time was right to bring the traumatic recall to a closure, the patient surprisingly objected and introduced a second trauma (A. 51).

52. I: [Looks at the patient, shrugs her shoulders with a questioning look and a hands-opening-up gesture, inviting the patient to talk]
    P: [Leaning forward] Tet is the name of the lunar new year. It's like Christmas for us. In '68, the North and the South agreed on a cease-fire for the holidays.
53. I: [Silent, attentive, and ready to listen]
    P: In '67, the North Vietnamese had a similar truce. This time, we saw activity everywhere, not just battalions. We saw entire divisions, which are three battalions strong. We radioed it back to headquarters in Saigon. They said they didn't think it meant anything. "But there is so much activity," I said. They laughed. "It's the lunar new year. It's Tet. Nothing is going to happen on the holidays."
54. I: [In listening pose, silent]
    P: [Squirming in his seat, leaning back, looking up to the ceiling, looking at his hands, his knees, leaning back again, sighing]
55. I: [Mirroring some back-and-forth movement] You sound helpless. You sound desperate.
    P: I was. And I was mad. What could we do? I couldn't convince our command that it was different this year, that something was going to happen. [Shrugs his shoulders] Why do they have us out there if they don't listen?
56. I: [Bending forward, with a frown on her face, pressing her lips together as if suppressing the perception of pain to come]
    P: [Also bending forward] We went back to our village where we had lived with the Montagnard people for 2 years. There were 27 women, 14 children, and some 35 men. We were real close to the men . . . and the children. [Eyes become wet]
57. I: [Closes her eyes]
    P: We had given every one of them an American name. We missed our own children at home, so we played with them. We never messed with their

women. They were proud people. They were highland people. You could trust them.

58. I: [Trying to look into the patient's eyes]

P: [Squirms in his chair, looks briefly at the interviewer, and then looks for some hold in the room, sighing] We checked out the hills around us and the jungle—North Vietnamese regulars were everywhere. We were outnumbered 1 to 10. We put the women and the children into the underground bunkers.

59. I: [Looking at the patient's mouth, still expressing pain that she anticipates to come]

P: [Angry, with a pleading voice] I called back to our command post, telling them we are surrounded, we expect to be overrun any time, please help us. We had promised the Montagnard people that we would get them out of there if things got rough. I could not get any action. [Eyes fill with tears]

60. I: [Reflecting sadness] You feel awful.

P: [Clinching his fists] Desperate. . . . We had modern weapons, powerful mortars, machine guns. . . . [Shaking his head]

61. I: [Swaying her head, making a fist with her right hand and holding it with the left as if it were a rifle]

P: But the Montagnards are proud people. They did not like our weapons. They liked the old French carbines: one shot, one man, one action.

62. I: [Throws her head backward and inhales]

P: [Exhaling with pressure] I called for help. Finally, they sent us some South Vietnamese rangers. The special forces didn't respect them—during the day they helped us, at night they turned into Viet Cong.

63. I: [Shrugs shoulders] You did not feel helped.

P: [Raises one eyebrow] I didn't at first. The North Vietnamese started attacking and shelled us for 2 days. I called headquarters for help. The answer: "Heavy fire everywhere. The north has started an offensive. They are overrunning us. You have to hold!" But there was no way.

64. I: [Bending forward as if feeling pain in her stomach]

P: [Looking at the office wall as if he sees the Vietnamese storming out of it] They stormed us. We counterattacked where the jungle was the thickest. All men in one spot. We broke through their line and escaped into the jungle.

65. I: [Breathes faster]

P: The Montagnards stayed back. They defended the village and the bunkers with their women and children.

66. I: [Looking at the patient, takes a deep breath and holds it in]

P: [Clinching his hands together as if holding a rifle] We fought our way out with our bayonets. I got a blow on my head. I went out. When I came to, I was laying in deep bamboo grass with my front teeth knocked out, blood running out of my mouth.

67. I: [Wetting her lips]

P: Then I saw the women. [Stares in fear, closes his eyes, shakes and bends down his head] No, that's all. . . . I can't go on with it. [Looks up]

68. I: [Opens her eyes in fear]

P: [Bends over]

69. I: [Slowly turning the expression of fear into an expression of pain, looking at the patient and waiting]

    P: [Stretches hands in front of him, palms up] The Vietnamese had all women strung up by their hands on bamboo rods connecting their huts. These dark-skinned women were hanging there naked. The Montagnard men were lying dead. The Vietnamese had grabbed the children by their hair—all 14 of them—and made them look at their mothers. [Biting his lips]

70. I: [Bent over, biting her lips with pain in her face]

    P: One Vietnamese officer pulled his machete and with one strike cut off their nipples . . . blood spurting out.

71. I: [Crosses her arms in front of her chest, leans over as if protecting her own body]

    P: The women were silent. No moaning. No screaming. Only the children were crying, trying to look away from their mothers. The North Vietnamese soldiers held them by their hair and their ears as if they were reins and made them look.

72. I: [Taking a deep breath and sitting up straight]

    P: Then, the officer jammed his machete into the vagina of each hanging woman, one by one, and turned it around . . . blood was shooting out of their bodies, but they made no sound, these proud women. There was only the screaming of the children.

73. I: [Bending over the side arm of her chair and breathing hard]

    P: The soldiers butchered the children. They crisscrossed their bodies with machete blows, cut off their fingers, their arms, their heads. No bodies were left, only blobs of blood.

74. I: [Swallows and wets her lips]

    P: Silence. Only the smell of blood and taste of my blood in my mouth. . . . [Pauses] Then the North Vietnamese marched off.

75. I: [Buries her head in her hands, then looks up, encouraging the patient to continue]

    P: Some of the South Vietnamese rangers came back out of the jungle, and our group came back too. I had lost only 5 of 25 men. But all the Montagnards were dead. We cut down the women. We had no time to bury them. In the past, the North Vietnamese would kill the men, cut off their dicks, and stick them into the mouths of the dead. They would kill the women and let the children go. Here they had tortured the children the most. They mutilated these proud women and just killed their men.

Early on, the interviewer tuned in to the patient's helplessness with mirroring (Q. 55–57). She guided (A. 56) and trailed him (A. 57) to the revelation of the conflict that marked another trauma. As an alternative, the interviewer could have used cathartic enhancement and asked the patient to express his anger about headquarters in Saigon. Such intervention could also have been appropriate at A. 59 and 63. However, such catharsis might have interrupted the patient's report and overwhelmed him. Therefore, the interviewer focused on the patient's helplessness and not on his anger. The patient verbalized his anger once (A. 55) and expressed it in his voice (A. 59), but returned to his feeling of helplessness.

The interviewer trailed the patient through the description of the traumatic event (A. 59–63). The patient picked up the interviewer's shoulder shrug with his own sign of helplessness—raising his eyebrow (A. 63). The interviewer stayed in a pacing mode through A. 66 and prompted the patient to talk. The patient began to image and reexperience the trauma (Q. 66) and remained in this state for several minutes (Q. 66–74). When the patient stalled (A. 67), the interviewer paced him through his blocking (Q. 69). She combined mirroring his pain and trailing with emotional reactions to the trauma (Q. 71, 73–75).

The interviewer allowed the patient to lead while she became an attentive, interested, and emotionally participating listener. Rapport was established by the interviewer's ability to accurately mirror the patient's pain, and by the patient's feeling comfortable enough to let *her* expression of pain amplify *his* expression of pain. The key element of rapport was the nonverbal exchange that brought the interviewer and patient in tune. Visualizing the scene the patient described, the interviewer reflected and anticipated his pain in her facial expressions and body postures. Her goal was to enable the patient to live through the experience again with her helping him to get in touch with his feelings. The barrier to recall was the patient's anxiety in becoming overwhelmed by his feelings. As he had reported, he had shut out his wife from his traumatic world, thus showing his degree of avoidance.

Step 5: Approve

76. I: Is that what you relive in your nightmares?
    P: I see the glasses of that officer. They reflect the sun rays right into my face. I can't see his eyes. I see his bony nose, and I hear him bark, "I'm in command."

         I hear the commander who told me to hold. . . . The hew sound of the machete as it cuts off the nipples. . . . And I see the blobs of meat that were children I knew. . . . And then I hear the moaning of my friends. Have you ever heard the moaning of the dying? People moan differently when they die than when they are wounded. And then I hear the dull pung of the bullets that hit the dying bodies of my own men. And then . . . the silence. Have you ever heard silence in your dreams? I scream and scream . . . but I can't fill the silence.

77. I: Why can't you get rid of these memories? What is haunting you? Why are they coming back?

P: I don't know. I should have shot that officer when we took off on the road. Then I wouldn't have had to shoot all our men. I knew he would get us all killed. Rank over experience. I should have convinced him to avoid the ambush. We knew how to take out guards with knives.

78. I: What a burden.

P: That's why I never wanted to have children with my second wife.

79. I: It crippled your life.

P: After the horseshoe ambush I swore to myself never, never again would I let people get close to me. But with the Montagnards it happened again. I loved those children and those people, and I could not protect them.

80. I: I sense how helpless you felt against your commanders—and how guilty.

P: [Tearful] There must have been something that I could have done. I should have just ignored the order and gotten the Montagnard people out of there.

81. I: You played by the rules; you followed orders.

P: But the orders were wrong.

82. I: You did what you could.

P: It killed everybody.

83. I: You can play back the past, but you cannot change it. The outcome is the same. You hear the moaning and groaning and then the silence; you hear the commander's voice, you see his glasses. . . .

P: What can I do?

84. I: Accept what you did—it is all you could do. The past is gone—you can't change the past from hindsight.

P: [Sits in silence]

85. I: I lived with you through your experience of having to shoot your friends because a green commander didn't listen; how your friends, the Montagnard people, got butchered because the high command didn't listen to your reconnaissance and did not prepare for the offensive. Your helplessness makes you hang on to the past.

As in the previous scene, it became obvious that the patient could not discharge his anger about headquarters because he was obeying an officer's order. For the same reason, he could not flee the death trap. He could not discharge his anger over the Viet Cong's cruelties because he had to face the trauma alone while laying in the grass. He could not scream out, grieve, or run away because the enemy would have killed him. Unfinished emotions appeared to be associated with his trauma—he continually reexperienced his unfinished anger and grief in his dreams (Q. 76).

The interviewer invited the patient to reflect why these events became his trauma (Q. 77). Mr. G. found a partial answer by suggesting that he should have killed the officer who led them into the trap (A. 77). Then he seemed to discard this idea and blamed himself that he should have done a better job convincing the officer to avoid the ambush (A. 77). Yet he failed. Thus, he took the road of avoiding close friendships (A. 79). Yet he became emotionally close to the Montagnard families, who were killed like his friends before. Again, the patient could foretell the disaster but not prevent it. It appeared that this event became a personal trauma for Mr. G. at the moment when his sense of control was challenged, thus setting him up for the development of posttraumatic stress disorder.

The interviewer interpreted the patient's flashbacks as an expression of his helplessness against authority. The patient agreed. She pointed out that he had described his feelings well but that he had never named them, that he suffered through experiences but did not reflect on them. Rather than cognitively accepting his helplessness as inevitable, he continued to protest against it and torture himself with a search for alternative solutions. In this brooding effort to rewrite the past, he did not find acceptable solutions. Instead, he coped by avoiding closeness, such as denying his wife the opportunity to have children and then divorcing her. This manner of coping only deepened his sense of helplessness. The interviewer addressed the patient's helplessness to prepare him for therapeutic cognitive integration of the trauma (Q. 85).

Diagnosis

Axis I

1. Posttraumatic stress disorder with delayed onset
2. Major depressive disorder, severe

Axis II.   Deferred.

6. Posttraumatic Stress, Imaging, and Active Listening in Psychiatric Disorders

Imaging and active listening can be used for interviewing patients with any disorder in which avoidance, repetitive and intrusive thoughts, or dissociation occur, such as in the following:

- Posttraumatic stress disorder, acute or chronic, with or without delayed onset.
- Avoidance behaviors related to agoraphobia, with or without panic;

specific phobias; social phobias; and avoidant personality disorder.
- Obsessive-compulsive disorder characterized by intrusive repetitions and obsessive-compulsive personality disorder.
- Panic disorder, generalized anxiety disorder, overanxious disorder of childhood, and possibly dependent personality disorder. Research shows that monozygotic twins are concordant for anxiety disorders but not for the specific type (Torgersen 1983). Therefore, it appears that a disposition for anxiety is inherited. External events may shape the development of the specific form that the anxiety disorder takes. Imaging and active listening may help to identify the avoided stressors.
- Dissociative disorders, such as derealization and depersonalization disorder, dissociative amnesia, dissociative fugue, dissociative identity disorder, acute stress disorder, dissociative disorder not otherwise specified, histrionic personality disorder, and borderline personality disorder. Patients who have histrionic personality disorder are suggestible and may therefore be prone to dissociation. Patients with borderline personality disorder respond to stress, especially to loss, with dissociative symptoms (DSM-IV criterion 9). The precipitating psychological factors may be explored with imaging and active listening.
- Adjustment disorder with anxiety, depressed mood, or with both are triggered by stressors. A minor "trauma" can be repeated in the patient's fantasies and dreams. It may not occupy the patient's mind at all times, but it may scar the patient. If untreated, it may destroy the patient's marriage and family, as well as his social and work relationships. Not the big bang of war but the small, sharp thorns of everyday living can cause such trauma. Here is an example:

George: Linda, you expect me to go to your brother's house at Christmas. You remember what your brother said to me when we got married 20 years ago?
Linda: That's long forgotten now.
George: Not for me. He told me I was a worthless, uneducated klutz, that I would never amount to anything, and he's sorry that I became part of the family. You didn't say a word to defend me. It still makes me angry.

Linda knows that at every family gathering the same story emerges. When George is angry, he will bring it up. He cannot process the disappointment he experienced from the comments of his brother-in-law, and it permanently mars their relationship.

What may be a minor stressor for one patient can be a major trauma for another, such as in the following example.

Rebecca, a rabbi's daughter, was rejected by her mother-in-law and her sister-in-law, who were both angry that she neither enriched the family wealth at the time of the wedding nor pursued a lucrative business career but instead took a low-paying but prestigious university job. Rebecca was enraged about and helpless toward this criticism. She loved her husband, but he did not stand up for her against his well-to-do but uneducated family. She relived the conversations with her in-laws and had nightmares. Insomnia, palpitations, and anticipatory anxiety set in when she had to visit the in-laws.

In Chapters 1 through 3, we use hypnosis, free association, and active listening to uncover traumas and precipitating psychological factors. In the following chapter, we demonstrate a technique that relieves the patient's anxiety and fear of not being taken seriously as being truly sick. This technique, which we call "validating of somatic symptoms," does not directly focus on coping deficits that turn ordinary life events into stressors for such a patient. Validating relates to the patient that her disorder is legitimate. The method allows the patient to release information about the stressors that she would otherwise deny in fear that her symptoms would be interpreted as excuses to avoid responsibilities.

CHAPTER 4

SOMATIZATION

Summary

In this chapter, we discuss how to recognize somatization disorder and how to counteract the patient's fear of being considered a "fake" through a technique we call *validation*. It turns the hostile and resistant patient into a cooperative ally who is willing to explore psychosocial factors, negative life events, and other psychiatric disorders that may be associated with developing somatization disorder and maintaining and aggravating its symptoms.

◆ ◆ ◆ ◆ ◆

Our bodies are our gardens, to which our wills are gardeners.

William Shakespeare
Othello (1605)

◆ ◆ ◆ ◆ ◆

119

1. What Is Somatization?

Somatization is a key component of somatoform disorders. We feature somatization disorder because it is the best-studied disorder in the somatoform group. Somatization disorder is a psychiatric disorder in which, starting before age 30 years, a patient reports multiple physical symptoms that are medically unexplained. These symptoms include pain perception throughout the body—in the head, abdomen, back, joints, chest, rectum, or during intercourse, menstruation, or urination. The patient reports disturbances of the autonomic gastrointestinal system with nausea, diarrhea, bloating, vomiting, and food intolerance and disturbances of the sexual and reproductive system with sexual indifference, impotence, vaginismus, and menstrual irregularity.

Pseudoneurological signs and symptoms that do not follow any known pathways and are not limited to pain occur; as stated in DSM-IV (American Psychiatric Association 1994), these are "conversion symptoms such as impaired coordination or balance, paralysis or localized weakness, difficulty swallowing or lump in throat, aphonia, urinary retention, hallucinations, loss of touch or pain sensation, double vision, blindness, deafness, or seizures; dissociative symptoms such as amnesia; or loss of consciousness other than fainting" (p. 446).

By definition, somatization includes pains arising from many sites. The pain symptoms wander around in the body; they occur at certain times and not at others; they change in quality from stabbing to throbbing to cramping to burning. We do not know what causes the pain (for sure, not a wandering uterus, which led to the name hysteria!).

The symptoms do not reflect any known physical illness but instead portray the patient's presumptive model of being sick. Thus, the disorder progresses by an increase in the number, severity, and duration of symptoms, and by a spreading of symptoms over more body sites rather than by a progression of the disturbance in one particular organ system, as is the case in most known physical disorders. But this progression is not associated with physical signs of structural abnormalities or with abnormal laboratory findings (Cloninger 1986).

At least three general medical disorders are associated with disturbances affecting multiple organ systems:

- Systemic lupus erythematosus affects connective tissue and the vascular system of all organs, including the brain.
- Multiple sclerosis leads to lesions at multiple sites in the central nervous

system, which in turn leads to associated symptoms and signs in the innervated areas.

● Acute intermittent porphyria leads to lesions in the central and peripheral nervous systems and, via concomitant severe hypertension, to extensive vascular lesions (Pincus et al. 1992).

Unlike somatization disorder, these three disorders can be confirmed by tissue and laboratory test abnormalities.

Somatization disorder is associated with other psychiatric symptoms, including conversion, dissociation, phobic anxiety, and affective symptoms (Feighner et al. 1972). Lifetime comorbidity with major depression (87%), panic disorder (45%), mania (40%), and phobic disorder (39%) raises the question of whether somatization disorder is a homogeneous or heterogeneous entity (Liskow et al. 1986). Nevertheless, recent findings may point to limbic kindling and/or neurobiological sensitization mechanisms as a basis for somatization disorder and its associated psychiatric disorders (Bell 1994). In the DSM-IV definition of somatization disorder, three types of somatic symptoms (i.e., pain, gastrointestinal, and sexual) and two types of pseudoneurological symptoms (i.e., conversion and dissociative) are included.

Somatization disorder is found primarily in women (Guze 1967).[1] According to DSM-IV (American Psychiatric Association 1994, p. 447), this disorder occurs only rarely in men in the United States. However, a higher reported frequency was reported among Greek and Puerto Rican men, suggesting that cultural factors may influence the sex ratio. Furthermore, in epidemiological studies in Los Angeles and Puerto Rico, Escobar et al. (1987, 1991) found that the abridged somatization construct (i.e., a lifetime presence of at least four medically unexplained physical symptoms for males and six for females) had a high prevalence (50–100 times greater than that of somatization disorder proper) without the gender bias (Escobar et al. 1987, 1991). In the Los Angeles Epidemiologic Catchment Area program, the prevalence of somatization symptoms was 4.4% in 3,132 community respondents (Escobar et al. 1987).

In somatization disorder, symptoms often arise during childhood. At this time, the patient misses school because of stomachaches, nausea, and vomiting. After menarche, a female patient may get medical attention for cramps, excessive bleeding, and irregular menstruation. During marriage, a female patient may refuse intercourse because of vaginismus. Finally, ab-

---

[1] Therefore, we use the female gender for patients described in this chapter.

dominal complaints may become so severe that the patient seeks a hysterectomy and abandons the possibility of childbirth and burdensome child rearing.

Families of patients with somatization disorder have a higher incidence of somatization disorder, alcoholism, and antisocial personality disorder (Arkonac and Guze 1963; Cadoret 1978; Cadoret et al. 1976; Cloninger and Guze 1970; Guze et al. 1967, 1986; Woerner and Guze 1968). Family studies show that somatization disorder is familial and possibly genetically transmitted. What appears to be transmitted is an inability to comply with rules and demands. These disorders may be expressed differently by males and females in the same family. Males may develop antisocial personality disorder—that is, they cope with rules by ignoring or breaking them. Female family members may develop somatization disorder—that is, they cope with rules and regulations by developing somatic symptoms and conversion symptoms (e.g., paralysis). These symptoms may also prevent them from following rules and meeting demands.

These multiple symptoms of somatization disorder were described by Briquet in 1859. Perley and Guze (1962) summarized them in their symptom list. They were condensed to 37 symptoms for DSM-III (American Psychiatric Association 1980). The authors of DSM-III-R (American Psychiatric Association 1987) included 35 of those symptoms. Othmer and Desouza proposed the Seven Symptom Screening Test (Othmer and Desouza 1985). These seven symptoms were listed in boldface type in DSM-III-R. In DSM-IV, the criteria require a minimum of four pain symptoms in different sites or functions of the body, two nonpain gastrointestinal symptoms, one sexual or reproductive symptom other than pain, plus one pseudoneurological "symptom or deficit suggesting a neurological disorder not limited to pain" (p. 449). Thus, at least a total of eight symptoms are required for the diagnosis.

2. Somatization in the Mental Status

The patient who somatizes may be recognized during the clinical diagnostic interview by one of the following characteristics.

Dramatic Presentation

The patient with somatization disorder presents with a history of vague symptoms. She resists specifying the symptoms and exaggerates their severity. This exasperating presentation often provokes rejection. Any sense on the patient's part that she is being rejected increases her drama, and may even make her become accusatory. When she feels pressured, she may obstruct the interview by claiming sudden onset of symptoms. Rather than negotiating different interviewing terms, she uses her symptoms spontaneously to divert, obstruct, interrupt, or terminate the interview:

I am too sick to sit here any longer and answer your questions.

My splitting headache is coming back. I can't think anymore.

My back is killing me. We have to stop the interview.

Poor Concentration

Poor concentration is in keeping with patients who have somatization disorder. Their right brain functions are more developed than their left brain functions. For example, Riley (1984) found that, in comparison with depressive and nonpsychiatric control subjects, college students with Briquet's syndrome (a forerunner of somatization disorder) performed relatively poorly on tests of left hemisphere functions (e.g., right field sensory perception, verbal comprehension, and right side motor skill and strength), but did well on tests of right hemisphere functions (e.g., left field sensory perception, visual and spatial comprehension, and left side motor skill and strength).

Suggestibility

Patients with somatization disorder are suggestible. They may endorse anxiety or affective symptoms, including manic ones. If asked for examples, they may describe increased energy, push of speech, and elated mood, but these symptoms are usually not severe enough to interfere with psychosocial functioning or to require treatment. Patients may also report pseudohallucinations that often seem to occur at night (e.g., seeing or speaking to dead relatives sitting at the patient's bedside). It is difficult to decide whether an affective disorder is present or not, as we do not have any way to test conclusively for a physical basis of their symptoms. Clinical experience shows that patients with somatization disorder frequently do not benefit from antidepressant treatment; they report side effects from medication instead. The point is not to overlook the possible diagnosis of somatization disorder in favor of a questionable affective disorder. Keep the question of a somatization disorder in focus. Identify somatic symptoms that are unconnected with each other and that do not relate to any known medical or psychiatric disorder. Because somatization symptoms start at least during the teenage years, use a historical approach. Trace patients' somatic symptoms back through their life; for example, with a female patient, start with her first menses and before.

Lack of Insight

Patients often are psychologically blind to cause and effect of their symptoms, and become irritated when asked about such connections, arguing,

> I'm not making up my pain. I'm really sick. Why can't anybody find out what is wrong with me?

They counteract social demands with a barrage of symptoms that are often presented in a passive-aggressive and defiant manner. Such patients may express their distress saying,

> Can't you see how sick I am?

> Don't you see that I can't do it?

> Can't you see how sick you have made me?

A somatization disorder patient replaces assertiveness with somatic symptoms. She swings between the poles of self-pity and angry accusation. There is seldom a direct link between the somatic symptom and the specific demands placed on the patient. In addition, the somatic pain response or dysfunction is not linked to a specific task or demand, but to a specific organ, as in the following example.

> A cook whose job it is to taste different types of foods for the chef objects to the task. However, her somatic symptoms do not involve nausea or vomiting, as one might expect. Instead they involve a general disability, including abdominal pain, headaches, back pain, and dizzy spells. In fact, her response to social pressure often involves abdominal pain. She states, "My stomach is my weak spot." She insists that she has a somatic problem that an internist or a surgeon should address and not a psychologist or psychiatrist. "My problem is not in my head. I have real pain. I'm not imagining it." Her disability is medically documented through her hospital-

izations and her agreement to undergo risky diagnostic and surgical procedures, some of which are only weakly indicated.

Besides risky and invasive diagnostic procedures, patients with somatization disorder appear to prefer physical therapy such as surgical interventions. Cohen et al. (1953) noted that the excess of operations in somatization disorder (hysteria) is maximal during the decade of ages 21–30 years. We interpret such history of frequent surgeries as the patient's attempt to validate her complaints as physical in nature.

Stressors

Stressors for the patient are demands to fulfill social expectations in a timely manner that she cannot effectively negotiate. Instead, she may respond with increase in pain and other dysfunctions. Her main stressors are work, children, spouse, and friends. These stressors are illustrated in the following hypothetical scenario.

Work as stressor.   As an employee, the patient faces a boss who demands performance. She craves attention and understanding, not simply rewards that she has earned. For her, it is so much more important to be esteemed and loved rather than to be judged only by the amount of work that she completes. The boss often criticizes her as being inconsistent. At times she works overtime and at other times she fails to complete the minimum. Her colleagues are cold. They don't understand that she is hurting. They demand that she carry her load and refuse to make allowances for her being a sickly person. Therefore, she often has crying spells and breakdowns.

Pain interferes with her ability to concentrate and pay attention. Her memory for details is poor. Nobody listens to her. She does not feel valued by others, even though she experiences herself as sensitive. She knows she is an emotional person. She can feel, laugh, and cry with others, but nobody feels, laughs, and cries with her. She has a hard time controlling her emotions, anger, and disappointments. Rather than caring, others turn their backs. When she complains, ears are deaf. She is at a loss. She cannot perform like others.

At home, she is plagued with dizzy spells and cannot possibly concentrate on housework and complete it in due time. In her view, her spouse is very demanding. He criticizes her and she has a breakdown, cries, and retires to her own room just to return to tell him all about her medical problems, the throbbing headaches, and abdominal pain; all of this finally makes him accompany her to the physician.

Motherhood as stressor. As a mother, the patient is easily irritable. Her children are too active, too loud. They neither listen nor obey her. The children don't study, and they are tardy and skip school. Their illnesses worry her. They do not understand that she is nervous and irritable. When she yells at them, the children just laugh or run away.

Spouse as stressor. As a wife, the patient is worn out. How can her spouse expect her to be up for lovemaking when she is overworked and hurting so much? With the abdominal pain she experiences, she cannot enjoy sex when he insists on it. Her husband appears to be insensitive, not taking into account her pains. He doesn't even seem to listen when she tells him about her nausea. However, she does not dare to speak up against him. She is afraid that he will criticize her even more and leave her. So, rather than negotiate in an assertive manner the rules and expectations that she can fulfill, she communicates through her pains and dizzy spells instead.

Friends as stressor. Socially, the patient considers herself able to make friends, but does not feel she has found the right people. Most acquaintances do not help out when she needs them. She feels she is always available for them, but right now she is too tired, worn out, and hurting to extend the expected amount of help.

In summary, the patient feels her list of stressors is too long and time pressures too harsh. Nobody understands that she is sick. They unfairly judge her even though she has told them about her medical problems. She experiences double anguish: from her somatic symptoms and from rejection by the people around her.

Vulnerability

Even under minimal stress, this patient reports irregular biological functions, which reflects a somatic vulnerability. She reports feeling sickly. She looks worried and appears preoccupied with her body. Her sleep problems interfere with her ability to be rested. Her appetite is disturbed. At times, she is ravenously hungry and gains weight. At other times, she cannot eat. Her energy level fluctuates dramatically: she may feel weakened and then report periods in which she needs little sleep and is full of energy. From many doctors she may receive multiple treatments, but claims none really help. From all the medications that she has tried, only pain medication, like propoxyphene hydrochloride (Darvon), is useful. All other medications, including regular doses of antidepressants and sedatives, have troubling side effects. Hypnotics do not work anymore. After multiple surgeries—appendectomy, hysterectomy, and gall bladder removal—the symptoms, especially abdominal pain, come back. Scarring leads to new discomfort.

She has the feeling that doctors do not care, cannot or do not want to help her, and do not take her medical problems seriously because they cannot find anything. These doctors seem to suggest that her problems are all in her head. Her husband and family seem to think so too. She resents being asked to see a psychologist or psychiatrist, because that proves to her that the physicians and her family believe she is fabricating her symptoms.

The patient misleads you diagnostically with her plethora of physical symptoms. Her complaints raise questions about whether she has

- A psychiatric disorder with somatic symptoms as coded on Axis I, such as major depressive disorder
- A somatoform disorder that has no known medical physical basis, such as somatization disorder
- A physical disorder that has taken on a psychogenic overlay (i.e., she appears to use her confirmed medical disorder to dodge her responsibilities)
- A physical disorder in which symptoms fluctuate, such as multiple sclerosis, that may be mistaken for a somatoform disorder

Demonstration of Physical Symptoms

The patient experiencing somatization complains dramatically about her pain and disability. However, the account of her history fluctuates. She is vague in answering the "what," "when," "where," "why," and "how" questions. She denies symptoms she endorsed only minutes earlier and reports new symptoms she previously denied. Her exaggerations and contradictions disgust her friends, family members, and caregivers alike. Instead of reaping the empathy she yearns for, she harvests rejection.

3. Technique: Validation of Somatic Symptoms

Patients who somatize are expressing their psychological, social, and biological inadequacies in terms of somatic symptoms and dramatic suffering. Validation utilizes this tendency by accepting the patient's complaints in the language of bodily dysfunctions.

Take, for example, the patient who complains about chest pain and palpitations, which she attributes to a heart disorder. You confirm her complaint by saying,

Yes. Obviously there is something wrong with the way your heart works.

Usually this confirmation comes as a surprise for the patient, because she is used to physicians assuring her that there is nothing wrong with her heart because her electrocardiogram, treadmill test, echocardiogram, arteriogram, and heart X ray were normal. Therefore, the patient feels relieved that you validate her complaints as a legitimate medical disorder, but she will bring up the issue other physicians raised:

My doctors have told me that there is nothing wrong with my heart.

Explain that the other physicians are right and wrong at the same time. They are correct in regarding the heart as a functioning muscle and assessing it as indeed working well. They are wrong in regarding the patient's perception of pain as false, because pain is a symptom—a subjective feeling—and therefore it is real for the patient. Explain to the patient that the heart, like any other organ of the body, is supplied by the brain with nervous impulses through the autonomic nervous system. In turn, the heart sends stress signals to the brain using the autonomic nervous system. The patient's weakness does not lie in a weakness of the heart muscle or its blood supply, but could lie in the autonomic nervous system that links the heart to the brain or in the brain itself.

Explain further to the patient that the autonomic nervous system does not malfunction for just one organ like the heart but frequently for several organs, such as the uterus and the stomach, and the joints. At this time, the patient may affirm that she has had joint pains and abdominal cramping for a long time, and even had surgery to relieve the discomfort, but nothing physical has ever been found to be wrong. You are the first one who seems to know about what is going on with her.

Now it is time for you to express surprise:

How come? The disorder has a well-recognized name: somatization disorder. It is a disorder that can cause disability and pain.

Brighter patients may ask why the heart, stomach, or uterus does not show any physical irregularities, such as an arrhythmia in the electrocardiogram, or upper gastrointestinal defects on the X ray. You may explain,

Sometimes the brain may refer pain to an organ such as the heart, even though the heart itself is not directly involved. Let me explain that. We all know about phantom pain that can occur after an amputation. Such a patient feels pain or itching in a foot that was amputated several years earlier. The pain is real even though the foot is gone. This tells us that our brain can be stimulated and can project that stimulation to a body part even if it is gone.

The patient may express relief that you disagree with her other physicians and family members who imply that her pain is imagined. Explain that the problem is indeed in the head—that is, in the brain, not imagined but real.

This education bridges a possible adversarial relationship between interviewer and patient and establishes an alliance by validating the communication system that the patient uses to express discomfort. After confirmation, you can then explore the stressors that aggravate her somatic symptoms. Let her list all the circumstances in which the pain was brought on or became worse. You will get a report of social demands, calls for responsible behavior, and duties. Unlike in a healthy person, where demands induce excellence, a person with somatization symptoms becomes aggravated. Family members, friends, employers, and some therapists recognize this pattern and adopt a punitive attitude—brushing off the patient and her complaints and telling her in so many words to stop complaining and start working like everybody else.

Once you have learned the circumstances in which the symptoms occur, establish a temporal, but not causal, relationship between stressor and symptom. During the interview and in the course of giving her history, the patient will offer many examples of how she has experienced increasingly severe symptoms as social pressure mounted. Yet, such a patient resents any suggestion that symptoms are an excuse to avoid tasks or demands. She resists the interpretation that her disabling pain disorder is the physical expression of an intrapsychic or interpersonal conflict, even when she provides ample evidence. She resists such an interpretation with anxiety, hostility, hate, avoidance, or escape. Freud's (1952–1955) early experience with such interpretive endeavors gave testimony to that fact. Therefore, if you want to explore the patient's conflict, talk about it without connecting it with her pain symptoms. She is sensitized because she has heard this "accusation" from family, friends, and foes alike. Make it clear to her that you accept her view that she is physically sick. You cannot interpret the secondary gain that a patient may derive from her disorder from a psychoanalytical viewpoint without incurring her wrath. Approach her primary and secondary gain from her point of view, not yours. Her insight—not yours—should dominate the interview.

4. Five Steps to Reassure the Patient

Step 1: Listen. Let the patient describe her pains to you. She will be detailed about all the sensations she feels. She may use comparisons to make you understand her type of pain, such as,

> My headache feels like a metal band is twisted around my head. It pulls tighter and tighter until my head will explode.

> I have this terrible pain in my belly as if a big hairy fist is squeezing my stomach.

> The pain on my right side feels like long steel knives stabbing me.

Listen to these reports and encourage the patient to tell you when the pain happened and what was going on in her life at the time. Do not suggest any cause-effect relationship between stress and pain unless the patient volunteers it.

Some patients refuse to talk to you unless you are a neurologist, internist, gastroenterologist, or gynecologist. They feel that a psychiatrist, psychologist, counselor, or social worker lacks expertise in physical illness and therefore will assume problems are not real but imagined. In that case, point out to the patient that you understand her complaints better than an internist because you focus on the autonomic nervous system that is involved with her pain. Thus, establish your expertise and express empathy for the misunderstandings that she has had to endure about the nature of her disorder.

Step 1 is not a passive maneuver to let a somatizing patient take her usual course of behavior. It is an active reassurance that the interviewer shares her point of view and knows that she truly experiences pain. This starts the process of validating her symptoms. As the patient continues to believe the physical locus of illness is where she feels the pain, the interviewer holds the view that the disturbance is located in the brain, but does not share this view with her yet. At the end of Step 1, rapport is established: the interviewer has shown empathy for her pain, shares her insight, takes her disorder seriously, and has joined her as an ally.

Step 2: Tag. Select the patient's most prominent symptom and explore the circumstances that surround it. The patient may be vague with dates. She may, however, be able to describe the stressors as long as you do not suggest that her symptoms were her way to avoid the stress. Following the same format, continue to tag other key symptoms. Tagging alerts the patient. It prepares her to consider that there may be a link between stress and somatic response. This is the key technique for Step 2, which paves the way for Steps 3 and 4 (confront and solve). Ask questions such as,

> When your problem started, what did you do immediately before the pain hit you?
> After what tasks do you seem to get sick?
> When was the last time you got sick?
> What preceded your pain?

Step 3: Confront. Attempt to juxtapose stressor and somatic response. The patient's reaction will give you a measure of the strength of her resistance to accept somatization as her way of managing stress. At this point, hostility can easily emerge in a patient who chronically somatizes, although it is usually short lived if you apply proper techniques.

When you encounter a patient with a host of medically unexplained symptoms, monitor your inner response toward her. Her anger and exaggerations may irritate you. If you brush her off or act irritated, you will compound the interviewing difficulties. If you feel like rejecting her, realize that the patient does not have the freedom to agree with your view. Her symptoms have been part of her lifestyle since preadolescence, and your rejection threatens your rapport with her. By accepting her history of changing symptoms as the highlight of her emotional life, the patient will reward you with cooperation.

Step 4: Solve. Start with the diagnosis. Tell the patient that she has a somatoform disorder. Explain step by step that the disorder involves the autonomic nervous system and that she was most likely born with that condition. Introduce the concept that a somatoform disorder is aggravated by outside stress. Then, trace her tendency to somatize throughout her life history and explore which symptom was aggravated by what demand. At the end of Step 4, you and the patient should know what type of demands she is most sensitive to and has the most difficulties mastering.

Step 5: Approve. Now, use role reversal. Thank the patient for making the effort in the interview to explain her condition to you. Express empathy about how difficult it is to live with her degree of sensitivity to stress. Thus, you have responded to two complaints that most patients with somatization disorder voice:

> Doctors don't know what's wrong with me.

You certainly have shown her your expertise and that you do know what is wrong with her.

> Doctors don't care.

You have demonstrated that you do.

If validation of symptoms fails, the other methods discussed in Part I of this book may help (i.e., hypnosis and free association), especially in those patients who have a history of conversion or dissociative symptoms on top of somatization symptoms.

5. Interview: Validating Somatic Symptoms

Ms. W., a 30-year-old, obese, African-American woman with hair dyed red and styled to perfection, is hospitalized on the gynecological service because of severe abdominal pain and frequent vomiting. The patient refuses to leave her bed, although in the gynecologist's opinion, she is not severely physically disabled. She had asked for Empirin [aspirin] with codeine for abdominal pain. Unable to find any medical basis for her distress, the doctor requested psychiatric consultation to evaluate the patient for psychogenic pain and narcotic abuse.

The patient is lying in bed at 11:00 A.M., dressed in a colorful nightgown and wearing meticulously applied makeup. (I = interviewer; P = patient)

Step 1: Listen

1. I: Hi, Ms. W. My name is Dr. O. Dr. X. asked me to see you.
   P: Who are you? Dr. X. didn't tell me about you.
2. I: I'm a psychiatrist. . . .
   P: Wait a minute! I don't want to talk to no psychiatrist.
3. I: Let me explain. I'm here to. . . .
   P: [Interrupting] I don't want you here. There's nothing wrong with my head. I don't need a psychiatrist. My stomach hurts and I'm nauseated and I have to vomit. The nurses can tell you. It's not in my head. Do you hear me? There's nothing wrong with my head. I don't have to. . . .

Even though there was no medical reason for her to be in bed, the patient remained there at 11:00 A.M. This was a clue that she might be using the bed to legitimize her sick role. She switched to hostility (A. 3) the moment she assumed that this interviewer, too, considered her problems to be fake. The patient equated psychiatric problems with unreal, imagined problems and put up her preemptive defense against such an assumption. At this juncture, the interview was in danger of being broken off.

4. I: [Interrupting] That's awful . . . that's terrible. [Looks up to the ceiling, and shakes his head using a nonverbal attention getter]

   P: [Startled; taking a breath] What's awful?

5. I: It's awful that people think the problem is all in your head.

   P: That's right. That's why I don't need you to tell me the same thing.

6. I: [Shakes his head in disbelief] Really? People think it's in your head? Who says such nonsense?

   P: My husband does for one. And my sister-in-law thinks I'm making it all up, that I'm pretending to get out of work.

7. I: They don't take you seriously? Your own family? It must be tough to listen to that when you feel bad and when you're hurting. You must feel a real letdown.

   P: [Starts crying] I really do. They laugh at me. But then they listen when my doctor tells me I need surgery again. I guess that's the only time they feel sorry about what they have done to me.

8. I: So they think it's in your head? Hasn't anybody figured out what's really going on with you? What kind of disorder you have?

   P: [Shakes her head] No. Nobody can find anything. I don't have an ulcer, and there's no tumor in my stomach. But something must be wrong because I vomit all the time.

9. I: So they really haven't figured out what causes your vomiting and your stomach cramps?

   P: No, they haven't.

10. I: That's why Dr. X. asked me to figure out what disorder you have. I believe if you are that sick you must have a real disorder.

    P: [With an arrogant tone] How would you know? You're a psychologist. You wouldn't know about the stomach.

11. I: Well, there are real disorders that can cause you to have stomach pain and vomiting without a tumor or an ulcer. You may be sicker than you think.

    P: Oh? Is that so? Nobody told me about that.

12. I: Let me tell you about it! [Takes one step closer to her bed, pulls up a chair to the bedside, and sits down] Psychologists and psychiatrists know about those disorders. And I'm a psychiatrist. I also studied medicine before I went into psychiatry.

    P: And you think I have a real disorder?

13. I: You are sick. You are not feeling well. We should try to find out what causes that.

P: [Frowning] How do you do that?

14. I: First, by talking to you.

P: [Disappointed] Just talking?

15. I: [Putting his hand on hers] And then we also may have to run a few tests to see what else is going on . . . we may also have to stick you with a needle to get some blood.

P: [Emphatically] Oh, that's all right; I'm used to tests. So what do you want to know?

16. I: Dr. X. has told me about all the pain you feel. He told me that not even pain medication gives you relief. You must have gone through a lot. [Presses her hand]

P: That's right. I have awful pains all the time, and then all that vomiting.

17. I: Can you tell me more about the pain?

P: Well, I have it right down here. [Patient points to the pubic area.] It's always hurting. I'm in so much pain. I'm really depressed about it. [Her eyes start tearing up.] My doctor called it urinary incontinence.

18. I: Tell me more about it.

P: Whenever I sneeze, some urine drips out. Isn't that terrible? [Tears start rolling] They ran some tests, but they can't seem to find anything.

19. I: So what do they want to do?

P: Well, they want to do some surgery. They want to lift my bladder and fix it that way. [Smiling]

20. I: Hmmm. Have you had surgery before?

P: Oh, yes, many times. I have spent many months in hospitals. It seems like I've been in hospitals all my life! [Shrugs her shoulders and smiles]

21. I: What other surgery did you have?

P: Last year my gall bladder was operated on; but I had many operations before that.

22. I: What kind of surgery?

P: Oh, I have always had problems. Also, I was pregnant five times, but I had two miscarriages.

23. I: So you have three living children?

P: No, just two. The other one died when she was a few days old, but now I don't have to worry about pregnancy anymore since my hysterectomy.

24. I: I'm sorry to hear about your child. [Pause] Can you remember the dates when you had surgery?

P: Oh, it was some time ago. I can't really remember when all that was and how it came about. [Sits up in bed, bends over, and presses her hands against her stomach] And I'm feeling nauseated now—I feel I have to vomit. Can you come back another time, when I feel better?

25. I: Oh, I'm sorry that you feel so bad. Let's take a little rest.

P: That's okay. We can keep going.

26. I: I'm impressed. Even though you feel so bad, you take good care of your makeup.

P: It's important to me not to show how bad I really feel.

27. I: Do you have an upset stomach now?

P: No, I guess I'm just upset.

28. I: Do you run a temperature?
    P: I don't think so. I feel fine.
29. I: Do you have any flu symptoms or diarrhea?
    P: No, I'm just upset.
30. I: You mentioned your hysterectomy. How did that come about?
    P: I had all that terrible pain. So they figured there must be something wrong. One doctor examined me and he found a real big lump down there. [Points to abdominal area] And then another doctor examined me and he could not find anything. Then they both examined me and all of a sudden the lump was gone. They did surgery because they thought they might have missed something. They thought it must have been a cyst that burst. So they took out one of my ovaries.
31. I: Was that when you had your hysterectomy?
    P: Oh no, that was the time before that.
32. I: When did they do surgery on your uterus?
    P: That was later.
33. I: What was the problem then?
    P: My uterus was four times as big as normal. It must have been the flu. And there was fluid in it.
34. I: Did the hysterectomy stop the pain that you had down there?
    P: Oh no, I was on pain pills for months.
35. I: Are you still on pain pills now?
    P: Yes, but I was off them for 2 months.
36. I: Hmmm, so you were off? How did you get off them?
    P: When I had all that pain, a lot of doctors examined me and one of them finally figured it out. He found a tumor and took it out. It had something to do with the scar tissue. It was affixed to my abdominal wall.
37. I: But now you have pain again?
    P: Yes, about 2 months after they removed the tumor, it acted up again. And now they think the bladder is sinking.
38. I: Do you have most of your pain in your abdomen?
    P: Yes, it's all down here.

Given their lifelong experience with medically unexplained, somatic symptoms, chronic somatizers (Goldberg and Bridges 1988) expect to be rejected, although they still hope to find acceptance. Therefore, in this case, the interviewer fed into the patient's hopes. Even though Ms. W. began by being hostile, the interviewer did not retaliate by becoming antagonistic himself. He removed himself as the target of her anger and joined her as an ally. He let her know, feel, and hear that he looked at her disorder from a somatic point of view (Q. 5–7). He expressed empathy for her problems (Q. 4–7) and showed interest in her history of changing symptoms (Q. 8–10).

He overcame her skepticism (Q. 10) and established his expertise by telling her that she had a real disorder (Q. 11–13). By putting his hand on hers, he gave her the impression of a somatic "hands on" process, underscored with the announcement of blood tests (Q. 15, 16).

When the interviewer tried to direct the patient to supply a specific history of her surgeries (Q. 20–22, 24), she gave a demonstration of somatizing to avoid this boring task (A. 24). In response, the interviewer backed off and complimented her on her makeup (Q. 25, 26). This positive feedback saved the rapport (Q. 27–38).

Ms. W.'s speech was fluent, verbose, and dramatic and showed exaggerations and vagueness with poor reference to time (A. 16, 20). Her affect was labile (A. 18, 19). She endorsed the following list of unconnected somatic problems: stomach pain (A. 3), nausea (A. 3, 24), vomiting (A. 3, 8, 16, 24) without abdominal infection (Q. 28, 29), abdominal pain (A. 38), pubic pain (A. 17, 34), urinary incontinence (A. 17, 18), fluid in uterus (A. 33), gallbladder surgery (A. 21), hysterectomy (A. 23), removal of an ovary (A. 30), surgery on scar tissue (A. 36), a bursting cyst (A. 30), two miscarriages (A. 22), and a sinking bladder (A. 37). The announced tests were to rule out thyroid disorder, endometriosis, and gallstones (Q. 15). Her vague and exaggerated description of her pain, her admission that physicians' physical findings were minimal, and her somatizing to avoid pressure would suggest a somatoform disorder.

Patients with somatization disorder usually come to the attention of an internist, general practitioner, surgeon, or gynecologist before they come to a psychiatrist, because they report mostly physical symptoms (Kirmayer and Robbins 1991). Patients with somatization who come first to a psychologist or psychiatrist usually seek help for affective and anxiety symptoms.

Step 2: Tag

39. I: When did your abdominal pain start this time?
P: It was there all the time.
40. I: But now you are in the hospital. What brought that about?
P: Oh, I had terrible fights with my husband. He just doesn't understand.
41. I: I'm sorry to hear that. Can you tell me more about it?
P: You see, I'm a nurse, but I stopped working because I just couldn't work being so sick.
42. I: And your husband could not understand that?
P: Well, he had no problem with that. But can you imagine? When I stopped working, he didn't want me to bring the kids to the baby-sitter anymore.
43. I: I see. . . .
P: That creep wanted me to take care of them all by myself. He said why should we pay for a sitter when I'm home anyway. [Biting her lower lip and becoming tearful]

44. I: So you had difficulties with that?
    P: [Turning her eyes up] Of course! You understand! [Nodding] You know I'm
        too sick to do that. [Shakes her head] Those little monsters get on my nerves.
        I got depressed and screamed and cried. Then my stomach acted up and
        I doubled over with pain. [Holds her stomach and bends over]
45. I: So it's because of the kids that you got into an argument with your husband?
    P: No, he put more pressure on me, that asshole.
46. I: Oh? What kind of pressure?
    P: Would you believe, he hollered at me?
47. I: About what?
    P: He said I'm a terrible housekeeper, that our place looks like a pigsty. He
        wanted me to be my own cleaning lady, that jerk. Do you believe that?
48. I: Oh?
    P: If I have to do that for that slave driver, I might as well keep on working.
        The job wouldn't be any worse than housekeeping.
49. I: So what happened? Take your time. Tell me how it really felt!
    P: My stomach got worse. It felt like a big knot that kept twisting and turning.
        I felt the pain right through my back as if it was shooting into my buttocks.
        I got diarrhea. I got nauseated and started vomiting as if the knot wanted to
        come out. I turned inside out.

By expressing empathy (Q. 41, 42, 49), the interviewer motivated the
patient to complain about her husband's demands and her ensuing physical
symptoms. Thus, he established a temporal connection between an outside
stressor (i.e., the marital discord [A. 40]) and the abdominal pain. By using
continuation techniques (Q. 41, 43, 44, 48, 49), he let the patient tell him
what events had preceded the onset of the severest symptom (Q. 39–41). He
assessed the chronology and not causality of the symptoms in order not to
annoy the patient or risk her falling back on her conviction that the
interviewer thought her pain and dysfunction were psychological and
therefore not real. Without overtly relating the fights to the patient's pain,
the interviewer tagged the fact that an increase in marital pressures brought
an increase in pain (Q. 42–49). Insistence on cause and effect could have
broken off the interview.

The patient displayed more dramatic (A. 41–43, 49) and labile affect,
changing from one extreme to another. She vented her anger about her
husband's demands on her (A. 42–47). She showed dependency by trying
to ensure the interviewer's approval (A. 44, 47). Her somatic stress response
(i.e., her seeking hospitalization) appeared on the spur of the moment
(A. 40). An upsetting demand affected her totally—she responded with
volatile emotion, crying, a display of devastating somatic symptoms, and
depression. She progressed from emotional to physical symptoms of abdominal pain (A. 44).

Step 3: Confront

50. I: So, when your husband asked you to take care of the kids, your stomach pain got worse?

    P: [Angry] I didn't say that. I'm sick, you understand? I'm sick to begin with! Why can't even you understand that? You make me really upset. [Pressing her fists into her stomach area]

51. I: But your pain did get worse! You're even hurting now.

    P: You make it sound as if I made it all up as an excuse. [Starts crying] You make my stomach feel worse.

52. I: No, I don't mean to do that. You just seem to be sensitive to the stress that you are going through, especially with your husband.

    P: [Stops crying] Yes, he's something else, isn't he?

53. I: Yes, he doesn't seem to help your stomach pain and your vomiting any.

    P: [With a firm voice and staring at the interviewer] He certainly doesn't.

54. I: You see, that's what I'm concerned with—how his criticizing you worsens your problems.

    P: [With a softening voice] But I'm sick to begin with. I'm not making it up. I really have pain.

When the interviewer confronted the patient with the relationship between her demanding husband and her increasing pain, their rapport became strained (A. 50). When the interviewer pointed out that the patient's pain increased in response to this confrontation (Q. 51), she rebuffed him. This denial made her appear naive and illogical and raised the question of whether she had a lower-than-average IQ. Her insight was poor. Her denial of the relationship between stress and pain demonstrated the psychological blindness that is characteristic of patients who somatize. Only after the interviewer deflected her anger (Q. 52) and joined her as an ally (Q. 53, 54) did her anger—and with it, her voice—soften. She still insisted that she had real pain (A. 54).

Step 4: Solve

55. I: I think you have a disorder that is called somatization disorder. Many doctors don't really know about it.

    P: Hmmm . . . You know, you're the first one who says there's really something wrong with me. All the other people think there is something wrong with my head. [Puts her head into her hands and shakes it] They say that stuff even when they know that I need surgery all the time. Isn't that something?

56. I: [Nods his head] And surgery doesn't even help you, right?

    P: [Suspiciously] What do you mean by that?

57. I: Well, your pain is still there after the surgery, isn't it? Think about your belly pain! You had surgery for it and the pain is still there.

P: [Nodding her head] It sure is. [Pulling up her nightgown] Look! I have all these scars here. I'm still hurting underneath them. [Points to her abdomen] All that hurting that I went through.

58. I: You see? That pain . . . that comes from somatization disorder. People are usually born with that disorder.

P: Oh? Yeah? Really? Wow! That's why I have all that nausea and hurting and vomiting. Now you told me what it is. Nobody has told me that before. Isn't that something?

59. I: You see, people with somatization disorder get pain and nausea when they have to do too much. Other people can straighten things out but you get sick instead.

P: How's that? I don't understand what you're saying.

60. I: Well, you get upset and depressed when things are getting too much. But you also get upset with your whole body. Your whole body gets upset and acts up. You speak up with your body. Because you can't say no, your body says no. It's just too much. Your body tells other people: "It's enough. I can't take it anymore."

P: Is that so? That's right. I can't talk to my husband. I'm scared he'll walk away if I tell him I can't do it. I try and try to do everything, but I just wear myself out.

61. I: It sounds as if you really have a kind of somatization disorder. Let me find out more about it. May we start at the beginning, if that's all right with you?

P: You think I can do it? I can give it a try. But I'm still hurting. I'll try to do it anyway.

62. I: Well, if it is too much let me know and we can take a little break. I'm anxious to know how it was when you had your first menstrual period.

P: Oh, that was a long time ago. I must have been 11 or 12. I didn't know what struck me. Nobody had ever told me, you know. All of a sudden there was all that blood in my panties. I really got scared. I didn't even know where it was coming from.

63. I: Did you talk to anybody about it?

P: I was so scared. So I told my mother. My mother gave me something to use.

64. I: Didn't she tell you what was going on?

P: Are you kidding? [Mocking] My mom? She never told me anything. [Rolls her eyes upward, and shakes her head] She never cared about what happened to me. [Shrugs both shoulders] I don't think she really cared.

65. I: Did you have regular periods after that?

P: Regular periods? Are you kidding me? They came for a few months and then they stopped and then they came back and they stopped again. And I finally told my mother. And you know what she asked me? She asked me if I was pregnant?

66. I: Were you?

P: No! What nonsense! I hadn't had any sex. I didn't even know what that was. Nobody had told me about sex.

67. I: Were your periods the same all the time?

P: You mean were they heavy sometimes? Yeah, they were real heavy. Other times . . . no, not at all; I only used two pads a day. There wasn't anything normal with me.

68. I: How did you feel then?
    P: Oh, I had terrible pains. I had cramps and back pains and headaches and I didn't know what to do. Sometimes I put my legs up on a wall because I was told that would help. And I was screaming with pain.
69. I: It really hit you hard! Did you ever go to a doctor?
    P: Oh yes, when I was still in high school, I had my first D & C [dilatation and curettage], but they didn't find anything and I still had that hurting and that cramping and that stabbing back pain. [Touches her abdomen, then her back, and moans]
70. I: Did you have some more D & Cs later on?
    P: I went through a lot. I had D & Cs and I had my two miscarriages after that and then I had some bleeding in between.
71. I: What did all that do to your sex life?
    P: Well, I wasn't interested anymore. When I got my hysterectomy I didn't care for that anymore. I just wanted to be left alone. I can do without it.
72. I: What about sex before the hysterectomy?
    P: It always hurt. I always had pain with it. I didn't care for sex.
73. I: You said one of your children died.
    P: Yeah. All of a sudden she just lay dead in her crib.
74. I: I'm sorry to hear that. How did you feel during those pregnancies?
    P: Oh, I was really, really happy. Those were the best times in my whole life, you know. [Smiling and beaming] For that time I didn't have any periods. And I didn't have the pain.
75. I: Really? Did you have any morning sickness?
    P: Oh, just for 2 or 3 months. But I felt really good, you know. I wish I would feel that good again. But it all stopped when I got out of the hospital. I couldn't walk. I was paralyzed. My legs just wouldn't move. They were stiff in the knee. They even had me see a nerve doctor. But he said that I didn't need any treatment. It would go away. I just needed a little bit of rest. I used crutches but then I got tired of them. And I guess my strength came back.
76. I: So you were really paralyzed. That's important to know. [Patient nods] Now back to the vomiting—did you have problems with vomiting any other time?
    P: Just now. Over the last few months. I vomit all the time. And the doctors can't tell me why I do that. [Looks sad and depressed]
77. I: Do you have any shortness of breath now?
    P: I haven't thought about it. But I don't remember. You know when you hurt that much, it seems that about everything is wrong.
78. I: Did you have this problem at any other time?
    P: Maybe when I go upstairs too fast.
79. I: Did you ever have the feeling of having a lump in your throat?
    P: Oh, I don't know . . . wait, yes, when I was young . . . whenever I was excited I had a hard time swallowing.
80. I: Besides pain, have you ever had any burning sensations in your mouth or vagina?
    P: Oh yes, I have a lot of that.
81. I: Did you go to a doctor?

P: Yes, I thought I had an infection. They took a culture but they said there was nothing wrong.

82. I: You seem to have had quite some experience with surgeons.

P: Oh yes. I've had surgery all the time. I can't even remember when I did and what was wrong. There is always so much going on. You know, my husband made me a list with all the surgeries on it. It's over there in my bag. You can take it and make yourself a copy. Oh no, I think it's over here. [Pulls a piece of paper from her nightstand drawer and gives it to the interviewer]

83. I: Okay. How was your health before all this surgery started?

P: I've never been healthy. I've always been sickly. When I was 7 years old, I had already had rheumatic heart disease. I had that special kind, the one that doesn't go in your heart. But they didn't find anything but I still always have pains in my knee joints.

84. I: Did you get any swelling in them?

P: I thought so but the doctor said no.

85. I: Did he take any X rays?

P: Yes, but he said he couldn't find anything. All he said was I should lose some weight.

86. I: Did he do blood tests?

P: How do I know what he draws all that blood for? But it doesn't make any difference. They never find anything anyway. [Grimaces]

87. I: Who told you that you have rheumatic disease?

P: My mom said that's what it was. You know, I think she has more common sense than all these doctors. Maybe she should have been a doctor.

88. I: What about headaches?

P: I never had problems with my head. It was all down here. [Pointing at her abdomen] But I had a lot of headaches when I had to take all that medication during my pregnancies. They didn't want to give me any but I felt so bad I took some from my mom and from my sister. They said it could hurt the baby. But when I had to vomit every day until the baby was born, what could I do? You know all that vomiting made my head hurt.

89. I: Ever have any problems with your thyroid?

P: Yes, for 2 or 3 years I took thyroid medication.

90. I: When was that?

P: That must have been before I had my stomach stapled to control my weight.

91. I: What was wrong with your thyroid?

P: I don't know. I couldn't tell you. The doctor gave the thyroid pills to me. He said my thyroid wasn't working right because I gained so much weight.

92. I: You saw a doctor for your weight?

P: No, I had gone in for the problem with my swallowing. I guess that was it. I couldn't swallow and then I had to vomit. I think it was also for my throbbing headaches and he started talking about my weight.

93. I: You went through a lot. I wonder whether you ever had periods of memory blanks, where you did not know what had happened?

P: I'm a scatterbrain, all right, but I was never that forgetful, I don't think.

94. I: Let's find out about your scatterbrain. Can you multiply 2 × 24 for me?

P: Oh, I was always poor in math.

95. I: I'm sure you know what 2 × 24 is.
    P: Isn't it 48?
96. I: Okay. Now, can you multiply 2 × 48?
    P: Oh no, I just did one. I need paper and pencil to do that.
97. I: Well, I'm sure you can do this one also.
    P: What did you say I should do?
98. I: Tell me what 2 × 48 is.
    P: [Writing numbers with her finger on the bedcover, keeps looking at the covers] Isn't it 86?
99. I: Well, try again.
    P: [Raises her eyebrows, blinks, looks at the bedcover again] I'm sorry, what was it?
100. I: 2 × 48.
    P: [Works on the bedcover some more] Oh, that's 96. And what did I say before?
101. I: You said 86.
    P: Oh, I see what I did. But I'm really getting tired.
102. I: Just relax. We are through with the math. All that's left is to check your memory. You said you had problems with it. I want you to remember four words that I'm going to tell you: tulip, eyedropper, yellow, and honesty. Can you repeat that?
    P: I can try. Tulip, eyedrop, yellow and . . . what was the last thing?
103. I: Was it justice, honesty, or equality?
    P: Oh, it was honesty.
104. I: Well, keep these four words in mind. I will come back to them later on.
    P: I don't know whether I can keep that much in my mind. I don't feel good.

The interviewer strove to become an expert ally who told the patient that he understood her condition. Therefore, he educated her about her disorder and validated her symptoms. He explained to her that a patient with somatization disorder responds globally to stress with emotional and physical pain (A. 59, 60) and communicates the stress to others by complaining about pain rather than being assertive. She then understood that she experienced negative emotions in terms of somatic symptoms (A. 60). The interviewer validated her complaints by giving her condition its proper name (A. 55, 59), which made the illness "real." He stayed on a descriptive level—that is, he did not interpret her somatic symptoms as having a merely symbolic meaning, nor did he suggest that they serve as an attempt to resolve her conflicts. The patient accepted the diagnosis like a present that nobody had offered her before. This deepened the rapport.

Next, the interviewer was able to take a history with a cooperative patient (A. 62–93). She tolerated his abrupt transitions (which saved the interviewer time) as he attempted to assess unrelated symptoms specific for somatization disorder.

As to mental status, some of the patient's statements contradicted each other (A. 64 versus A. 87, A. 74 versus A. 88, A. 79 versus A. 92, A. 88 versus A. 92). She admitted that her pregnancies were the only time when she enjoyed herself (A. 58, 59), yet later she stated that she vomited all the time during them (A. 88). Her thought associations were generated by feelings rather than logic (A. 91, 92). Her answers appeared vague and circumstantial (A. 62, 77, 82, 86). She underlined her speech with gestures and intense facial expressions when she talked about the neglect by her mother (A. 64). Her affect changed dramatically in accordance with the content of her speech, which gave the impression of lability (A. 64 versus A. 74). She was oriented but described herself sometimes as confused. Her insight and judgment were poor. She could multiply 2 × 48, but with some difficulty, which showed that her intelligence was at least borderline. Her immediate recall seemed to be disrupted by poor concentration, as was her multiplication.

In Step 4, the interviewer was able to take the patient's history and overcome the challenges posed by this type of patient and make a diagnosis. The key question concerns the presence or absence of a psychiatric or a medical disorder other than the somatization disorder.

To make the diagnosis of somatization disorder, it is recommended in DSM-IV that four specific patterns of complaints be assessed, each of which Ms. W. met:

- A history of pain in at least four different sites or functions—the patient endorsed stomach, menstrual, head, and joint pains and pain during intercourse.
- A history of at least two gastrointestinal symptoms other than pain—the patient endorsed vomiting and the feeling of a lump in her throat.
- A history of at least one sexual or reproductive symptom other than pain—the patient endorsed having had a hysterectomy and the feeling of not caring for sex.
- A history of at least one symptom or deficit suggesting a neurological condition not limited to pain—the patient endorsed paralysis (A. 75).

Given the patient's vagueness and circumstantiality, such a review may be a formidable task. The Seven-Symptom Screening Test (Othmer and Desouza 1985) for somatization disorder can help. These seven symptoms are

- Shortness of breath
- Dysmenorrhea

- Burning in mouth or sex organ
- Lump in throat
- Amnesia
- Vomiting
- Pain in the extremities

If a patient endorses three of the seven symptoms, suspect somatization disorder. If you suspect somatization disorder, you should establish that the symptoms

- Started before age 30 years
- Interfered in some way with the patient's life
- Were medically unexplained

Ms. W. endorsed all seven symptoms: dysmenorrhea (A. 68), vomiting (A. 76), shortness of breath (A. 77, 78), lump in throat (A. 79), burning in sex organs (A. 80), pain in joints and extremities (A. 83), and memory blanks (A. 93).

Step 5: Approve

105. I: I have to thank you for helping me understand your problems, even though you didn't feel too well.
     P: Oh, that's fine. You really seem to care and understand what I'm going through.
106. I: Well, I try to understand your point of view. You are so sensitive to pressure, and your body starts hurting when you have pressure. This is important to know.
     P: But nobody understands. They don't believe me when I hurt.
107. I: It's important that you understand, because that may help you to handle stress better in the future.
     P: Will that make my pain go away?
108. I: No, I think your body will always respond with pain, but if you recognize stress better, you can handle it better. You will get some control. And you can avoid surgery.
     P: But my husband won't understand that. He only believes me if a surgeon finds something wrong and operates on me.
109. I: I think we can make your husband understand what your condition is like without going for more surgery. When you are under pressure, your body responds with real pain. In this interview we have both come to understand this. And we will help your husband understand it too.
         Remember, I asked you to keep four words in mind. Do you still recall which ones they were?

P: Well, one was tulip, and one was yellow. I don't remember the other two.

110. I: Just try!

P: [Wrinkles her forehead] Eyedrop, . . . yeah, that's what it was. But the other one I don't remember. It was kind of a weird word.

111. I: Well try.

P: [Shaking her head] It's gone.

112. I: Well, let me give you a choice of three words again. Maybe you can pick the right one: justice, honesty, or wisdom.

P: Hmmm, honesty! Wasn't it honesty?

113. I: Yes, that one is more difficult for you to remember. But you did real well. Even with all that pain and being nauseated you spent a whole hour with me. I will tell your doctor what we talked about and what we discovered.

P: You really listened to me. You made me feel better.

The technique that worked here was role reversal. The interviewer thanked the patient rather than waiting for the patient to thank him. He told her that she helped him understand her condition. He made the patient feel good about the interview by

- Repeating several times that he believed her pain and problems were real (Q. 105–109).
- Summarizing how both he and she understood what types of pressure brought on or worsened her symptoms—knowledge that would help in therapy.
- Attempting to tell her that her pain would get worse if she did not negotiate her needs with others. He assured her that such a negotiation could improve her relationships (Q. 107, 108). At the same time, he told her that her understanding her illness might not resolve her symptoms, that she might remain a sensitive person who responded in a special way to people and circumstances. He ended by emphasizing his professional role.

This technique provided closure to the patient's two main complaints about health professionals: 1) that they did not understand her, and 2) that they did not know what was wrong with her.

Diagnosis

Axis I. Somatization disorder.

6. Somatization and Validation of Somatic Symptoms in Psychiatric Disorders

Seven somatoform disorders are listed in DSM-IV (Table 4–1). These somatoform disorders can only be considered if a general medical condition or the direct effect of a substance cannot fully explain the symptoms. The common feature of somatoform disorders is that patients report physical symptoms suggestive but not truly attributable to a chronic or acute somatic ailment. Significant impairment in social or occupational functioning with marked distress must occur to warrant the diagnosis.

Patients who complain about physical symptoms that cannot be verified by organic findings often experience rejection by family and physicians. Such patients often express the feeling that they are not taken seriously. Validation takes the patient's problems at face value and accepts that a symptom is a subjective report and, therefore, has clinical significance in itself, regardless of whether it is explained by psychological trauma or by a general medical condition. The overall approach is to recognize that the patient is experiencing pain and that she expresses her pain not directly but indirectly by somatic symptoms. In our culture, somatic symptoms are indeed an acceptable way to express dysfunction and pain. Therefore, it is recommended that you not reject the patient's pain by proving to her that there is no basis for her symptoms. The basis for the patient's somatic symptoms is her sense of subjective pain and impairment and not a subjective marker of a general medical condition. By validating the patient's somatic complaints you are not validating the presence of a somatic disorder but the patient's pain and its legitimate expression by somatic pain. It is inappropriate to prove to the patient that you are too smart to be fooled. As interviewer, you should not feel as though you are in a competition where you pitch your medical knowledge against the patient's imitation of a general medical condition. On the contrary, you are responding to the patient's distress with professional empathy. This is a universal principle in handling patients. Thus, the patient's somatic pain should invite you to search for the source of her complaints. Even the malingerers—usually— will have a functional impairment that prompts them to pretend. Therefore, your task is not to stop at proving malingering, but to identify the possible despair that makes the patient malinger.

This position raises the question of whether J.-M. Charcot was medically and politically correct when he stated, "This brings me to say a few words about malingering. It is found in every phase of hysteria and one is surprised at times to admire the ruse, the sagacity, and the unyielding tenacity that

Table 4–1. Characteristics of DSM-IV somatoform disorders

Disorder	Claim	Subjective evidence	Differential diagnosis
Somatization disorder	To be medically ill	Multiple pains and autonomic symptoms	Other somatoform disorders, major depression, anxiety
Undifferentiated, somatoform disorder	To have an acute physical illness	Acute onset of multiple physical symptoms of more than 6 months' duration	Somatization, conversion, pain disorder
Conversion disorder	To have an acute neurological illness	Sudden dramatic "neurological" deficit symptoms	Dissociative disorder, neurological disorders, especially multiple sclerosis and acute, intermittent porphyria
Pain disorder	To have an acute or chronic disease	Localized nonremitting pain in one or more organs	Conversion, somatization disorder
Hypochondriasis	To have a serious disease	Inability to find an explanation for "sense of being seriously ill"	Delusional, mood, obsessive-compulsive disorder
Body dysmorphic disorder	To have a chronic physical defect	Awareness of unaccepted, chronic, physical features	Delusional disorder
Somatoform disorder not otherwise specified	To experience onset of a physical illness	Onset of some somatic symptoms of less than 6 months' duration, such as being sick or fatigued; pseudocyesis	Somatization or pain disorder, hypochondriasis

especially the women, who are under the influence of a severe neurosis, display in order to deceive . . . especially when the victim of the deceit happens to be a physician" (as quoted in Guillain 1959, p. 138).

The interviewing techniques discussed in Part I were applied to Axis I nonpsychotic disorders that rarely show psychotic features. These nonpsychotic disorders were referred to as "neurotic" disorders in DSM (American Psychiatric Association 1952) and DSM-II (American Psychiatric Association 1968). In Part II, "Psychotic Communication," we introduce techniques for difficult patients with psychotic disorders.

PART II

PSYCHOTIC COMMUNICATION

PSYCHOTIC COMMUNICATION

Psychosis or psychotic-like symptoms, as defined in DSM-IV (American Psychiatric Association 1994), occur in a wide variety of Axis I psychiatric disorders. These include the cognitive disorders, schizophrenia and other psychotic disorders, mood disorders, some anxiety disorders, and somatoform disorders. Even though not mentioned in DSM-IV, psychosis is suggested in factitious disorder, in which it is feigned, and in dissociative disorders (especially in dissociative identity disorder), in which it appears to be mimicked. Such widespread occurrence of psychotic, pseudopsychotic, and feigned psychotic symptoms poses a special challenge to you.

According to DSM-IV, a psychotic disorder manifests itself in four cardinal symptoms or signs (compare schizophrenia and other psychotic disorders), of which at least one should be present to make the diagnosis:

- Delusions
- Hallucinations
- Disorganized speech (frequent derailment or incoherence)
- Catatonic or grossly disorganized behavior

In addition, psychosis may show one or more of the following three signs (which, however, are not required in DSM-IV for the diagnosis of psychosis or of psychotic features):

- Lack of insight
- Disturbed affect
- Irrational actions

In DSM-IV, psychosis is on center stage in one group of disorders and plays only an intermediate or peripheral role in other groups. In the group of Axis I disorders called "schizophrenia and other psychotic disorders," psychosis is a necessary but not sufficient component. This group includes

- Schizophrenia, with its types of paranoid, disorganized, catatonic, undifferentiated, and residual
- Schizophreniform disorder
- Schizoaffective disorder
- Delusional disorder
- Brief psychotic disorder
- Shared psychotic disorder (folie à deux)
- Psychotic disorder due to a general medical condition, with delusions or hallucinations
- Substance-induced psychotic disorder
- Psychotic disorder not otherwise specified

Following the DSM-IV concept of psychosis, schizophrenia and other psychotic disorders may be on the incline. First, psychotic disorders due to a general medical condition may become a rapidly growing group because of the population's increasing longevity. Second, psychoses induced by substances such as alcohol, amphetamines, cannabis, cocaine, hallucinogens, inhalants, opioids, phencyclidine, sedative-hypnotics, and anxiolytics may increase in proportion to the increase of substance use. We expect this increase even though the above-mentioned general medical conditions and substances produce a psychosis only part of the time. Third, a portion of the cognitive disorders are also associated with hallucinations and delusions. Because cognitive disorders are age related, increased longevity of the general population will lead to an increase of psychotic symptoms too.

The interviewer faces special differential diagnostic problems when he encounters psychotic symptoms that are substance induced or due to a general medical condition. If the impact of the substance or of the general medical condition is severe enough to cause the psychotic symptoms, it is usually also severe enough to cause the symptoms and signs of a delirium, a dementia, or an amnestic state. Therefore, the interviewer has to assess cognitive functioning carefully to make an accurate differential diagnosis between a cognitive disorder with delusions and/or hallucinations (see Part III, "Cognitive Impairment") that is due to use of a substance or a medical condition and a psychotic disorder due to use of a substance or a medical condition without cognitive impairment.

In mood disorders, psychotic symptoms play an intermediate role. They indicate severity. If a major depressive disorder or bipolar disorder is determined to be severe with psychotic features, it is coded in the fifth digit as a "4"; the psychotic nature is then further specified as being mood congruent or mood incongruent. The clinical significance of this distinction does not seem to be fully explored at this time. The specifiers "with psychotic features" and "with catatonic features" are also used to describe the current or most recent episode of a mood disorder.

Apparent psychotic symptoms play a more peripheral role in one of the anxiety disorders—posttraumatic stress disorder—and in some somatoform disorders. In posttraumatic stress disorder, criterion B states in part: "The traumatic event is persistently reexperienced in one (or more) of the following ways: . . . (3) acting or feeling as if the traumatic event were recurring (includes a sense of reliving the experience, illusions, hallucinations, and dissociative flashback episodes, including those that occur on awakening or when intoxicated)" (p. 428).

Psychotic-like symptoms may occur in some somatoform disorders. For example, patients with conversion disorder may report hallucinations even though the DSM-IV criteria for conversion disorder do not explicitly mention hallucinations as a symptom. In such instances, reality testing is usually preserved—that is, the patient knows that the hallucination is a misperception. Criterion A for hypochondriasis states that the patient has "preoccupation with fears of having, or the idea that one has, a serious disease based on the person's misinterpretation of bodily symptoms." Criterion B states that "the preoccupation persists despite appropriate medical evaluation and reassurance." These two criteria seem to indicate that the preoccupation with a serious disease is both fixed and false, which is the definition of a delusion. However, Criterion C qualifies these criteria, in that "the belief in Criterion A is not of delusional intensity. . . . " (p. 465). In DSM-IV, a similar approach is taken toward body dysmorphic disorder, in which the key symptom is a preoccupation with an imagined defect in appearance that causes clinically significant distress or impairment in social, occupational, or other important areas of functioning. However, if the physical preoccupation is held with a delusional intensity, an additional diagnosis of delusional disorder, somatic type, is made.

Here is the challenge for the interviewer—symptom by symptom in the order of increasing difficulty:

- *Hallucinations* can interfere with your interview because voices may tell the patient not to talk to you. Once you suspect such a command hallucination in your patient, you can directly ask her about it and she usually admits it.

- *Disorganized speech* may make your interview impossible. However, after you have identified the patient's speech as psychotic—and not caused by an aphasia as a result of a neurological disorder—you may conduct a limited mental status examination, obtain a history from outside sources, and initiate treatment before continuing with your interview.

- *Delusions with or without hallucinations* can become a challenge if the patient acts on these delusions, has no insight, and even includes you in his delusions, especially if they are persecutory in nature. Although European psychiatric textbooks have held that actions taken on delusions are infrequent (Anderson and Trethowan 1973; Bleuler 1916; Fish 1967; Jaspers 1963; Merskey 1980; Slater and Roth 1969; also, compare Wessely et al. 1993), in a recent empirical study, Wessely et al. (1993) reported that 50% of subjects with delusions act on them, according to outside informants. This increased to over 80% if actions reported by the patients were counted. Furthermore, Wessely et al. found that roughly 70% of delusional patients had taken aggressive actions toward themselves or others, and 10% had taken defensive actions. Only 20% claimed to have never taken any action. Obviously, such a patient acting on his delusions can be pretreated with a neuroleptic before the interview. If verbal methods fail, you have no choice but to tranquilize the patient, especially if he is physically dangerous. However, you can establish better rapport and avoid involuntary treatment if you are familiar with the principles of interviewing such a patient (discussed in Chapter 5, "Psychotic Acting Out").

- *Catatonic or bizarre movements* are frequently combined with a state of excitement or withdrawal. Often you have to sedate the excited, catatonic patient and then use the interviewing principles for psychotic acting out if she is delusional and hostile. Many times catatonic bizarre movements are followed by a state of motoric immobility, as evidenced by catalepsy, waxy flexibility, stupor, or extreme negativism, including muteness. By definition, such a patient does not respond to you. You need special preinterview interventions with amobarbital, lorazepam, stimulants, or neuroleptics to interview such a patient. The principle for such an interview is described in Chapter 6, "Catatonia."

Psychosis with these extreme presentations is easy to detect but difficult to overcome in the interview—the ultimate challenge for you.

CHAPTER 5

PSYCHOTIC ACTING OUT

Summary

In interviewing a patient who acts on her delusions and hallucinations, you must support her acceptable goals and means and diffuse the destructive ones. Help the patient to substitute her socially unacceptable behaviors (such as wanting to harm a family member) with acceptable ones, such as having a family conference. This guidance creates rapport and prepares the patient to accept medication treatment.

◆ ◆ ◆ ◆ ◆

Force has no place where there is need of skill.

Herodotus (c. 485–425 B.C.)

◆ ◆ ◆ ◆ ◆

155

1. What Is Psychotic Acting Out?

Psychosis is a mental state in which a person's reality testing is impaired. Your patient may reject your version of reality and see you as her worst enemy. However, most patients, even when controlled by lifelong delusions and hallucinations, do not act on them continuously. For example, a patient who believes she is Queen Victoria may—instead of calling in her servants—clean up after dinner, in observance of the routine of her psychiatric ward. If confronted with her "irrational" behavior, she may explain that she is here in disguise to check on her subjects. Such a patient can be easily interviewed because she does not act on her delusions and refuse to grant you an audience.

In contrast, the grandiose, acutely excited patient may act on her delusions and may pursue goals that are elusive, unrealistic, or destructive. She may take irrational actions harmful to others (18%) and self (14%) (as indicated by patients' self-report presented by Wessely et al. 1993). For example, a patient with persecutory delusions and hallucinations attacked her brother because he did not answer her when she sent him a message through extrasensory perception. You must both accept your patient's experience as her reality and try to persuade her to express herself in less harmful ways. She may quickly turn you into her foe, especially when you confront her with reality. She may not even wait for such a confrontation but launch a preemptive strike to scare you off because from the outset she assumes that you are an agent of her enemies. Her explosive, hostile, and defiant behavior prevents you from exploring any topic in depth because even harmless questions may infuriate her.

Thus, excitement and hostility jam your rapport with her, block standard interviewing techniques, inhibit mental status exploration and testing, and obstruct the pathway to diagnosing. Because the patient resists exploration and testing, you cannot assess which diagnostic criteria for which disorders she may meet. Therefore, major parts of the history remain unexplored.

2. Psychotic Acting Out in the Mental Status

Acting on delusions and hallucinations only occurs in a segment of patients who are psychotic. For example, in their study of a mixed sample of delusional patients—62% with schizophrenia, 9% with delusional psychosis, 26% with affective psychosis, and 3% with other psychoses—Buchanan et al. (1993) found that only 42% had acted on their delusions during the last month. Every single patient within the 42% who took action cited evidence that supported their delusion, whereas only 84% of the remaining 58% who did not take action cited such evidence (Buchanan et al. 1993). Of those who did take action, 57% actually searched for information that confirmed or refuted their delusions, whereas only 16% of those who did not take action did; in addition, 83% of those who took action stated they felt frightened by their delusions, versus 46% of those who did not take action.

Patients with delusions and hallucinations show three different profiles of actions: aggressive (73%), defensive (11%), and no action (16%). The proportions of these action profiles is, of course, affected by the mixture of diagnostic entities included in the base sample (Wessely et al. 1993).

Aggressive Action Profile

Patients who show an aggressive action profile may show one or more of any of the following behaviors: hit others (18%), claim that they need to protect themselves (25%), break things (19%), harm themselves (14%), or try to leave their living area (12%) (Wessely et al. 1993).

Clinical observation teaches us that patients who may take action during the interview, whether based on delusions or not, show two key signs: excitement and hostility.

Excitement.   The grandiose, excited patient is easily identified by *observation* (Othmer and Othmer 1994). All of her symbolic movements and gestures—reactive, grooming, facial, postural, and goal-directed movements—are increased. She may jump up, walk around in the office, or try to take the chart away from you and enter notes. Usually she can be engaged in *conversation* as long as you can follow her changing topics, push of speech, and flight of ideas.

Systematic *exploration* of her mental status is more cumbersome than conversation—she ignores your questions or gives erratic answers. She allows you to listen but not to question. If she comprehends your questions, she may still be too distracted to answer them. When you interrupt and redirect her, her anger may flair up. She tries to take control of the interview by attempting to interview you. She acts out her ideas and sees you as her audience.

The psychotic patient has no insight into being sick. Her uninhibited, blind acting-out behaviors make it difficult to identify her pain, empathize with it, and ally with her against the source of her problems. She rejects the patient role and may assume a bossy posture. She feels that she can fire you as the interviewer if you do not support her delusional goals. You become her foe when you oppose her opinions or restrict her activities.

She may reject *testing* or, if she agrees, may not complete the test but ridicule you with silly, playful, or irrelevant answers. She may skip to a more attractive topic and become intrusive, overbearing, and pushy.

Hostility. Outside *observation* links patients' delusional actions to delusions of persecution (Buchanan et al. 1993). However, patients themselves link their actions to delusions of catastrophe. This discrepancy between outside observation and self-observation may shed light onto the nature of persecutory delusion. Usually, the patient has no insight that his delusions are perceived as persecutory in nature. He feels much more threatened by a catastrophe to which he may respond with fearfulness. As an outside observer, however, you may notice the persecutory thought content and an affect that is often a blend of fear and hostility. Such a patient watches you continuously. His eyes become narrow, tracking you, staring you down, wanting to intimidate you. He is guarded, vigilant, and tense. He clenches both fists, opens and closes them rhythmically, grinding his teeth. His body may curl up, ready to attack you if you appear critical.

In *conversation,* he may discharge his anger and hostility in an unrestrained manner. His speech may become pressed, urgent with latency of response. He screens his words carefully so as not to give you any clues to use against him. Clearly, this patient does not trust you. Initially, he may hide his suspicion and hostility, feign cooperation, deny hallucinations and delusions, or lie to you. He sees empathy as trickery and accuses you of being intrusive, nosy, and abusive.

When you *explore* his problems, you encounter a minefield of sensitive topics. His hostility warns that you are invading sacred territory. It is difficult to explore the suicidal and homicidal potential of such a high-risk patient, who may act on his hostile delusions. If you point out to him his aggressive and self-defeating behavior, he may stiffen his resistance rather than feel understood. He may abruptly tell you that he has no problems or, if he feels you are coming too close, he may decide to mislead you. Often hostility is paired with suspicion or anxiety about being hurt. You cannot establish stable roles for the patient and you. He does not accept the role of one who is experiencing pain, nor of an adult afflicted with an illness, nor of the VIP who hired you as a consultant. You are neither expert, guide, authority, nor healer but a threat. His responses are unpredictable. He may alternate between fleeing the scene or attacking you—flight or fight.

Formal *testing* of cognitive functions becomes obstructed by his hostility. You may feel physically threatened and lose your composure. Frustrated, you may resort to administering a sedative or major tranquilizer rather than continuing with the interview.

Defensive Action Profile

The defensive action profile appears to fit only a minority of patients if you are faced mainly with schizophrenic patients, as was the case in Wessely and Buchanan's studies (Buchanan et al. 1993; Wessely et al. 1993). The proportion of defensive actions may increase if you are faced with bipolar or unipolar depressed patients. These patients report that they are trying to escape from, protect themselves from, or stop what they delusionally fear. In their self-reports, these patients do not link their actions to delusions of reference, delusional memories, religious delusions, delusional jealousy, grandiose delusions, delusions of guilt, or sexual or persecutory delusions, even though outside observers feel that it is these types of delusions that are motivating their actions (Buchanan et al. 1993; Wessely et al. 1993).

To facilitate understanding patients who act on delusions, we describe the transcendence from a nonpsychotic to a psychotic state.

> An engineer, transferred from a small town to a metropolitan area, feels uncomfortable in his new environment and rejected by his co-workers. He wonders why. He starts to ruminate about the fact that his unionized co-workers could have learned that 10 years earlier he accepted assignments outside of his job description. He also wonders whether he has annoyed somebody. Also, he worries whether that weakness of his—masturbating once at age 17 years at a construction site—has become known to his colleagues. He becomes anxious and excited. He hears his colleagues make remarks and hum songs about how nice it would be to be age 17 again. They even bring the kind of lumber to the job that he worked on when he accepted the assignment outside of his job description 10 years ago. Convinced that he has found the key to his rejection, he asks for meetings with his co-workers to resolve the issue. However, they do not admit that they reject him or know about his shortcomings. Before he can take any further action, his wife brings him to a psychiatrist.

This patient's progression from worries to delusions and hallucinations shows how psychotic symptoms can develop from guilt, concerns, or conflicts. The psychotic patient reverses his reference system. He replaces the external reality, previously shared with others, by his personal, internal reality that is accessible only by him. His fears and hopes become fixed convictions difficult to correct, even when faced with contradictory evidence. His thoughts may become loud, intrusive, and uncontrollable and take on the quality of actual voices. He projects this internal world of delusions and hallucinations into his environment and starts to react to these mirrors of his internal world as if they were reality.

This transcendence from an inter- or intrapersonal conflict to psychotic signs and actions seems to occur frequently in a patient with a psychosis other than schizophrenia. Our example is not meant to show that conflicts cause psychosis, but that the rudiments of a prepsychotic conflict can become the thought content of a psychosis if the patient is so predisposed. This conflict can be recovered, addressed, and solved.

3. Technique: Facilitate Realistic Actions and Diffuse Psychotic Ones

Patients who act on their delusions are more likely to change their delusional convictions than those who do not act on their delusions. In Buchanan et al.'s study (1993), 57% of those who took action modified their delusions when confronted with contradictory evidence, whereas only 20% of those who did not take action modified their delusions when faced with such evidence.

Clinical experience and neuroanatomical considerations elucidate the basis for this finding. In patients who take action, you can mainly modify the action and, to a lesser extent, the delusional thought content itself. If we accept that both verbal thoughts and delusional verbal thoughts originate in the vicinity of Wernicke's language center and its associated areas, we can understand Buchanan et al.'s (1993) findings. To make the delusion an action, it has to be transmitted to the frontal lobe. Thus, this transmission may occur from a disordered to a nondisordered area of the brain. Therefore, we can redirect the transmission to the frontal lobe but cannot modify the original delusion that was formed in the disordered supramarginal gyrus or its vicinity. Regardless of the correctness of this theoretical consideration, you can target your interviewing technique toward the patient's delusional action, as described below.

Often, the patient's goals of pathological action contain one aspect that the interviewer can support. Identifying this goal and facilitating realistic and diffusing destructive actions are the key techniques for interviewing the psychotic patient.

Support Socially Acceptable Goals

Get to know your patient's delusional system. Because the psychotic patient is firmly convinced of his internal reality, do not challenge it. Accept it and make it the basis of your communication with him. Explore his internal world and learn about his hallucinatory and delusional perceptions, conclusions, means, and goals.

Then, restate his delusional goal in broader and socially acceptable terms. For example, if the patient says,

> My mother lied to my employer. She told him that I stole more than $1,000 from his cash register over the last 3 months. I will get her for that lie.

restate this in a more socially acceptable form:

> You suspect that your mother betrayed you. You are angry about that. You don't know why she did it. And you want to get even with her.

Express your support for the part of the goal that is socially acceptable (e.g., in this example, the patient's need for justice). Let the patient verbalize the unacceptable part of his goal and discharge his anger. Listen to how he wants to push, strangle, or even hit his mother, and just feed back to him that you notice his anger and disappointment. The patient's verbalizations of his anger may become a substitute for any destructive actions because the patient perceives his delusional impressions and thoughts with a strong sense of reality, yet may act on them with a weaker sense of conviction.

Examine with the patient the premises of his goals. For example, in the above case, help the patient find out that the employer, and not the patient's mother, detected a theft from the cash register and that the employer merely informed the patient's mother about the theft. The delusional patient may still remain hateful toward his mother, but now he has a second target for his hatred—namely, the employer who accuses him wrongfully. The new information broadens the patient's field of attack: now he has to deal with the hatred for his mother and the employer, maybe even other employees, such as the cash register clerk or the bookkeeper. In this way, diffusion decreases the patient's hostility toward a single target.

Support Socially Acceptable Means of Action

Examine the appropriateness of the patient's means of action. Often the link between hallucinations and delusions and specific means of actions is weak.

This weak relationship is the target of our interviewing technique. Although it is difficult to change the content of a hallucination or delusion by verbal arguments, it is possible to persuade a patient to give up one course of action in lieu of another by introducing new information. Thus, you can deflect the destructive actions by offering an alternative plan. For example, say you are on a mountain hike with a friend. Bad weather breaks unexpectedly. Panicked, your friend wants to rush back to the cottage on a wet, slippery, dangerous mountain pass during the storm. You cannot change his panic. You cannot change his goal—to find shelter and safety. But you can offer alternative means to reach his goal by pointing out, for example, that you could stay in a nearby cave and wait out the storm.

This same technique works with delusional or hallucinatory patients. Propose an action plan with appropriate means based on new insights that are acceptable to them despite their delusions. In the case of the man accused of stealing money from the cash register, suggest,

> Let's invite your mother and have a conference with her. Discussing with her what she has done to you may help you and her more than attacking and hurting her.

Such guiding of the patient toward a constructive action often convinces the patient that you truly want to help him and he may go along with you.

Alternatively, you may have to resort to committing a homicidal patient or using a neuroleptic if he becomes violent. However, court-ordered and involuntary treatment will make it more difficult for you to establish rapport later.

Address the Conflict

Because the patient's delusions may have originated from conflicts that were not all fixed and false, attempt to address the conflict that preceded her delusional state. For example, a patient may feel jealous toward her sister and feel that her mother favors her sister as she turns against her other daughter, the patient. Discussing that sibling rivalry may help the patient understand why she is delusional about her mother. Now she may see her suspicions in a broader context, even though nothing has changed about her delusion. Develop a plan of action based on the patient's acceptable goals and means and on the nondelusional part of her conflict, such as inviting both the sister and the mother to a family conference. This type of diversion and substitution works because it does not challenge the patient's delusion, yet it does invite action.

Bypass Disruptive Actions

You may not always be able to diffuse a patient's psychotic hostility. You may have to bypass it. For example, bypass disruptive threats, such as a threat to leave the interview situation. Apologize to the patient that you touched on a point that he is sensitive to, and tell him you will leave this discussion for later because there are more important topics to cover.

You can also bypass a patient's delusional goal and thinking by simply focusing on the desired action without justifying it logically. For example, a patient, ignoring the fact that she had threatened other people, tells you that she does not want to see her father during visiting hours in the hospital because he committed her unjustifiably. You just tell her,

> I understand your anger, but your father is here now. We will meet with him. I am getting him now.

To your surprise, the patient may receive him kindly, thereby contradicting her previous intent.

This works because delusional perception and thinking are not tightly coupled with the ensuing action in the psychotic patient. Thus, you have two methods to modify the actions of a psychotic patient: 1) support a justifiable part of the patient's goals, and 2) ask for a specific action directly without becoming entangled in reasoning.

4. Five Steps to Guide the Patient to Constructive Actions

To substitute the patient's pathological means with acceptable ones, follow the five-step approach.

Step 1: Listen—identify the source of acting out. Allow the patient to display his delusional thoughts, hallucinations, perceptions, anger, or excitement. Gauge where it is coming from. While you allow the patient to ventilate, observe delusional goals and ideas. Encourage him to express himself openly. As you are talking with him, determine a working diagnosis. Many psychiatrists will use a sedative-hypnotic or a neuroleptic agent before engaging in a diagnostic interview. Provided the environment is safe for you and the patient, we suggest you learn to verbally manage the grandiose excited and paranoid hostile patient without the help of drugs.

Step 2: Tag. Reformulate the patient's goals and means in a socially more acceptable form. Use the patient's anger, hostility, and excitement to propel the interview in a solution-oriented direction. Negotiate with the patient a statement of his goals and means. This accomplishes two objectives: 1) the patient notices that you are making an effort to understand him, and 2) he is less likely to use you as a target of his hostility because you keep him focused on his original goals. Do not challenge any of the psychotic patient's goals as unrealistic or, even worse, as psychotic.

Step 3: Confront. Determine which part of the goal is realistic so that you could support it if it were not enmeshed with delusional thinking. The problem is the patient's strong emotional investment in his pathological means. Therefore, you have to allow him to vent and discharge his anger and excitement first. If possible, transform motor activity and hunger for action into verbal discharge. However, if the patient remains tense, invite him to stand up, pace, or walk the hallways. Continue the conversation while walking with him. You may say,

> I realize that you are excited and very nervous. If it helps you, let's walk around while we are talking.

Then, slowly transform this space to walk into a space to talk. Urge the patient to talk about his planned activities. Whenever he wants to take action, redirect him to verbalize instead. A teenager may need to hit a punching bag or ride an exercise bike before he can verbalize.

When the patient refuses to answer your question in favor of another topic, bypass that objection by assuring the patient that you will discuss all other topics in detail later.

Step 4: Solve. Support the patient's realistic goals. Then work out with the patient the means that the two of you want to take to reach that goal. It is your task to transform his delusional goals into a realistic action plan. Insist on reality-oriented action. Although the patient is not able to recognize his beliefs as delusional, usually he can realistically examine whether a certain plan of action has merits or not as long as your realistic plan does not interfere with his delusional ideas.

After you have stated your support for the patient's realistic goals, he may calm down because he sees you as an ally. You then proceed with your next intervention. If he remains hostile, allow him to vent his anger again; then repeat your support for his realistic goals. By adopting the realistic part of the patient's goal, you avoid becoming or remaining the target of his hostility. Now you may address the interpersonal conflicts that preceded the psychosis.

Step 5: Approve. Praise the patient for leveling with you and agreeing to an effective course of action. Offer to further explore the background of his conflict. Ask whether he had similar problems in the past with similar types of emotional response. Explore his psychiatric, medical, and social history in the form of excursions centering around his current conflict.

5. Interview A: Delusion of Grandiosity

Here is an example of verbal management of a patient's psychotic state of grandiose excitement.

Mr. S., a 72-year-old white man, is accompanied by his wife and daughter. When they enter the examination room, Mr. S. refuses to sit down. He stands close to the door and wipes the palms of his hands on his pants, giving the impression that his hands are wet. He stares out the window and does not look at the interviewer. (I = interviewer; P = patient; W = wife; D = daughter)

Step 1: Listen

1. I: Hi, Mr. S. My name is Dr. O. How are you?
   P: Terrific. Just fine. If it wasn't for them over there. [Pointing at his wife and daughter while staring the interviewer in the face] They've robbed me of all control. No say over my own life! Just 'cause I'd prostate surgery. Heh, now I'm not a man anymore, they think. [Bites his lips and paces] She [pointing at his wife] tells me what to do now. Unbelievable! Unbelievable! Every school child gets an allowance. No! Not me. Bean counters! They restrict my own money. I just can't get it! I will set an end to that. [Hits his fist on the interviewer's desk]
2. I: Tell me more about it!
   P: [Positions himself in front of the interviewer] A human being has basic rights, right? [Talking faster and faster] Mine are taken away. I'm degraded. I'm a nobody. I want to go to the bank, get some money, buy new engines for my Cessna. No. That little favor is denied to me. By them. Unbelievable! [Pacing back and forth] How can I conquer the skies? With them around? They don't understand a goddamn thing! I have a higher mission in life. [Cynically] You hear? You ladies with your cooking pots!
3. I: Hmmm. You sound angry and frustrated.
   P: Damn right, I am. I need to get gas for my motor saw. I want to clean out

my 10 acres. But no! Nobody goes with me. They won't let me work outside. They say [mocking his wife's voice], "It's 15°F outside. It's after midnight. You'll catch a cold. You need more sleep." [Jumps up and down and paces in anger] It's none of their damned business. I'm not cold. I'm not tired. You hear? You purring pussies! Sticking by the fire. [Slams both hands on the desk] I say it again! It's none of their darn business! And it's none of your darn business either, Doc. [His head getting red, droplets of saliva spouting from his mouth]

4. I: Well, Mr. S., I understand how upset you are. Please, sit down so that I can help you get over your anger.

P: [Shakes head and remains standing]

D: [To the interviewer] Do you think you could treat my father as an outpatient?

W: [Panic-stricken, shaking her head behind her husband's back, hissing] No, no, for heaven's sake, I can't handle him at home. He's crazy. Don't you see?

P: [Glances hatefully at his wife] I'm enlightened, woman! Some people become enlightened but not you! I know that much.

5. I: How's that?

P: Think of Einstein. For 2 years he did not start a fire in a cast-iron stove because he thought there were five people living in there. [Looking hatefully at his wife again] And Einstein was not crazy. We all admire Einstein.

6. I: Certainly, Einstein was a great man. It seems we have lots to talk about, Mr. S.

P: I can't believe you. You just don't get it at all. You don't understand a thing of what I'm saying. You think . . . you don't get it! [Sitting down]

7. I: I want you to . . .

P: [Interrupting, getting up, and positioning himself in front of the interviewer, talking rapidly] Do you know what it says in the Bible, in Genesis? [Pausing and waiting for an answer] Go out and multiply. And we certainly do that. But it also says something else. Do you know what that is?

8. I: [Acts stunned, silent]

P: Genesis 3:23. Of course, you wouldn't know. It says, go out and subdue the earth. I heard the Lord's voice. And I'm doing just that. I obey God. Nobody will stop me obeying my God. [Shaking his finger in the interviewer's face]

9. I: Of course, you should obey God.

P: You're darn right, I will. Let me tell you something else. I have that creek going through my land, and no grass is growing there because of the mud. I heard God's voice, "Subdue the earth!" So I brought in wood, put peat in between the slabs and black dirt on top and now the grass is growing where nobody ever thought it would. But do you think these serpents appreciate what I did? No way! They never wanted me to do it in the first place. They objected that I serve the Lord. For that they'll burn in hell. Thou shall not challenge thy God or his dutiful servant.

W: [To the patient] That was last summer.

P: [Irritated] Just let me finish, woman! Your gender brought enough misery to this world. Read the Bible! Read Genesis! [Shaking a fist toward her; turns to the interviewer] Now you hear, this fall I started to work on the engines for my plane.

D: That's right, but his pilot license has expired.
10. I: [Standing up] Well, Mr. S., . . .
P: [Interrupting] I don't believe this. You don't listen. I have no basic rights.
I was not told that I came here for admission. They told me you would
check my medicine. But I should have known better. When both of them
[pointing with his head toward his wife and daughter] showed up, I knew
something was brewing. I just didn't think that they wanted me in the
hospital that bad. These serpents! And I'm not going. Keep *them* here.
[Pointing to his wife and daughter]
11. I: Well . . .
P: [In protest] Last year, I spent my birthday in a hospital. And that time is
coming up again in a month. I'm not going to do that again, you hear? No
way! That's it.
W: [To patient, begging] You couldn't sleep last year. You were pacing and
screaming and laughing all the time. You couldn't relax. And we all came to
visit you a lot in the hospital.
P: I give you this—you were good visitors.

The interviewer's opening question was designed to elicit the patient's
chief complaint. Because the patient appeared to be agitated, the interviewer avoided the question, "What kind of a problem brought you here?"
Instead, he used a less leading question (Q. 1), which prevented the patient
from answering "I don't have any problems," an answer common for an
agitated patient who may lack insight. The open-ended question made the
patient talk. The excited answers (A. 1–11) revealed the patient's view that
his problems were induced by his family.

The interviewer made two attempts to focus on the patient's psychopathology (Q. 3, 4). However, the family members prevented the patient's
response with concrete, somewhat irrelevant interjections. Despite these
interferences, the interviewer retained the family in the room because they
kept the patient involved in the interview by providing a target for his
irritation.

The patient sought eye contact only when he expressed his anger to
either the interviewer or his own family members. He paced and showed
brisk expressive and reactive movements. His speech showed increased
production, speed, and push, with intolerance for interruptions (A. 10, 11).
His associations were flighty (A. 8, 9). He showed perseveration on a
delusional topic (A. 7–9).

The patient's affect was labile, bright, excited, and angry. His mood was
elated (A. 1). His anger originated from the perceived restriction of his
grandiose expansive thinking and actions, but his delusions lacked a fixed
enemy. He called his wife and daughter "serpents" only when they restricted

or tricked him (A. 9, 10). They were not his persecutors per se, but became friends when he recalled their visits at the hospital (A. 11). His delusion of grandeur and his hallucination of hearing God's voice (A. 9) were congruent with his elated affect.

Through listening, the interviewer was able to ascertain the patient's mental status and the source of his excitement and anger—namely, his being controlled by his family (A. 1–4, 9–11). The patient strove to be in control over his actions. Uncovering the patient's goals enabled the interviewer to support these goals (Q. 9). However, the patient wanted to accomplish these goals in an inappropriate manner, congruent with his disorder: fertilizing a muddy area in a creek, working outside in freezing temperatures after midnight, spending money on an airplane without having a license to fly it. The detection of these inappropriate means showed the necessity of letting the patient discharge these urges verbally and in action (i.e., by pacing). At a later time, the patient would need to be enticed to substitute his activities with socially acceptable ones, such as regular farming and selling his broken airplane.

Step 2: Tag

12. I: Mr. S., you want your basic rights back and control over your life.
    P: Darn right, I do. [Pointing at his wife and his daughter] They won't let me do what the Bible tells me to . . . what God's voice tells me to.
13. I: You won't tolerate your family's mingling with your rights any longer. You won't let them hinder you any longer in your mission to subdue the earth.
    P: [Hostile] Isn't this what I'm telling you all along? I obey God. And I will do it again and again. But listen to them serpents! They want me to obey them. Adam, that fool, did it once and it cost us the paradise. [Turning to the women] You want to tell me what to do, hey? When to come inside, hey? When to go out, hey? Even what to buy, hey? Oh, no, what not to buy, right?
    W: [To patient] But, . . .
    P: [Interrupting and turning to the interviewer] Listening to their stuff? I couldn't buy anything. [Turning back to the women] Not anything? Anything! Isn't that right? For that, you'll burn in hell.
14. I: So you feel your family should leave you alone and let you buy what you want? Otherwise they will burn in hell? You feel there is really nothing wrong with you?
    P: That's right. I follow a higher order.
15. I: And you absolutely don't want to be here for your birthday.
    P: Who says that I need an adjustment of my medication? All I need is to be in control of my life. You hear? My control! [Looking hatefully toward the women] Not your control! [Hissing like a serpent] The Lord be my witness! [Looking upward]

The interviewer was empathic to the patient's feeling of being restricted and manipulated by his family (Q. 12–15). He tagged the patient's two realistic goals, one of which was abstract (A. 12) and the other concrete (A. 15). He also tagged for the patient the two unrealistic means to exercise his rights (Q. 13, 14). With this feedback, he offered a verbal outlet for the patient's unrealistic means for establishing control—farming during the winter nights and investing money in a broken airplane when he had no valid pilot's license. The patient's response to the tagging of his unrealistic means (Q. 13, 14) confirmed that he had no insight into his actions. He was not able to correct his poor judgment.

Step 3: Confront

16. I: You are really upset and angry, Mr. S.
    P: I am. They turn right into wrong and obedience to God into an illness. They make me mad. Very mad. And it is against my belief to be mad against my own flesh and blood. I pray God may punish them for that.
17. I: And you said your own flesh and blood may burn in hell.
    P: Did I say that? But that's right. They may! [Walks in front of his wife and daughter and points a hand at each of them] God will destroy you. You oppose him. He is working through me. And there is nothing I can do to save you. Nothing. Nothing. You are just paying for your sins. Not that I want it to happen. You brought it on yourself. [Breathing heavily, then sighing and finally walking backward and dropping into an armchair]

The interviewer tagged the patient's inappropriate means (Q. 16, 17). He let him ventilate his anger. This acceptance of the patient's emotions seemed to neutralize the situation and led to a voluntary rather than involuntary admission. The interviewer did not confront the patient with his grandiose, delusional arguments; his preaching; and the reported hallucinations. However, he confronted him with his unrealistic means by intentionally overstating the patient's revenge: eternal punishment for his family. Often such overstatements prompt a patient to soften an extreme position. In this case, Mr. S.'s extreme anger and concurrence with the interviewer's statement confirmed his lack of insight and his poor judgment.

Step 4: Solve

18. I: I'm glad you got out your anger and frustration. I agree you should be in control of your own life. And I'll help you to get it back.
    P: I don't need any help. I can take care of that myself.

19. I: I agree. You have to control your life yourself. All I can do is help you sleep better and give you peace of mind. And you should be home for your birthday next month. So the earlier we get started, the better. You need control over your life back.

   P: [With resignation, pointing to his wife and daughter over his shoulder without looking at them] They should have told me that they wanted me in here. I don't need any change in my medication. I've never felt any better.

   W: [To patient] You need to tell the doctor you wouldn't even take your medicine. You wouldn't listen to any of us.

   P: [Shrugging his shoulders and turning his back to his wife, talking to the interviewer] My doctor retired last month. I retired from being his patient or anybody else's patient. You hear me, Doc? A man has his basic rights, and God asked him to take control over the earth. And as I told you I'm doing just that. Nobody should stop me. God did not say that woman should subdue man.

20. I: Mr. S., I understand your feelings. I will record that you don't want to be here. Okay. [Writing on an intake sheet] But I'm looking forward to talking to you about Genesis. We have a lot to talk about. And we will start right now. [Stands up, signals the patient's wife and daughter to stand up too] We will go to the admissions office and get started.

   P: [Gets up too, takes his hat and coat, and goes along]

21. I: [In the admissions office] Mr. S., please read this.

   P: [Reads the forms without protest]

22. I: Do you understand what you are reading?

   P: Yes. It says I agree to voluntary treatment.

23. I: Yes. That's right. Do you agree that you have lost control over your life? That you don't sleep? That you are up all the time? And that you try to buy all kinds of things? And that's the reason why your wife is scared to let you have any money?

   P: That's right. But there's nothing wrong . . .

24. I: I know your feeling about that. You and I will take care of that. Please sign here so that I can adjust your medication and give you back your sleep and your control over your life. We'll try everything we can to get you out of here before your birthday. Please, sign here.

   P: [Signs the admission papers]

Step 5: Approve

25. I: I'm looking forward to listening to you about Genesis. [Gets up and walks the patient to the ward]

   P: They! [Pointing over his shoulder to his family] They never want to hear about it. They walk away.

26. I: We'll get that all straightened out. And at your birthday you'll be home and back in control. We'll work it out together.

   P: It's ridiculous that a psychiatrist has to show them how to listen and to let me be in control.

27. I: Mr. S., I think you did the right thing to get it all worked out.

The interviewer supported the patient's goals to give him back control over his life and try to have him home by his birthday (Q. 18, 19, 26). However, his and the patient's vision of the means by which that would be accomplished differ. The patient envisioned "control of his life" as unrestrained realization of his delusional plans (A. 19). In contrast, the interviewer envisioned "control of his life" as elimination of the delusions and adherence to reality. The interviewer bypassed the patient's determination to go home and to clean out underbrush in 15°F weather. He substituted the patient's delusional desire for action with goals that he could support—namely, making the patient feel in control and inviting him to talk about religion (Q. 20). Assessing the latter would be important for continuous monitoring of the patient's thought content.

The interviewer kept the patient focused on these common goals during Step 5. The patient accepted the interviewer's wrap-up of his problems: loss of control, loss of sleep, and loss of frugality. Thus, rapport was maintained. Also, the patient did not express doubt that the interviewer could restore those lost functions in him, even though at this point he did not value sleep and frugality highly.

The only action the interviewer encouraged the patient to take was to talk about his delusions in detail. To do that, he had to be in the hospital. The promise to spend time with him on his delusional topics gave the patient some feeling of satisfaction (A. 25).

The interviewer turned the patient's lack of insight, poor judgment, and objection to being interviewed into cooperation by identifying and empathizing with his main source of discontent—restriction by his family. Once the patient believed that the interviewer would help him to feel less restricted, he submitted himself to being interviewed.

The patient had had a similar state of elation a year earlier, from which he recovered.

Differential Diagnosis

Axis I

1. Bipolar disorder, most recent episode manic, severe, with mood-congruent psychotic features.
2. Rule out preexisting delusional disorder, mixed type, grandiose and persecutory.
3. Rule out beginning dementia of the Alzheimer's type, with late onset,

with delusions and hallucinations, with predominantly manic, not depressed, mood.
4. Rule out beginning vascular dementia, with delusions.
5. Rule out substance-induced persisting dementia; consider possible
chronic fertilizer, herbicide, and pesticide exposure.

5. Interview B: Delusion of Persecution

In the following case, the patient considers the interviewer as her enemy
and directs her hostility toward him. Her rejection challenges the interviewer
to get enough information to identify the patient's source of discomfort and
to create a therapeutic alliance.

Three police officers are crowding around the information desk in the
emergency room. They are holding onto a middle-aged female who is yelling
at a man and at a couple. (I = interviewer; P = patient; O = police officer)

Step 1: Listen

1. I: [Looks at the patient]
   P: [Looking away from the interviewer, shouts at the man who came with the
       police] You fucking asshole! I'll pay you back! I'll have my lawyer sue your
       ass off. You just wait! I'll get your lawyer too. Fuck him! You both lied to the
       judge!
2. I: [Introduces himself] Is there any way I can help?
   P: [Stares the interviewer in the eyes] I don't want to talk to no fucking
       psychiatrist. It's my ex [pointing at the man] who needs to talk to a shrink.
       He's a manic depressant [sic].
   O: We have a court order for Mrs. B. She pawned her jewelry to get money for
       a handgun.
   I: [Studies the court order, which reads that Mrs. B. bought a gun and told her
       friend that she would use it to take care of her problem, indicating that she
       might shoot her ex-husband. She also said that afterward she would go into
       the woods and shoot herself because she would not want to die next to her
       ex. The ex-husband stated that Mrs. B. had accused him of betrayal. The
       dentist for whom she was working as a hygienist had called and told him
       that she was complaining to the patients about him, crying in front of them,
       and claiming that he read her mind and messed with her thoughts.
           After the patient's involuntary admission to the hospital, the interviewer
       approaches Mrs. B. again. She is sitting in her room with a mental health
       worker who is observing her as a precaution against suicide.]
3. I: Mrs. B. I'd like to know how to get you out of this mess.
   P: [Stares the interviewer in the eyes and with a hostile, sharp, cold voice] Save
       your breath. The only person I'll talk to is my lawyer.
4. I: Is there any way that I can help you now?

P: [Her eyes narrow to a slit] Open this darn door and let me out of here. If not I'll break down the elevator door.

5. I: What got you in here in the first place?

P: Goddamnit! Can't you hear me? Save your breath! [Presses her lips together] You don't fool me, you're in with them. Don't use your silver tongue on me! I'm not talking to you. End of conversation! [She gets up, leaves her room, and walks down the hallway toward the lounge. The mental health worker follows her.]

The patient was alert and oriented to place and person, as she understood immediately that the interviewer was a psychiatrist. She responded to his empathy with hostility, angry affect, absence of social graces, and insults (A. 2–5). Her unrestrained anger was directed toward the man who had come with the police (A. 1, 2). That she was being involuntarily admitted augmented her irritable, angry affect and persecutory ideas (A. 3). She saw the psychiatrist as a persecutor and incorporated him into the delusional plot against her (A. 5). The interviewer could not establish rapport with this patient. She avoided eye contact and rejected the interviewer's help (A. 2–5). Her hostile stare (A. 2–5) expressed defiance.

So far, the interviewer could identify two acceptable goals of the patient: 1) she strove for justice in the conflict with her ex-husband (A. 1), and 2) she wanted to get out of the hospital (A. 4). The interviewer also identified two unacceptable means she had for accomplishing her goals: 1) she would break down the elevator door (A. 4), and 2) she would shoot her ex-husband for his alleged betrayal and then herself (information was garnered from the court papers).

Differential Diagnosis

1. Delusional disorder
2. Major depression with psychotic features
3. Bipolar disorder with persecutory delusions
4. Substance-induced psychotic disorder
5. Borderline personality disorder
6. Antisocial personality disorder

Step 2: Tag

The interviewer follows the patient.

6. I: Mrs. B., you want to get out of here.

P: [Abruptly getting up from the couch in the hospital ward lounge and

walking past the interviewer down the hallway toward her room] I told you, I'm not talking to no shrink.
7. I: You want to get justice in your struggle with your ex and his lawyer.
   P: Leave me alone! I'm not listening to you.
8. I: You want to use violence to get out of here—break down the door! You sounded ready to jump at your ex out there in the lobby.
   P: Save your spit! I know what I said.

Tagging of the patient's acceptable goals (Q. 6, 7) yielded the same hostile response: Mrs. B. was fixed in her hostile affect and in her hostile perception of the interviewer (A. 6–8). She neither confirmed her claims nor agreed with the goals that the interviewer restated.

Step 3: Confront

9. I: [Walking behind the patient] Well, Mrs. B., you said your ex-husband brought you in here under false pretenses. He and his lawyer lied to the judge and the police just to get you committed.
   P: [Keeps on walking down the hall without looking back to the interviewer] Yes, they did. These bastards really did. And he's friends with the lawyer . . . the lawyer's behind it. They plotted to get me out of the way.
10. I: You feel that they should really pay.
    P: [Stops, turns around, and makes a fist] They shall and they will. [Points her finger at the interviewer] You can't put me away forever. I'll get to these bastards. [Starts walking again]

The patient's tense and abrupt movements indicated agitation. She acted out her impulses (A. 9). Her speech was fast and peppered with derogatives (A. 9, 10). She discharged her hatred and anger in short sentences. Her responses showed that she was indeed listening to the interviewer, comprehended the content and intent of his statements, and could give a response in line with her persecutory thought content. Because neutral tagging of the patient's goals and means did not solicit confirmation, the interviewer next restated her persecutory feelings, which converted her previous rejection of the interviewer's statements into acceptance. She even elaborated on her answer (A. 10).

The interviewer enabled the patient to discharge her anger about being persecuted. This discharge neutralized her feelings so that she could be receptive for Step 4, when the interviewer would offer her his alliance with her socially acceptable goals.

Step 4: Solve

11. I: If they brought you in here under false pretenses, I will help you nail them. I'm not their man. Your ex and the lawyer don't have me in their pocket. I will not do their dirty work for them if indeed that's their plan.

    P: Oh yes, it is. They wanted me out of the way. Just lock me up. [Stops walking, stands facing down the hallway] I just look at him. I can tell.

12. I: [Standing behind her, talking to her back] If that's so, they made a big mistake. You will be out of here in no time. I will help you to get them if they gave false testimony. I want to help you.

    P: [Sighs and turns around, facing the interviewer for the first time]

13. I: Do you want to nail your husband?

    P: [Emphatically] You bet your boots. The court appointed a lawyer for me. I tried to call him already. I'll catch my ex, that asshole.

14. I: And I will help you do that.

    P: [Looks at interviewer in disbelief and grunts] Hmmm.

15. I: Think about how we can best do it.

    P: [Hostile, staring at the interviewer, with rapid speech] You should know! You are holding me against my will. You want to help me? Hey! Just let me go.

16. I: I will. But I have to prove that your ex lied. And you have to help me do that. I can't do it by myself. I need your help.

    P: [Hostile] How's that?

17. I: You know what all went on. I don't. We have to prove that your ex lied to the court, distorted the facts, and put you in here against his better judgment. Can you help me with that?

    P: [Less hostile] How?

18. I: [Slowly starts walking toward an open interview room] He testified that you pawned jewelry to buy a gun. Is that true?

    P: [Following him] No, that's a lie. I took my ring to a jeweler to get the diamond reset.

19. I: Can we prove that?

    P: Yes, you can call the jeweler. [Firmly] I did not pawn my ring.

20. I: [Sitting down in the interview room] Okay, we have the first point in our favor. [Patient nods her head with satisfaction] Now, your ex claimed that you said, "I may get a gun and go into the woods and kill myself." Is that true?

    P: [Sitting down too] No, it's a lie.

21. I: But your ex had a witness for that. Was the witness lying?

    P: [Looks at the interviewer and does not answer]

22. I: Can we prove that the witness is lying?

    P: [Keeps looking at interviewer]

23. I: If we want to prove that they are lying, you have to tell me what you really said.

    P: I said, "If my ex treats me like this, I may as well get myself a gun and take care of my problems."

24. I: So you said that to your friend?

P: Yes.

25. I: And your ex heard it?

P: No, she told him.

26. I: And did you repeat it to your ex?

P: Yes, I wanted to shake him up.

27. I: What happened then?

P: I was exhausted. I went to bed and slept. Next thing I knew the cops are knocking at my door. They got me here.

28. I: You slept during the day? You must have felt poorly.

P: Yes, I did. I was exhausted. I hadn't slept well for the last 8 weeks. I always woke up and could not get back to sleep. [Starts crying]

29. I: Hmmm. You must have gone through a lot.

P: [Sobs] I'll get the bastard for that! I didn't know what was happening. All of a sudden, the cops are there to pick me up. [With hostility] The asshole wanted me out of the way and he has to pay for that.

30. I: What did you want your ex to do?

P: I wanted him to sit with me, listen to me, and show me some understanding.

31. I: But could he know that you didn't mean it?

P: Of course, he could. He should have known, he should have tried at least.

32. I: Were you angry when you mentioned the gun?

P: You bet I was. I slammed the door in that ass's face and went to bed.

33. I: So you did with him as you did with me—just walk away.

P: Yes, but he could have tried. You tried, didn't you? He just doesn't care, the asshole. I hate that bastard.

34. I: I don't believe you. I think he cares about you. He wouldn't have gone through the trouble to get you here if he didn't care.

P: [Tears running down her cheeks] How can he care if he puts me here? [Biting her lower lip] He's a conniving asshole.

35. I: Well, he said that you were upset over the last few weeks, that you argued a lot and that you cried at your work. Is that a lie?

P: What would you do, if your spouse has it in for you? I heard him whispering even at work. Psss!

36. I: Hmmm. I think he's worried about you. Do you want to get back at him for that?

P: [Angry] Bull, if he loved me, this asshole didn't have to bring me here.

37. I: Maybe he worried about you and just did the best he knew how.

P: Oh, baloney, he knew better.

38. I: You said you'd use a gun. And you said you had been upset for some time. Let's say he didn't mean to lie or get you out of the way but that he did the best he could. What do you think he felt about you?

P: [Pause, then frowning] He was scared. [With a softer voice] That asshole was scared.

39. I: You're right. I want to help you to get out of this mess. I want to work with the two of you not against you. Do you think he would come here?

P: He might.

40. I: Do you want him to come? I think he still cares for you and I want to find that out.

P: [Silent]
41. I: Will you talk to him if he comes?
P: I'll let him have it then.
42. I: I understand. You're angry and disappointed that he shoved you over to the police and the court and did not handle it himself.
P: You bet.
43. I: It looks like he was scared.
P: [Shrugs her shoulders]
44. I: I don't want to do his work for him. I want him to make it up to you. And I want to work with you and I want him to take care of what he has started.
P: Hmmm.
45. I: I don't want you here by a court order. I want to work with you, find out how depressed you are, how I can make you feel better and get you out of here. Is that okay?
P: What do you want me to do?
46. I: First of all, I want you to stay in this hospital voluntarily, and I want to tell the court that you are here voluntarily. I don't want you to have a commitment on your records.
P: What if I just sign out and leave?

As the key intervention for rapport, the interviewer adopted the possibly delusional claim of the patient as being real. This broke the ice. It formed the beginning of the therapeutic alliance with her (Q. 11). He slipped into the role of an advocate for her rights. This fit the patient's goal. She indicated she would like to use a lawyer against her ex-husband (A. 13). He took the lead in helping her to pursue her purpose—namely, to nail her ex-husband for false imprisonment, if indeed it was false imprisonment. And just as a lawyer would, he asked her for assistance in this pursuit (Q. 14–29). Thus, in the patient's perception, he switched roles from the prison guard in the service of her ex-husband to the attorney prosecuting her enemies for the injustice she was suffering (Q. 14). Strong, direct, repetitive statements (Q. 11, 12, 14) made it simple for the patient to understand that the interviewer had adopted her goal as his own. It was less likely that he would become a victim of her delusional misinterpretations. From the position of ally, he addressed her suffering (Q. 29). He soothed her perception of neglect by her ex-husband by pointing out his caring (Q. 34, 36, 37) and his anxiety (Q. 38).

In three moves, the interviewer diverted the patient's hostility against himself and the ex-husband by 1) becoming an ally in joining the patient in her goal; 2) changing the ex-husband's image as a rejecting, plotting persecutor to a scared person who needed to ask the police for help; and 3) reformulating her legal accusation of false imprisonment to a communication problem that could be solved by cooperation.

The interviewer could have taken a less supportive and more neutral approach that would have allowed the patient to ventilate but would not have necessitated him supporting her goals; this strategy might have worked in the long run. However, often a patient with delusions of persecution sees herself as isolated and believes that others band together against her. To shake this delusional perception, a very clear message of support is necessary to help the patient overcome her suspiciousness against the interviewer and consider him as a possible ally.

Mrs. B.'s labile affect ranged from angry and hostile to sobbing and crying, which occurred when she finally accepted the interviewer's empathy (A. 28, 29). She reported that her mood had been depressed for at least 8 weeks (A. 28).

Step 5: Approve

47. I: I don't think you will play a trick on me. I trust you.
    P: Why? You don't know me. You don't know how horrid I can be.
48. I: I know you some—I know you were honest with me about your ex. You could have told me that you never made the threat with the gun, that you never were upset, or never cried. But you admitted all that.
    P: So?
49. I: You were mad as hell but you didn't lie to me.
    P: Hmmm.
50. I: You know that, by law, I have to hold you if you are suicidal. And you yourself told me how depressed you were.
    P: But, I wouldn't have done it . . . I don't think.
51. I: I don't know that. I can't read your mind. I don't have a crystal ball. And I think your ex did not know either. I think he brought you here because he cared for you and believed what you said.
    P: [Starts sobbing, then becomes angry] That man and his lawyer . . . they have something up their sleeves!
52. I: [Calls the nurse to bring the admission papers] This really has gotten to you. [Stands up and puts his hand on her shoulder] Now, I want you to help me and find out how depressed you have become.
    P: How's that?
53. I: I will do a clinical interview with you, and the psychologist I work with will give you a structured interview and a depression scale.
    P: Hmmm . . . But you will see my ex and his lawyer? They are really sneaky. I know they plotted all this.
54. I: Let's find out. We will meet with your ex and we'll have things worked out pretty soon.
    P: I hope you're right. [Nurse enters with the voluntary admission forms. Mrs. B. reads and signs them.]

The interviewer raised the patient's self-image, which had been damaged by her perceived conjugal rejection (Q. 47–49). This positive feedback established rapport and allowed the patient for the first time to admit some falsehood in herself (A. 47). The interviewer confronted her with the reality of the situation (Q. 50–54), and she objected only faintly (A. 53). He satisfied her secret need—namely, to hear that her ex-husband still cared for her (Q. 51). Thus, the interviewer tried to make the patient feel good about dismissing hostility and revengeful plotting in favor of cooperating with the interviewer to reach a mutual goal—to straighten out the patient's relationship with her ex-husband.

This case example demonstrates an interviewing strategy with a delusional patient without putting her on a neuroleptic first.

Differential Diagnosis

Axis I

1. Major depression with psychotic features
   Pro: The patient claimed that she had maintained a stable relationship with her husband even after her divorce, that she was still able to work as a dental hygienist, and that she had a clear onset of depression 8 weeks earlier (as noted in the commitment papers).
   Con: The patient's increased psychomotor activity, intense hostility, rapid speech, and labile mood point to bipolar disorder.
2. Bipolar disorder, depressed
   Pro: The patient's degree of agitation, her rapid speech, and the spontaneity in her actions support this diagnosis.
   Con: The patient had no volunteered history of clear mania.
3. Delusional disorder
   Pro: The patient had prominent delusions that were difficult to shake with logical arguments.
   Con: The patient had labile affect, a succinct onset, and then decrease of delusional and hallucinatory thinking in response to positive feedback, and some auditory hallucinations.
4. Schizophrenia, paranoid type
   Pro: The patient had persecutory delusions, some auditory hallucinations, and an initial coldness and hostility toward the interviewer.
   Con: The patient had worked for many years, she had maintained her relationship with her ex-husband, and she had a recent onset of her

persecutory thinking. She also was able to submerge her delusional and hallucinatory thinking in response to positive feedback.

5. Substance abuse—such as alcohol abuse (alcohol-related jealousy) and amphetamine-induced persecutory delusions

Pro: The patient had persecutory delusions with a recent onset, labile mood, and delusional jealousy.

Con: The patient showed no evidence of a history of substance abuse.

6. Hostility and Facilitating in Psychiatric Disorders

Hostility derives from a number of psychiatric disorders (see the differential diagnosis in Table 5–1).

A patient's hostility may stem from cognitive impairment (delirium, dementia, or amnestic state), intoxication, or a severe attention-deficit disorder. You will be struck by her inability to follow your train of thought. She acts frustrated. Questions aggravate and irritate her. With the exception of the patient with attention deficit, the cognitively impaired patient also may report hallucinations and delusional thinking. She requires a simple, concrete, and calm interview approach because any stimulation overload leads to decompensation and explosive discharge.

The patient experiencing manic excitement and hostility appears to be overactivated, expansive, and ready to rebel against any perceived constraints. His thinking is expansive and grandiose, and—in the more severe cases—lacks organization and goal direction. Distraction is often the way to handle such a patient in the interview.

In contrast to the patient with mania, the patient with a delusional disorder usually shows more circumscribed goals and proposes more specific, exaggerated and destructive means. Such goal direction is also seen in patients whose delusional hostility presents in conjunction with major depressive disorder or schizophrenia. These are the patients whom you can redirect to take acceptable action and to merely verbally ventilate their assaultive plans, as shown in this chapter.

In dissociative disorder, the hostile patient usually lacks the perplexity typical of cognitive dysfunction disorders, the attention deficit and excitement typical of the manic patient, and the intense determination typical of the persecutory delusional patient. The patient cannot explain her hostility, which occurs in response to a trigger that induces the dissociation. The suddenness and the lack of obvious provocation alert you to the possibility

Table 5–1. Hostility in psychiatric disorders

Disorder	Patient's impairment	Patient's perception of the interviewer	Patient's reaction	Patient's goal
Cognitive disorder	Understanding context	Aggravator	Feeling frustrated, overwhelmed	To remove stimulus overload
Substance abuse	Filtering information, understanding context, controlling impulse	Aggravator, irritant	Feeling overwhelmed	To reduce stimulation
Attention-deficit/ hyperactivity disorder	Filtering information	Irritant	Having temper tantrums, hitting objects, screaming	To remove distraction
Mania	Controlling excessive energy	Obstacle	Protesting against imposed limits	To transform energy into action
Delusional disorder	Interpreting social relationships accurately	Persecutor	Becoming suspicious, feeling anxious, making accusations, expecting malice	To eliminate perceived enemies
Dissociative disorder	Integrating rejected impulses	Interrogator	Acting out	To protect secrets
Antisocial personality disorder	Respecting rules	Despot, authority, rule enforcer	Protesting against rules and authority figures	To eliminate rules and authority

that the patient is dissociating. You overcome her hostility by hypnosis (see Chapter 1, "Conversion"), free association, or hypnotic switching (see Chapter 2, "Dissociation").

The patient with hostility based in antisocial personality disorder rebels against your imagined authority and imposed rules. His hostility develops out of the interaction with you, not another target, as is the case with the persecutory delusional patient. You may use the plus-minus approach for such a patient, pointing out the negative consequences of his hostility (see Chapter 12, "Concealing").

In this chapter, we applied the facilitating technique to the management of psychotic forms of hostility. We identified the patient's goals that were acceptable. We looked behind the patient's hostile outbursts, hallucinatory experiences, and delusional thinking for the impulse that represented the patient's legitimate interest. We supported the patient in reaching his objective. Thus, the principle of facilitating is universal—namely, it is being an empathic and supportive ally who helps the patient accomplish his goals. If the patient experiences the interviewer indeed being on his side, the patient is more likely to discuss and give up destructive, inefficient, or inappropriate means.

CHAPTER 6

CATATONIA

Summary

In catatonia, the patient ceases to respond to his environment. Interpersonal interaction seems to be discontinued. Medication can alleviate this expressive block: in depressive catatonia, amobarbital or lorazepam enables the patient to talk; in excited catatonia, haloperidol works. By temporarily reversing the catatonia, the interviewer can diagnose the underlying condition and determine further workup and treatment options.

When faced with danger, an opossum feigns death until danger has passed. Humans, too, can become mute and stuporous when faced with a dangerous situation.

1. What Is Catatonia?

In DSM-IV (American Psychiatric Association 1994), catatonia is defined as a subtype of schizophrenia in which the essential feature is a marked psycho-motor disturbance characterized by two or more of five clinical criteria:

1. Motoric immobility, either catalepsy or stupor
2. Excessive, nondirectable, apparently purposeless motor activity
3. Extreme negativism or mutism
4. Peculiarities of voluntary movements, such as posturing, stereotyped movements, mannerisms, or grimacing
5. Echolalia or echopraxia

Criteria 1 and 2 appear to be mutually exclusive. Therefore, clinicians distinguish catatonia as either a stuporous state or an excited state. How-ever, patients may fluctuate between the two states. In both states, the patient is alert but may not appear that way, which distinguishes catatonia from a comatose state. A catatonic state may also accompany neuroleptic-induced parkinsonism, a general medical condition, or a manic or major depressive episode.

An excited patient may become mute and paralyzed in response to his hallucinations and delusions. For example, one patient with schizoaffective disorder sat in the corner of his room with the blinds down; he was smiling and elated, as the Virgin Mary is often portrayed. As he explained later, he did not move or talk so that he would not disturb his pregnancy with the baby Jesus.

In the literature, this separation between a catatonic stuporous state and an excited state is implied but not always explicitly noted. Furthermore, there is a third state preceded by irrelevant, illogical thoughts, as is sometimes seen in catatonic schizophrenia. Cases of catatonia may therefore be diagnosed as schizophrenia, catatonic type; bipolar disorder with catatonic features; major depressive disorder with catatonic features; and catatonic disorder due to a general medical condition (American Psychiatric Association 1994).

In most types of catatonia, the patient's receptive language areas and the associated areas are intact; that is, the patient can receive but not express communications. This is important for rapport. It is essential not to treat such a patient according to how she acts but how she perceives. A patient's perception can be quite keen while showing reduced or nonresponsive, expressive psychomotor and verbal behavior. Two vignettes illustrate the catatonic patient's awareness of her surroundings.

Professor Bürger-Prinz of the University of Hamburg Medical School in Germany was making inpatient rounds together with a visiting professor. He pointed to a chronic patient with cataleptic catatonia: "Here is one of my patients in a terminal catatonic state." This patient eventually recovered. Months later, Professor Bürger-Prinz received a postcard from Switzerland which this former patient had signed as "your terminal catatonic state."

The following is an even more striking and graphic story.

Two catatonic patients were sitting side by side in a hospital ward. An instructor pointed out their bizarre postures to the medical students, waving his finger in front of the patients' faces. Suddenly, the instructor let out a scream. One of the patients had bitten off a segment of his right index finger and swallowed it. Immediately the patient fell back into a stuporous, emotionless state. The act happened so rapidly that the instructor never found out which patient had done it. (Rubin 1974)

Catatonia occurs not only in bipolar disorder and schizophrenia but also in neurological diseases, including dementia (Abrams and Taylor 1976; Altschuler et al. 1986). To evaluate the patient's mental status and chart the course of the most effective workup, the interviewer has to reverse the catatonic state. For example, if the patient is disoriented or shows other signs of dementia after the reversal of the catatonia, a brain scan and magnetic resonance imaging scan are indicated.

Rigidity may occur in response to general medical conditions. For example, extrapyramidal rigidity or "lead-pipe" resistance occurs as the result of lesions of the basal ganglia and their connections. Decerebrate rigidity occurs with loss of cortical connections. Gegenhalten (counterholding) may be seen in elderly persons without being a sign of negativism (DeJong and Haerer 1992). Akinetic mutism that mimics stuporous catatonia may result from severe communicating hydrocephalus, partial destruction of the diencephalic and midbrain reticular formation, and bilateral frontal lobe processes involving orbital, septal, and cingulate cortices (Edwards and Simon 1992). Furthermore, therapy for catatonia depends on the diagnosis. Treatment may range from neurosurgery of a tumor in the frontal lobe to electroconvulsive therapy (ECT) for a depressive catatonic state to treatment with psychotropic drugs, the choice of which depends on the patient's thought content.

2. Catatonia in the Mental Status

The mental status examination is limited to observation and physical and neurological examinations. During the examination, distinguish between two forms of catatonia: catatonia with motoric immobility or catatonia with excessive, nondirectable, apparently purposeless motor activity.

Catatonia With Motoric Immobility

This form of catatonia is frequently associated with muteness. The muteness is preceded by a change in the speed of mentation, seen in thought slowing and loss of goal direction, which eventually lead to monosyllabism, increased latency of response, and, finally, cessation of speech.

Preceding a total stupor, the patient's movements become slow, heavy, and deliberate and he ignores new stimuli. These slow or missing reactive movements point to depressive stupor, in which motor movements decrease in amount and speed. The patient complains that his limbs feel heavy, as if he is walking hip deep through mud, or he says he is freezing to immobility. He does not respond by turning his head toward you when you address him. This decrease in motor activity results in a motionless state, a stupor.

Seven so-called catatonic symptoms or signs are frequently associated with mutism and stupor: catalepsy, stereotypy, posturing, automatic obedience, negativism, echolalia, and echopraxia (Fish 1967). Mutism and stupor caused by a neurological disorder, such as a stroke, present only infrequently with these seven symptoms (Abrams and Taylor 1976).

Because the patient cannot give a history, you are limited to interviewing informants, who may report that the patient's movements and speech gradually became slower and more belabored until he stopped talking and moving altogether. Yet bizarre posturing, grimacing, and echolalia or echopraxia may still occur.

Catatonia With Excessive Motor Activity

This type of catatonia is on the other end of the activity continuum from immobile catatonia and is frequently preceded by thought racing, push of speech, flight of ideas, tangential speech, and fragmented sentence structure. Such a patient may claim she thinks in paragraphs. This process may begin with unconnected thoughts and a jumping from topic to topic until the patient's speech sounds completely disorganized. Like a speed reader, the patient picks up fragments of her own thoughts and produces an unintelligible word salad. Finally, the movements of her mouth become too slow to express the flood of thoughts. She may repeat only the last word of a question (echolalia) before she becomes mute. Yet comprehension is preserved. Such increase in thinking is often accompanied by an elated and excited mood and sets catatonia with excessive motor activity apart from immobile catatonia.

The same history of speeding up is present with respect to the patient's motor functions, which establishes the diagnosis of catatonia with excessive motor activity. Like speech, motor activity can increase or become disorganized, bizarre, and unresponsive to environmental stimuli. Persistent increase in motor activity leads to an excited state. The patient paces and remains in a constant state of motion. Her movements may lose fluidity and become awkward (e.g., she may walk as if she were riding a bicycle). Ritualistic movements may accentuate the motoric bizarreness. She may then be unable to keep up with her own pace and may fall into a state of muscular tension and rigidity. Masseter, anterior neck muscles and the mastication muscles tense up and lead to the so-called snout spasm. She may show catalepsy and incontinence. Yet she often tracks new stimuli attentively with her eyes. In contrast, the patient with immobile catatonia may lack all response to outside stimuli.

Inappropriate affect and mood, detached from thought content, may precede muteness and stupor. Social feedback is often ignored. The patient may respond to others in an irrelevant and inappropriate manner; for example, he may giggle about the death of a person he is close to or cry over a recent accomplishment. Respect the patient's affect and mood and treat it as appropriate for his state of mind. Such empathy is essential to establishing and maintaining rapport.

Informants may report that the patient became increasingly irritable, hostile, tense, and monosyllabic, claiming people were observing her, plotting against her, wanting to poison or otherwise do away with her. Then, they report, she deteriorated into a state of tense, angry, obstinate defiance and muteness, throwing hostile looks, ready to throw a temper tantrum any time, or ready to burst out in violence (excited stupor).

3. Technique: Amobarbital or Lorazepam for Immobile Catatonia

With current pressures for patients to be only briefly hospitalized, it is essential that when facing an alert but stuporous and mute patient, you are familiar with effective interviewing techniques. Furthermore, untreated catatonia may lead to peripheral thrombophlebitis with pulmonary emboly and sometimes pneumonia with fatal outcome. The excited form of catatonia can also be lethal and lead to exhaustion, hyperthermia, coma, cardiovascular collapse, and death. Urinary retention with increase in blood urea nitrogen and creatinine levels has also been reported (Salam and Kilzieh 1988).

To our knowledge, no author has yet described a reliable, verbal technique that can interrupt the mute and stuporous state without the help of medication.

Choice of Medication

The amobarbital interview is a diagnostic inquiry of a catatonic patient under the influence of an intravenously administered barbiturate with rapid induction and a moderately long time of action. This drug makes a mute patient talk and some amnestic patients remember (Kwentus 1981). You may also use amobarbital for the diagnosis of dissociative and conversion disorder (Baron and Nagy 1988; Hurwitz 1988; Marcum et al. 1986).

As an alternative to amobarbital, intravenous lorazepam was success-fully used in 1983 for neuroleptic-induced catatonia (Fricchione et al. 1983). Another benzodiazepine, intravenous diazepam, was used to relieve catato-nia not induced by neuroleptics (McEvoy and Lohr 1984). Subsequently, lorazepam 2 mg iv or im or 2.5 mg po was successfully used to alleviate different forms of catatonia (Harris and Menza 1989). Rapid response after 1 minute occurred with intravenous application, whereas oral application took 50 minutes. Investigators have agreed that catatonia is only temporarily relieved and returns after the effect of lorazepam wears off (Carroll 1992; Fricchione et al. 1983; Greenfield et al. 1987; Harris and Menza 1989; Rosebush et al. 1990; Salam and Kilzieh 1988; Salam et al. 1987).

A benzodiazepine antagonist, such as flumazem (Romazicon), reverses the effect of lorazepam on catatonia (Harris and Menza 1989). Thus, the associated disorder has to be successfully treated to alleviate catatonia permanently. Because lorazepam can be administered orally or intramuscu-larly, you may use an injection if the patient refuses oral administration. Lorazepam may fail in a number of cases (Salem and Kilzieh 1988). In those cases, amobarbital infusion may be tried. Regardless of whether you use amobarbital or lorazepam, the interview procedures are similar.

Procedure

Assume that the patient understands and perceives everything in detail. Explain the procedure to him as if he could answer you. Read the consent form to him and ask him to nod if he can understand you. If he nods, tell him to nod again if he will permit you to go ahead with the infusion that may restore his speech. Some patients, although not talking, may follow your instructions and sign a paper; others may not. If the patient remains mute and stuporous, ask his closest relative to sign the consent form while the patient is looking on. Make sure the person who conducts the interview is privileged to do so by the medical staff of the hospital where the interview takes place.

Next, insert an indwelling catheter in a cubital vein, and attach a syringe with 10 cc of a 5% amobarbital solution. For legal reasons, some psychiatrists may use a minor surgery room and the help of an anesthesiologist for the procedure. It may even be advisable to keep the patient fasting from midnight of the preceding day to ensure that the stomach is empty because, in very rare cases, the barbiturate can induce vomiting.

Slowly inject 1 cc per minute; stop when the patient appears drowsy or yawns, or by the fourth minute of the infusion in case of muteness (McCall et al. 1992). After he starts talking, stop the medication if he shows slurred speech or becomes light-headed. The titration of the amobarbital is highly individualized. You can easily miss the very light state of narcosis appropriate for the interview. Either the patient may not be sufficiently sedated and become excited and agitated, or he may become oversedated and fall asleep during the procedure. This problem arises because amobarbital crosses the blood-brain barrier slowly—within a matter of minutes—and, therefore, oversedation may lag behind the injection by some minutes. To prevent sleep, Rothman and Sward (1956) have used a combination of thiopental sodium followed by 5–15 mg of methamphetamine hydrochloride. Because most states ban intravenous administration of stimulant drugs, you may try to stabilize the mild narcotic state and give 10–20 mg of dextroamphetamine sulfate or 15–30 mg of methylphenidate 1 hour before induction of the narcointerview. Alternatively, reversal of depressive catatonia can be achieved with ECT.

4. Five Steps to Disinhibit

Step 1: Assess. Determine whether the patient has depressive or catatonic-excited stupor. Examine the patient's mental status, including the seven catatonic signs or symptoms (see above), and perform a neurological examination, including the papilla to exclude a papilledema.

Step 2: Tag. Express empathy and allegiance for the patient's state. You may tell her,

You do not move and you do not talk. I cannot hear you. I'm concerned that something is bothering you. Please, try to answer me. Nod your head if you can hear me.

If the patient nods, you may ask yes and no questions. However, most stuporous patients may not respond (negativism).

Step 3: Confront. Tell the patient that you cannot receive her thoughts:

Unfortunately, I cannot hear your thoughts. I cannot hear the voices that you may be able to hear. If you care to tell me, please do so.

Offer the patient paper and pencil to write down a message. If she ignores you or withdraws her hand, remember that the mute and stuporous state blocks the patient's expression but not her perception. Your behavior determines whether the patient perceives you as empathic, as a guide, as an authority and healer, or as rude and inconsiderate.

Step 4: Solve—the amobarbital or lorazepam application. If you feel that the patient is in a depressive stupor, proceed with the amobarbital or lorazepam interview. In case of a catatonic-excited stupor, you may choose either the amobarbital or lorazepam interview or neuroleptic treatment. (However, note that for subsequent treatment you will have to continue a neuroleptic drug; see example below.)

Reassuring. With a mute and stuporous patient, you cannot presume to know her thought content. When the amobarbital infusion or lorazepam application restores speech, her thought content will emerge. Now you can reassure the patient. You may reduce her anxiety and explain to her that she is safe, that the medication may relax her and make her alert (lorazepam) or sleepy (amobarbital), and that she will be able to talk more. Tell her that whatever she says is confidential and that you would like to know about all of her problems so that you can help her.

Opening the interview. When the patient starts to yawn (amobarbital) or looks around (lorazepam), ask her whether she can hear you. If she nods, ask her to talk. Ask her whether she feels safe. Repeat the question if you do not get any response. It is important that she breaks the silence. Her first words may be softly spoken, whispered, or limited to one word.

At the beginning, ask closed-ended, yes-or-no questions such as,

- Do you remember when you stopped talking?
- Did you know what was going on after you stopped talking?

After the patient has answered several yes-or-no questions, introduce open-ended questions such as,

- What happened when you stopped talking?
- What did you hear?
- What did you see?
- What did you think?
- How did you feel?

Gradually assess the most recent history of the patient's thinking, perceptions, and feelings before and after she became mute. Then assess her cognitive functioning to exclude any neurological disorders, keeping in mind that amobarbital as a barbiturate or lorazepam as a benzodiazepine may interfere with recent memory and with learning.

Step 5: Approve. Obviously, the mute patient has felt ambivalent about opening up and talking. The combination of medication and psychological approach has temporarily encouraged her to talk. Assure the patient that she made the right choice talking to you. Depressed patients experience self-doubt, guilt, and suspicion, all of which you want to reduce as specifically as you can in the hope of keeping the communication channels open.

In the following example, we present a patient who experienced muteness and stupor.

5. Interview: Major Depressive Disorder, Single Episode, With Psychotic and Catatonic Features

Mr. D., a 69-year-old, white, married male, is brought to the emergency room by the police after his wife had called them for help. Mr. D. had spent most of the last week in his bedroom, insisting on having his gun with him and keeping the door closed and all window blinds closed. He would peek through the blinds and check the door at regular intervals. He often muttered sentences such as, "All these hoodlums are moving in." During the previous two nights, he had stayed up all night, refusing to eat or drink. He had looked at his wife in a strange way. On the previous day, he had stopped answering questions and seemed confused. The wife felt that he must have had a stroke because he had to be pushed along when walking and his face had become expressionless as if paralyzed. He had become incontinent.

History.   His wife said Mr. D. had been tense and anxious most of his life. He was always very orderly and took regulations very seriously. As a young man in the service and in his 40s he had periods of drinking, but suddenly had stopped because "he did not want to get addicted." He had not been drinking since.

Family history.   The couple had two children, a son age 31 years and a daughter age 29 years. The daughter was prescribed diazepam off and on by her family physician for insomnia and nervousness.

Medical history.   Mr. D.'s medical history was uneventful, except for cataract surgery 2 years earlier. His physical examination, including vital signs, was normal. The electrocardiogram was normal, with no signs of arrhythmia. The patient had no history of kidney, liver, or cardiopulmonary disease. There was no evidence of upper respiratory infection, a history of porphyria, or an allergy to barbiturates.

Step 1:   Listen

When the interviewer enters the room, Mr. D. does not look up but follows him out of the corners of his eyes. When the interviewer introduces himself and tries to shake hands with him, the patient remains seated with his hands in his lap, motionless. (I = interviewer; P = patient)

  1. I: Your wife told me that you stopped moving and talking 2 days ago. She is
         concerned about what may be bothering you. Can you tell me?
     P: [No response; looks at interviewer and then blinks]
  2. I: Please nod if you can hear me.
     P: [Appears to look through the interviewer]

    When the interviewer asks whether he may touch him, there is no response. When the interviewer asks whether he could mildly squeeze his chest muscles to see whether he would feel it, the patient does not respond. When the patient is asked to stand up, he does not respond. When the interviewer repeats his request, no response. Supported at the elbows with the nurse's help, Mr. D. can be pulled up slowly. When asked to walk across the room to check his gait, he just stands there. His face remains motionless.

When asked to smile, he keeps the frown on his forehead, forming the omega sign. When the interviewer claps his hands behind his head, the patient shows eye blinking and a mild startle reaction, indicating that he can hear.

Examination for catatonic signs. The interviewer holds a needle in front of the patient's mouth and asks him to stick out his tongue. He does not oblige—this indicates an absence of negative obedience. The interviewer takes the patient's arm and moves it over his head, bending the hand inward. The patient slowly lets the arm drop down—this indicates an absence of catalepsy. Thus the patient shows only stupor and muteness, but none of the other symptoms of catatonia.

Neurological examination. In the examination of the 12 cranial nerves, the patient is uncooperative. He withdraws his face when a swab with ammonia is held under his nose, showing that his olfactory nerve (I) is intact. Because he stares into space, his eye background can be viewed; a papilledema is excluded. Because the patient visually tracks the interviewer, it appears that the optic nerve (II) is at least partially functioning. His spontaneous eye movements suggest that the oculomotor (III), the trochlear (IV), and the abducens (VI) nerves are intact.

Mr. D. does not withdraw when the interviewer uses a pin on his facial skin, but when his cheek is touched with an ice cube wrapped in gauze, the patient frowns, flinches, and withdraws—this indicates that the trigeminal (V) and the facial (VII) nerves are intact. The patient shows an eyelid and masseter reflex—this indicates that at least the upper part of the facialis is intact. Facial movements are symmetrical. When the examiner claps behind his back, Mr. D. startles. Thus he appears to have at least a partially intact auditory (VIII) nerve. He has a gag reflex, and withdraws his tongue when a lemon drop is squeezed onto it. He also swallows when water is squeezed into his mouth, and resists when his shoulders are pushed down. Therefore, it appears that the glossopharyngeal (IX), vagus (X), accessory (XI), and hypoglossal (XII) nerves are grossly intact. Mr. D.'s reflexes are symmetrical and 2+. He has no snout or palmomental reflex. His Babinski reflex on both sides is negative.

The patient is uncooperative. He appears to perceive sound but does not answer questions. The interviewer makes an effort to be reassuring to the patient but receives no feedback. The patient remains mute and stuporous but has no other signs of catatonia. His affect is depressed. His thought content is unknown.

Step 2: Tag

3. I: I cannot find any nerve damage that may have silenced you. I'd like to find out what made you stop talking and moving so that I can help you.
   P: [No answer]

Step 3: Confront

4. I: You don't speak, and I cannot hear your thoughts. I don't know what bothers you. Please tell me.
   P: [No response]
5. I: I cannot hear the voices that you may hear. If you care to tell me, please do so.
   P: [No response]
6. I: Please take a pencil and write down what's bothering you.
   P: [Does not take the pencil]
7. I: I know you can hear me. Unfortunately, I cannot hear you. Help me! Please nod if you can hear me.
   P: [Looks down]

The interviewer continued to treat the patient as if he expected him to answer any time. He offered alternate ways of communication (Q. 6, 7). He provided feedback to him because a delusional and possibly hallucinating patient often does not realize that his thoughts cannot be heard and that others are unable to engage in telecommunication (Q. 4, 5, 7). Throughout this section, the interviewer presented himself as a helper. He addressed the patient on an adult level without patronizing him.

Step 4: Solve

Even though the patient does not respond, the interviewer reads him a consent form for an amobarbital interview and explains that the infusion may help him to talk. During the explanation, the patient stares into space. The wife signs the consent form in front of her husband.

Mr. D. receives the infusion by slow drip in his left arm. After approximately 4 minutes, he yawns. Alternatively, the interviewer could have offered the patient 2.5 mg of lorazepam and asked him to swallow it with a sip of water to help him move and talk again. If the patient did not respond, the interviewer could have then explained that the nurse would give him an intramuscular or intravenous injection to help him talk and move.

8. I: Mr. D., you are safe. You are perfectly safe. Can you hear me?
   P: [Faintly] Hmmm.

9. I: Mr. D., I'd like to talk to you. Is that okay?

P: Hmmm.

10. I: Can you hear me clearly?

P: Yeah. [Closes his eyes]

11. I: Do you remember? I read the consent form to you? Your wife signed for you. You couldn't.

P: Yeah.

12. I: Do you agree with her signing?

P: Hmmm. I . . . guess.

13. I: Is it okay? Can you sign now? [Gives patient a clipboard and a pen]

P: [Signs the form while sighing] Ahh. . . . Just . . . just do it . . .

14. I: The medication will help you. Help you feel safe. You will feel relaxed and tired. I want you to feel safe. Do you feel comfortable?

P: I'm scared. Don't hurt me!

15. I: I will not hurt you. You are safe. Tell me, what makes you scared?

P: [Anxiously looking around] Don't hurt me!

16. I: I want to help you. Are you hurting anywhere?

P: No. [Closes his eyes]

17. I: [Stops the infusion] Mr. D., are you sleepy?

P: [Yawns] Yes. Why don't you get it over with?

18. I: Get it over with? How do you feel?

P: Bad.

19. I: Do you feel safe with me?

P: [No answer, swallows]

20. I: I want you to feel safe. Do you feel safe here?

P: [Opens his eyes, starts crying]

21. I: I'm trying to help you. [Takes patient's hand] I want you to feel safe. Your wife may hold your hand. [Motions the wife to come over and hold the patient's hand] Do you feel safe now? Is this okay?

P: [No answer, stiffens up]

22. I: Are you still scared?

P: [Looks away from his wife] Yes.

23. I: Tell me what you are scared of.

P: [Whispering] They'll kill me.

24. I: Who are they?

P: [Looking at his wife] I don't know. [Yawning]

25. I: Do they talk to you?

P: You know . . . they do.

26. I: I can't hear them. Please tell me, what do they say?

P: "Mr. D., you have to go." [Yawning]

27. I: Mr. D., are you awake?

P: I'm tired. Doc, get it over with.

28. I: I won't hurt you, Mr. D.; what will *they* do to you?

P: Kill me.

29. I: You are safe here. I can help you.

P: [Looks to the side, bites his lip] Doc, why don't you do it now? Let's get it over with. Do what they tell you. Please, get it over with!

30. I: Mr. D., I'm not going to hurt you. You are safe. I want to help you. I want to make you feel better again.
   P: Just get it over with.
31. I: Mr. D., I want to help you. I want to find out what bothers you. I'm on your side. How long have they been trying to kill you?
   P: I don't know.
32. I: How did you find out?
   P: They came to my house . . . at night . . . funny noises.
33. I: When did you first notice?
   P: Some weeks ago.
34. I: Do you remember what day it was?
   P: I'm not sure.
35. I: Do you know what day it is today?
   P: No.
36. I: Just guess.
   P: Friday.
37. I: That's right. Do you know what month it is?
   P: November.
38. I: That's right, too. Do you know what date in November?
   P: No.
39. I: Guess.
   P: Maybe the 18th.
40. I: Yes, you're just one day off. So, they came some weeks ago?
   P: [Closes his eyes, sobbing]
41. I: Are you okay?
   P: I'm so scared. [Interviewer starts infusion again.]
42. I: Did they hurt you?
   P: They switched her on me. [Withdraws his hand from his wife and points at her] She's not my wife.
43. I: When did you find out?
   P: Two days ago.
44. I: How?
   P: She wanted me to eat and drink. It tasted funny.
45. I: What did you think it was?
   P: Poison.
46. I: Did you eat or drink it?
   P: No.
47. I: What else has she done to you?
   P: She brought me here.
48. I: For what?
   P: To get me killed.
49. I: Mr. D., this is a hospital. Your wife brought you here to get help for you. I'm your doctor and I want to help you. You are safe here.
   P: They make it look like a hospital. They'll get me.
50. I: Why will they want to get you?
   P: For what I've done.
51. I: What have you done?

P: Something awful.
52. I: Like what?
P: I don't know. But they know.
53. I: How do you know that you have done something awful?
P: Because I feel awful.

Step 5: Approve

54. I: You will be safe here. Nothing will happen to you.
P: They'll kill me because I talk to you.
55. I: You did the right thing. Now I know what bothers you and now I can help you. I will give you something that will strengthen you and help you to be less anxious.
P: [Looks around fearfully]
56. I: You have not talked for 2 days. Let's see how well your mind is still working. [The interviewer estimates the patient's intelligence with the Kent Test (Kent 1946). He tests the patient's recent memory by asking him whether he can recall the details of the neurological examination; however, he omits the four-word test that measures recall immediately and after 10 minutes because the barbiturate would possibly interfere with storage of new material. After about 20 more minutes, the patient becomes sleepy and the interviewer terminates the infusion.]

Amobarbital was the facilitator in blocking the patient's psychotic anxiety and disinhibiting him. The interviewer complemented this effect of amobarbital with reassurances in order to keep the patient talking. The patient remained in a somnolent state of reduced alertness. However, his speech was not slurred. He was attentive enough to grasp the meaning of the questions and answered them in a goal-directed way. The interviewer offered statements of safety and support (Q. 8, 14–16, 19–21, 28–31, 49, 54) and respect for the patient (Q. 9) and asked for the patient's consent to the interview (Q. 10–13). The interviewer then explored the patient's thought content and tested his cognitive functions.

Thought content. It became apparent during the interview that Mr. D. misinterpreted the infusion as an attempt to kill him (A. 17). Because the patient remained nearly mute and responded mainly emotionally, the interviewer explored the reason for his anxiety (Q. 19, 22, 23). The patient's predominant affect was delusional suspiciousness and the fear of being killed. Underlying that fear was guilt, which was driving the patient to surrender himself for "execution." The patient reported auditory hallucinations (A. 25, 26). He demonstrated delusions of persecution that involved his own wife and the interviewer, both puppets of an unidentified group of persecutors.[1] The patient's delusional interpretation eventually began to unfold (A. 23). Throughout the discussion, the interviewer stayed with the patient's central emotion—his suspiciousness about being killed.

Cognitive functions. The patient was oriented to time (A. 35–39), to his own person (A. 26), and to the doctor's role (A. 27, 29). He was oriented to place; however, he misinterpreted the hospital as a place for execution (A. 49). During his stupor, the patient was aware of his surroundings. He recalled that his wife had signed the consent form for him (A. 11). He also signed the consent form himself (A. 13). His signing has two explanations: 1) the patient showed negative obedience, or 2) he had delusional guilt and wished to be punished.

Diagnosis

With the help of amobarbital, the interviewer confirmed the diagnosis of major depression, severe, with mood-incongruent psychotic and catatonic features, with hallucinations (A. 32), guilt (A. 50–52), and delusions of persecution (A. 23, 28, 31–34) and of his wife being an impostor (A. 42). Thus the patient is diagnosed with acute Capgras's syndrome, which makes him see the psychiatrist and the wife as persecutors.

During the interview, the patient gave no indication of stupor with mania. Also, his history was negative for bipolar disorder. A dementing process was unlikely, as the patient was oriented and could give a coherent account of his behavior, even though it was based on hallucinatory perceptions and delusional thinking. Because the patient signed the consent form (with his right hand), agraphia could be excluded, along with all forms of aphasia (A. 13).

6. Technique: Rapid Tranquilization for Catatonia With Excessive Motor Activity

As in the above interview, establish a working diagnosis (i.e., catatonia with excessive motor activity) with these patients and indicate whether the

---

[1] It is typical of the early stage of a persecutory delusion that its driving forces are still faceless. After a delusion becomes more chronic, the affective component usually vanishes, whereas the thought content becomes more organized and elaborate.

amobarbital interview was successful. If it was not, an alternative method is necessary to reverse catatonia.

First, ask informants about the patient's psychiatric history, especially episodes of muteness and stupor and treatment interventions and their outcome. Second, focus on the patient's behavior before the onset of stupor and muteness. These symptoms and signs indicate whether the patient is presently in a depressive or manic state of muteness and what his present thought content might be. Third, choose the appropriate pharmacological or somatic treatment before the interview, as discussed below.

Amobarbital. Amobarbital intravenous infusion breaks muteness in 60% of patients (McCall et al. 1992). It is not clear whether the response depends on the diagnosis or not; therefore, you may include amobarbital infusion as one of your options of intervention.

Methylphenidate. In our own clinical experience and a few case reports, there is the suggestion that methylphenidate infusion may succeed in breaking muteness when amobarbital has failed (Frost 1989). In Frost's study, methylphenidate was effective only at an infusion rate of 40 mg over 90 seconds. A slower rate failed to break the muteness. Because intravenous infusion of dextroamphetamine or methylphenidate is banned in the United States, a higher-dose oral application may be an alternative. As the lowest starting dose, consider methylphenidate 30 mg po or dextroamphetamine 20 mg po. You may increase the dosage in 10-mg increments up to methylphenidate 60 mg po and dextroamphetamine 40 mg po. We have used this method successfully in depressed patients with psychomotor retardation but not yet with mute patients.

Rapid tranquilization. The literature describes rapid tranquilization with hostile and excited patients who are not mute (Donlon et al. 1979; Dubin 1988; Dubin and Feld 1989; Dubin et al. 1985, 1986; Neborsky et al. 1981; Salano et al. 1989; Sangiovanni et al. 1973; Tupin 1985). Rapid tranquilization may be attempted with patients for whom amobarbital has failed. The advantage of this method is that you can continue rapid tranquilization until the patient becomes communicative.

Here is a modified protocol (Dubin 1988; Mason and Granacher 1980) for rapid tranquilization. The original protocol was designed to tranquilize an excited (i.e., centrally overstimulated) patient. We recommend it to reverse stupor and muteness, which may also represent a dopaminergic overstimulation of certain brain areas. Give haloperidol 10 mg im per hour.

Repeat every hour until the patient starts to walk and talk. If there is no response after 60 mg im, stop the injection. Then, beginning with the next day, continue with 30 mg po tid on the following days until catatonia resolves. If response occurs on the first day prior to a maximum dosage of 60 mg, give 1.5 times this dosage as a concentrate, divided in three equal parts po, on each following day. For example, if a patient responds to 20 mg on the first day, give 10 mg of concentrate po tid on the following days until catatonia and hallucinations and delusions disappear and the patient develops full insight into the morbid nature of his hallucinations and delusions.

This protocol is recommended if the patient is seriously ill and does not take in fluids, is incontinent and sleepless, and is at risk for dehydration. If the patient's vital signs are stable and he takes in fluids, you may start haloperidol concentrate 5 mg po tid and increase the dosage daily by 15 mg (i.e., 10 mg po tid, 15 mg po tid) until the patient receives 20 mg po tid.

Electroconvulsive therapy. Pretreatment with ECT is helpful if the patient is in acute distress. Because this treatment requires general anesthesia, you need written informed consent by next of kin, a court order, or sometimes both.

Verbal approach. Pointed questions can make the difference between breaking through the muteness during amobarbital infusion or after treatment with haloperidol. With a manic-stuporous or catatonic-excited patient, use repeated invitations to communicate in words rather than in thoughts or by extrasensory perception (ESP). Mix statements of reassurance with invitations to communicate verbally. Remember, bipolar patients can present in a mixed state and can switch from a depressive to a manic state. Likewise, grandiose thinking may switch into persecutory thinking and vice versa. In the following section, we describe how to attempt to communicate with a stuporous, catatonic, excited patient.

7. Five Steps to Return to Reality

Step 1: Listen. Conduct a neurological and a mental status examination. Assess the presence of reactive movements, intense muscle tone, a snout spasm, and spontaneous posturing that points to a catatonic, excited, mute, and stuporous state. The more of the seven catatonic symptoms you can identify (see above), the more likely it is that the patient has a catatonic-excited stupor associated with a bipolar disorder, manic state, or catatonic schizophrenia.

Step 2: Tag. Summarize your findings to the patient. Tell her you do not find any nerve damage and that you feel she can and will answer with words when she is ready. Ask her whether she is ready now. If she remains silent, move on to the next step.

Step 3: Confront. The catatonic-excited patient frequently has grandiose delusions and delusional perceptions. She may believe that she can hear other people's thoughts, that others can hear her thoughts, and that she can communicate by means of ESP. Therefore, she experiences speech as superfluous for communication. Her history before her muteness—if available—helps you here. This point is illustrated in the following case description.

> Ms. M. is age 24 years. While mute, she had an outburst of violence that ended in her throwing objects at her parents' heads. When later questioned regarding this behavior, she says she became frustrated with her parents because they did not respond to her thoughts and pretended instead that they could not hear her thoughts.

Therefore, you should prompt your patient as follows:

> Can you hear my words? Are you answering me with your thoughts? Please, answer me with words. I'd like to communicate with you in words, not just in thoughts.

If the patient does not answer, tell her it is important that you find out what may be bothering her. For example, if she is dehydrated, tell her you are concerned about her life and that you will give her some treatment, and explain it to her. Dehydration from a refusal to drink can be an early symptom of physical distress in a catatonic patient. Such a patient may fear that the fluid contains poison, as you may learn after the patient starts talking.

Step 4: Solve. Because the patient may be delusionally convinced that you can hear her thoughts, do not challenge her fixed false beliefs directly when you initiate the interview; instead, reiterate,

> Let's communicate on all channels with our thoughts, our emotions, and our words. Will you communicate in words with me also? Why don't you like to use any words?

She may explain suddenly that words are not fast enough:

Words do not convey the hologram of my impressions. I prefer to transmit to you directly my panoramic holistic views. Why don't you tune in on extrasensory perception now?

Then, you may tell the patient,

Do you feel that I can read your mind? Do you feel we are connecting?

If she says yes, you may say,

I'm not sure. Let's confirm what you are thinking. What is your thought right now?

Then say,

Can you read my thoughts? Let's compare what I'm thinking with what you are receiving.

After the patient responds verbally, explore her delusional thinking and perception, her degree of insight, and her orientation. Focus on the symptoms that preceded and followed the onset of her muteness. When her delusional perspective is explored, her entire history may open up.

Step 5: Approve. Emphasize that you are glad that now you can communicate on all channels with her and that you would like to keep all channels open so that you can communicate through mind, emotions, and words. Obviously, nonverbal communication has a different meaning to you than to the patient. However, at this point the patient is not able to realize the difference between nonverbal and extrasensory communication.

8. Interview: Bipolar I Disorder, Most Recent Episode Manic, With Catatonic Features

Mr. C. is a 22-year-old, white, 6'1", slim, blond, single man. The patient's mother reports,

My son has quit talking. We went through this once before when he was 17. It started the same way. He appeared as if somebody was winding him up, more and more. He moved faster, he talked a lot, he didn't sleep at night, and then, all of a sudden, he got this grin on his face and you couldn't get through to him. He stands in the middle of the room like a pillar.

His mother relates that in high school he was a good student, especially in science and math, and had an active social life. He never smoked, drank, or used any illegal drugs. Then Mr. C. stopped sleeping. He talked continuously and moved around a lot. Suddenly, he seemed to make only incomplete, hinting remarks, smiled, took strange postures, and talked to himself. Mr. C.'s mother continues with her story.

> When I took our son to the doctor way back, she told me he had catatonic schizophrenia. They hospitalized him and he snapped out of it. He took haloperidol for $2\frac{1}{2}$ months but refused to go back to the doctor after his prescription ran out. After his first hospitalization he changed; he seemed awkward, often somewhat silly, even though he graduated with honors. He attended college for 18 months, studying computer science, then left to do consulting. All of a sudden, he got all wound up and then stopped talking.

Mr. C.'s mother describes Mr. C.'s father as "having the traveling bug." Twenty years earlier, when the patient was age 2 years, the father had stopped working, talked about a great invention, became very energetic, and then disappeared. The family had had no contact with him since that time. Mr. C.'s mother, an X-ray technician, had supported the family. She never had any psychiatric problems, nor did Mr. C.'s 24-year-old sister, who is married.

Step 1: Listen

Mr. C. walks into the office looking edgy and jumpy. When the interviewer addresses him, Mr. C. glances at him, then looks around and ignores him. The interviewer calls his name again. Mr. C. takes a quick look at him, then continues to look around in the room. When asked to sit down, Mr. C. keeps standing. The interviewer takes him by the arm and tries to lead him to a chair. Mr. C.'s arm stiffens. He resists being led, but then suddenly goes along and sits down, staring at the wall. The interviewer takes Mr. C.'s hand, pulls it up, and bends it over the patient's head. The patient keeps this posture. His mouth is half open and forms a faint grin. His affect appears to be amused, as if Mr. C. is elated.

The interviewer conducts a neurological examination. It does not reveal any focal symptoms. The cranial nerves are intact. Reflexes are 2+ and symmetrical. When the interviewer bends Mr. C.'s arm, the patient resists and then allows the arm to be bent without resistance (clap knife rigidity). Mr. C. allows a neurological examination without active participation and also without showing hostility. He is not responding in any way to the interviewer's interventions. His behavior gives the impression that he is in a different sphere.

Mr. C. is mute and alert, but not stuporous. He shows catalepsy. He has no echolalia. His mother described some posturing. Automatic obedience is not evaluated. His affect appears blunt, but not depressed. Mood, thought content, memory, orientation, insight, and judgment cannot be assessed.

Differential Diagnosis

1. *Bipolar disorder, manic.* Mr. C.'s history of a manic-like episode points toward an affective disorder. The father's history supports this diagnosis.
2. *Schizophrenia, catatonic subtype.* Mr. C.'s social behavior does not seem to have fully recovered from his previous catatonic episode, as it generally does in bipolar disorder.
3. No evidence for drug-induced muteness.
4. *Neuroleptic malignant syndrome.* This diagnosis is excluded because the patient has not taken any neuroleptics during at least the past 5 years.

Step 2: Tag

(I = interviewer; P = patient)

1. I: Mr. C., you are not talking. I cannot help you if I don't know what you are thinking. I worry you are hurting somewhere. Please, tell me.
   P: [No response]

Step 3: Confront

2. I: Mr. C., I cannot hear your thoughts. Can you think and use your mouth and tell me your thoughts?
   P: [No response]
3. I: Mr. C., your mother told me you didn't speak for a while, when you were 17. It seems to me that the same thing is happening to you now.
   P: [No response]
4. I: If you cannot start talking, I would like to hospitalize you and give you some medication to help you talk again.
   P: [No response]
5. I: Mr. C., I have some papers here that I would like for you to read.
   P: [Ignores the papers]
6. I: If you can't read them now, I'll ask your mother to sign them. As soon as you are ready, I would like you to sign them too.

Step 4: Solve

Because Mr. C. has had a similar previous episode, and because he is not in any obvious distress but has stopped drinking and eating, the interviewer decides against amobarbital and instead opts for rapid tranquilization, with the goal of interviewing him after 24 hours, as is recommended for manic patients.

The patient is hospitalized. After 18 hours of rapid tranquilization with haloperidol, Mr. C. starts to eat and drink. The nurses report that he maintains eye contact, but does not speak. When the interviewer enters his room, the patient sits on his bed with a dystonic reaction, with his head moved to the right and both eyes wide open and rolled upward. The patient is given benztropine mesylate (Cogentin) 1 mg im; after 1 hour his neck muscles are softened and his eyes are in normal position.

7. I: Hi, Mr. C. My name is Dr. O. I am trying to get in touch with you and find out what's going on with you and how I can be of help.

P: [Looks at him and grins]

8. I: I'm glad you look at me. I'm glad to sense your feelings. I'm glad you can hear me!

P: [Keeps grinning]

9. I: I'd like to hear you too.

P: [Keeps grinning]

10. I: Say what you are thinking with your mouth!

P: [Grinning] You know.

11. I: How's that?

P: You hear my thoughts.

12. I: I'd like to hear your thoughts by listening to your words . . . as you use your mouth.

P: [With normal speed] No, no. . . . They are flying by. Thoughts are racing, running, jumping . . . away from words.

13. I: I talked to you yesterday. Do you remember?

P: [Grins] The window without windows.

14. I: You didn't answer me.

P: You heard me.

15. I: How can I? I can't hear your thoughts.

P: Thoughts are so loud.

16. I: They are loud for you. Do you remember? Remember what I asked you?

P: You shared with me. You put up, up in the space, holding up to the space, putting my hand above me.

17. I: Why did you not answer me?

P: Unconnected . . . in the fourth dimension. We shared thoughts. Thoughts share the space.

18. I: What do you mean?

P: It doesn't matter.

19. I: How do you feel now?
    P: Great.
20. I: Can you tell me?
    P: Flying. Skying. No weight highing.
21. I: Can you tell me what date it is?
    P: It doesn't matter. Dates are time and time is timeless.
22. I: Do you know it anyway?
    P: [Grins] The one hundred and fourteenth day of the fourth month, the fifth day of the fourth week.
23. I: [Looking up the day of the year in his calendar, smiling] You are right! It's Friday, the twenty-fourth of April.
    P: And 1990 years real B.C., which is 3 years before B.C.
24. I: You did not eat or drink yesterday.
    P: [Grins] It doesn't matter. Matter turns into mind. Mind turns into matter. [Humming] Matter doesn't matter. Matter matters not. Matter matters for mindless minds.
25. I: Do you remember when we first met?
    P: The large windowless office that opens all windows. To open the windows, have no windows. No windows open the windows of the mind. Close your windows to open the windows of the mind.
26. I: Mr. C., does anything bother you?
    P: Anything, everything. To fill out the space of the universe with my mind. To flow out and to fill out. Filling the endless space with mind.
27. I: I'm glad that you share thoughts and words. I will keep you on haloperidol to help you slow down your thoughts so we can keep talking. [At this point, the interviewer must decide between proceeding to Step 5—approve—and terminating the interview, and assessing the patient's thought content, other mental status functions, and history.]

Because the patient displayed eye contact and emotion, the interviewer built on this nonverbal interaction and fed it back to the patient. He invited him to put his thoughts into words (Q. 9, 10, 12) and Mr. C. followed through (A. 10), even though he was convinced the interviewer could hear his thoughts. The interviewer did not contradict his belief but invited Mr. C. to use words also.[2] To keep the patient talking, the interviewer used the patient's reference system and words whenever possible. He avoided confronting the patient with reality in order not to drive him back into muteness.

The patient used opposites (A. 13, 21, 24, 25), riddles (A. 21, 24, 25), and symbolic grandiose wordings (A. 16, 17, 20, 22, 23, 26). Yet his answers

---

[2] Contradictions restrict an excited, possibly manic patient, whereas use of additional means, such as words, empower him and build on his expansive tendencies.

referred to accurate observations. The conference room was indeed without windows. The interviewer had placed the patient's hand over his head. Even though Mr. C. reported racing thoughts, he talked in a near-normal rhythm. Only the lack of articles and conjunctions portrayed his racing thoughts.

The patient's affect was bright and nearly ecstatic. He was experiencing an elated mood (A. 20). His thought content was delusional, symbolic, and grandiose. He appeared to feel that he had to fill the universe with his mind (A. 26). He was oriented to time, but used an unusual way of expressing the date in a playful, punning way (A. 22). His short-term memory seemed to be intact (A. 13, 16, 25). The interviewer did not test Mr. C.'s insight. However, Mr. C. recognized his racing, loud thoughts and unconnectedness without evaluating them as symptoms of an illness (A. 12, 15, 17). His muteness documented that his judgment was impaired.

Diagnosis

The patient's mental status supports a diagnosis of bipolar disorder, manic, with mood-congruent thought content. His awkward formulations might prompt some clinicians to consider a schizoaffective disorder or schizophrenia, because Mr. C. became a loner and had some residual symptoms after his first episode at age 17 years.

9. Catatonia, Amobarbital or Lorazepam, and Tranquilization in Psychiatric Disorders

Listed in Table 6–1 are differential diagnoses of catatonia (Abrams and Taylor 1976; Altshuler et al. 1986), adapted to DSM-IV. In some of these disorders, catatonia may serve a purpose, as we have seen in our two patients. In Mr. D., muteness was a sign of persecutory fear and suspicion as he withdrew into himself. In Mr. C., muteness occurred during a state of elation (Abrams and Taylor 1976; Altshuler et al. 1986). In manic stupor, in contrast to depressive stupor, which often develops slowly, a patient can suddenly switch into a state of hyperalertness and muteness. In Mr. C., muteness indicated a state of ecstatic elation in which he indulged in an autistic world of pantheistic connectedness but was completely withdrawn from reality. Muteness may serve a third function—as anger control. Keeping all emotions and thoughts bottled up may prevent the patient from hurting somebody.

As to the mechanism of action of amobarbital and lorazepam, psychological factors such as disinhibition and anxiety reduction have been discussed above. A direct effect on the dopamine receptors D_1 and D_2 in the mesolimbic and mesostriatal systems may be of importance because gamma-aminobutyric acid (GABA) regulates dopamine neurons in these systems and lorazepam facilitates GABA activity (Salam and Kilzieh 1988). In addition, the GABAergic system reduces the synaptic transmission in a wide variety of stimulating and inhibitory pathways. The net effect of amobarbital and lorazepam appears to be disinhibition. Therefore, both have been applied to modify behaviors in which the patient voluntarily or involuntarily holds back information.

Amobarbital reverses muteness temporarily in over 60% of cases (McCall et al. 1992). Patients who do not respond to amobarbital or lorazepam may respond to stimulants or to rapid neuroleptic tranquilization. You may try a stimulant drug such as methylphenidate hydrochloride in a dosage of 30 mg for adults or dextroamphetamine sulfate in at least a 20-mg dosage.

If drug treatment fails, you may consider emergency ECT. This is especially indicated if the patient is dehydrated. To use this therapy, you

---

Table 6–1.   Differential diagnosis of catatonia (using DSM-IV diagnoses)

- Schizophrenia
    Paranoid type
    Disorganized type
    Catatonic type
- Schizophreniform disorder
- Schizoaffective disorder
- Brief psychotic disorder
- Mood disorder
    Major depressive disorder
    Bipolar disorder, most recent
    episode manic
    Bipolar disorder, most recent
    episode mixed
    Bipolar disorder, most recent
    episode depressed
- Dementia
    With delusions
    With depressed mood
    Substance-induced persisting
    (e.g., phencyclidine)

- Somatoform disorder
    Conversion disorder (hysterical
    aphonia)
- Dissociative disorder
- Factitious disorder (malingering)
- Disorders of childhood
    Autistic disorder
    Selective mutism
- Substance-induced catatonia
    Neuroleptic agents
    Phencyclidine
    Maprotiline hydrochloride
    Corticosteroids
    Antihypertensive agents
    Alcohol
    Mescaline
    Morphine
    Aspirin
- Coma vigilante

Source. Adapted from Abrams and Taylor 1976; Altshuler et al. 1986; Strub and Black 1977.

have to exclude increased intracranial pressure (which would be signaled by the presence of a papilledema).

Indications and Contraindications of the Amobarbital or Lorazepam Interview

The amobarbital or lorazepam interview is a diagnostic tool for mute, catatonic, or regressed psychotic patients. It is used for the following purposes:

- To assess orientation, memory, reasoning, and the presence of hallucinations and delusions in noncommunicative patients, patients with depressive stupor, or patients with a history of psychosis (Hoch 1946; Lindeman 1932). However, there could be a problem with the validity of testimonies obtained under the influence of amobarbital. For example, patients with posttraumatic stress disorder may report events that never happened.
- To reverse amnesia in patients with fugue states, dissociative states, or dissociative identity disorder (multiple personality disorder).
- To reveal the suppressed purpose of pseudoneurological symptoms, such as paralysis, pseudoseizures, anesthesias, and other so-called conversion symptoms.
- To identify lying. Under the influence of amobarbital, the patient may reveal things that he later regrets. Furthermore, there is no guarantee that his revelations are indeed factual; they may be a mixture of fact and fiction. Also, the patient may later have difficulties remembering what he said while medicated. Therefore, results should be confirmed by family members and after the patient has recovered.
- To identify the emotional trauma of events, such as rape, physical abuse, or torture. Limiting amobarbital's use to overcoming catatonia is less problematic than its use for lie or trauma detection, because the main goals in the former usage are to make the patient talk and assess his orientation rather than to identify a trauma. In addition, it is more important to know whether a patient *has* delusions and hallucinations than it is to know the specific kind he has. Thus, the application of amobarbital in catatonia is not dependent on detection of the truth or a lie.

Overall, the amobarbital interview should be used in the patient's best interest to help clarify symptoms with his consent and in confidentiality. The principle of the Hippocratic oath "Do no harm!" should always prevail.

As we have seen, psychotic disorders may interfere with the interview because the patient's perception of the interview situation and of the interviewer is distorted by hallucinations or delusions. Furthermore, catatonic features may render the patient unable to respond because she is mute or has increased mobility to such an extent that she cannot be redirected and successfully addressed. Widespread neurotransmitter systems are overstimulated or overinhibited in these psychotic disorders.

A neuronal malfunction or loss is also associated with the next group of disorders that can interfere with the interviewing process: the cognitive disorders.

PART III

COGNITIVE
IMPAIRMENT

THE LANGUAGE OF
THE FAILING BRAIN

COGNITIVE IMPAIRMENT
THE LANGUAGE OF
THE FAILING BRAIN

◆ ◆ ◆ ◆ ◆

Habet cerebrum sensus arcem.
The brain is the citadel of the senses.

Gaius Plinius Secundus (A.D. 23-24–79)
Historia Naturalis

◆ ◆ ◆ ◆ ◆

Elements of Cognitive Dysfunction

When the functioning of the brain falters, perceptions become disrupted, memory fails, and conclusions and predictions do not follow the premises on which they were based. Patients perceive, remember, conclude, or predict erroneously. We call disturbances of this process *cognitive dysfunctions*. Cognitive dysfunctions frequently result from a demonstrable lesion of brain tissue (e.g., death of specific neurons, like the death of cholinergic neurons in dementia of the Alzheimer's type [DAT]) or from reversible metabolic disturbances. The signs and symptoms of such lesions include changes in

213

- Level of consciousness
- Perception
- Attention
- Concentration
- Orientation
- Immediate, recent, and remote memory
- Ability to recognize familiar objects (gnosia, opposite of agnosia)
- Ability to comprehend spoken or written language and express thoughts by speech or writing (phasia, opposite of aphasia)
- Ability to perform simple tasks (ideomotor praxis, opposite of apraxia) and more complex acts (ideational praxis)
- Executive functioning (i.e., planning, organizing, sequencing, abstracting)

Cognitive Impairment as an Obstacle to the Interview

Cognitive impairment can disrupt your communication with a patient because of the patient's decreased awareness, inattention, distractibility, disorientation, amnesia, confabulation, aphasia, agnosia, apraxia, perseveration, mental retardation, and social indiscretion. Cognitive impairment can also lead to hallucinations, delusions, and catatonia, all of which may disrupt rapport. However, the symptoms and signs of cognitive impairment are so obvious in these cases that most interviewers recognize, diagnose, and manage them correctly.

Difficulties in interviewing patients with cognitive dysfunction arise from the following four sources.

Mild impairment.   If symptoms and signs are mild, cognitive impairment may escape your detection. Furthermore, if the patient lacks the insight to recognize his impairments, he cannot complain about it, or, when a patient does recognize impairments, he may hide or deny them. If confronted with his impairments, he may rationalize them as loss of interest rather than as an inability to perform. Thus, the patient's lack of insight, rationalization, and resistance to face his deficits may impede the interview.

Concealment of impairment by other symptoms.   A patient's impairment can be concealed by symptoms that appear to belong to noncognitive psychiatric disorders. Clinically, we expect that, in cognitive disorders, intellectual defects dominate over affective symptoms and signs, and that in mood disorders, the reverse is true. When the primary cognitive impairment becomes obscured by the severity of the affective or behavioral symptoms, signs, and behaviors, you may become distracted by the latter and fail to detect their cognitive underpinning. At times, clinicians fail to spot cognitive dysfunctions because they have prematurely established a diagnosis before 1) a comprehensive mental status examination of cognitive functions, and 2) a differential diagnosis of the key symptoms have been completed. Common clinical errors include classifying patients as manic, delusional, depressive, or schizophrenic when they have frontal lobe or other brain damage. For example, a middle-aged veteran was judged by the busy clinician to be an uncooperative schizophrenic patient because he stammered his answers and did not follow simple requests, such as sitting down. Later, a thorough examination showed that a left-sided frontal brain tumor interfered with the patient's ability to express himself (destruction of Broca's area, which is Brodmann area 44) and caused ideomotor apraxia.

Diagnosis obscured by social history. A patient's social history may suggest a psychiatric disorder other than a cognitive disorder. The patient may have high intelligence and a high social status. If she develops depression in conjunction with beginning dementia, her intelligence and her ability to rationalize may conceal her dementia and she may be seen as merely depressed. If she is not reevaluated neuropsychiatrically and physically, the dementia may remain concealed.

Cognitive dysfunction misdiagnosed as recurrence of another psychiatric disorder. A patient's psychiatric history may suggest a relapse of another preexisting psychiatric disorder, thereby obscuring the concomitant occurrence of a new cognitive disorder. Patients who have an established psychiatric history with an intermittent course (e.g., major depression or bipolar disorder) may thus only be diagnosed as having a relapse of that documented disorder when they become symptomatic again. The clinician may miss diagnosing the new cognitive disorder because he failed to thoroughly test the patient's neuropsychiatric functions.

Profile of Cognitive Deficits in Cognitive Disorders

A comprehensive yet focused neuropsychiatric mental status examination allows you to correctly identify the symptoms, signs, and behaviors of a cognitive disorder. Such an examination contrasts with a nonindividualized routine examination of cognition, which may neglect to take into account the patient's age, education, intelligence, and coexisting psychiatric disorders. History taking complements a comprehensive mental status examination but cannot replace it. For example, if a wife complains that her husband no longer seems able to operate his tractor, the cause could be a cognitive or affective impairment. The interviewer needs to discern which of the two sources explains the patient's impairment best.

In handling cognitive dysfunction, you have three tasks:

1. Obtain a detailed history from the patient or the informant to identify which symptoms and signs preexisted and which coincided with the recent problem.
2. Detect cognitive deficits in the patient's history and mental status, such as problems in rapport and inattention or lack of comprehension or forgetfulness.
3. Select the best mental status tests for the problem by identifying the brain functions presumably affected by the suspected disorders.

In Tables III–1 through III–3, a profile of cognitive dysfunctions as observed in the patients presented in Chapters 7–11 is given. This group does not constitute a statistically representative sample of cognitive impairment disorders, but indicates possible pitfalls in mental status assessment and diagnosis if cognitive functions are not tested. The + and − signs in Tables III–1 through III–3 are provided as if impairments were clearly and categorically present or absent. This approach is taken for its heuristic value and to avoid confusing hedging by using too many gradations such as +/−, ++/−, +/− −, etc. The severity of the measurable cognitive impairments is dependent on the location and size of the lesion, which determines the stage of the disorder. Thus, the + and − signs provide a relative comparison among the disorders at an early stage.

Inattention and lack of concentration.   Attention-deficit/hyperactivity disorder (ADHD) and two cognitive disorders—delirium and DAT—present with inattentiveness. For such patients you have to repeat the digits of the digit span test or the brief word list used for immediate recall. The attention of a patient with dementia due to Pick's disease often depends on the severity of the patient's motor restlessness. Inattention may be secondary to motor restlessness or to a tendency to perseverate.

Table III–1. Deficits in the early stages of disorders with cognitive dysfunctions—attention, orientation, and memory

Disorder	Attention		Orientation			Memory		
	Serial 7s, 3s	Digit span	Time	Place	Person	Immediate	Recent	Remote
Attention-deficit hyperactivity disorder[a]	+	+	−	−	−	(+)	(+)	−
Amnestic disorder	−	−	+	+	−	−	+	(+)
Delirium	+	+	+	+	−	+	+	−
Vascular dementia	−	−	+	−	−	−	+	−
Dementia due to Pick's disease	+	+	−	−	−	−	−	−
Dementia of the Alzheimer's type	+	+	+	+	−	+	+	−
Mental retardation	(+)	(+)	+	−	−	−	(+)	−
Affective[b] disorder with cognitive impairment	(+)	(+)	(+)	−	−	−	(+)	−

Note. − = cognitive impairment usually absent. + = cognitive impairment usually present. (+) = cognitive impairment caused by factors other than system-specific brain lesions.
[a]Attention-deficit/hyperactivity disorder is not listed under cognitive disorders in DSM-IV. However, it is a chronic condition that shares attention deficit, impulsivity, labile affect, and, frequently, disturbances in motor activity, learning, and social judgment with the group of cognitive disorders.
[b]Includes mania and depression.

Pseudoinattention.   The patient with mental retardation appears inattentive if a test exceeds his intellectual capacity. Test his attentiveness on *his* performance level. Affective disorders may have a secondary effect on attention. The manic patient is too distracted and the depressed patient too unmotivated and slow in mentation to do well on serial 3s and 7s and digit span. But if the interviewer can eliminate distraction in the manic patient or encourage the depressed patient, the performance of these patients is usually adequate.

Disorientation.   Of the three subtests (orientation to time, place, and person), orientation to time is the most sensitive. All patients with DSM-IV (American Psychiatric Association 1994) cognitive disorders are disoriented to time, except patients in the early stages of Pick's disease and patients with milder forms of mental retardation (classified under disorders usually first diagnosed in infancy, childhood, or adolescence). Disorientation to place is

Table III–2.   Deficits in the early stages of disorders with cognitive dysfunctions—focal neuropsychiatric signs

| | Neuropsychiatric sign | | | | |
Disorder	Aphasia	Agnosia	Apraxia	Shift sets	Pathological reflexes
Attention-deficit/ hyperactivity disorder[a]	–	–	-	–	–
Amnestic disorder	–	–	–	–	(+)
Delirium	–	–	–	–	–
Vascular dementia	–	–	+	–	+
Dementia due to Pick's disease	+	–	–	+	+
Dementia of the Alzheimer's type	+	–	+	–	–
Mental retardation	–	–	(+)	–	–
Affective[b] disorder with cognitive impairment	–	–	–	–	–

Note.   – = cognitive impairment usually absent. + = cognitive impairment usually present.
(+) = cognitive impairment caused by factors other than system-specific brain lesions.
[a]Attention-deficit/hyperactivity disorder is not listed under cognitive disorders in DSM-IV. However, it is a chronic condition that shares attention deficit, impulsivity, labile affect, and, frequently, disturbances in motor activity, learning, and social judgment with the group of cognitive disorders.
[b]Includes mania and depression.

characteristic for patients with delirium, amnestic states, or progressed Picks disease and DAT. Disorientation to person may occur in the delirious and amnestic patient and in a late state of dementia of any type.

Pseudodisorientation. Patients with severe major depression may appear disoriented to time because of psychomotor retardation and lack of motivation. Patients with mania may appear disoriented because of their distractibility. Encouragement and patience can overcome the patient's negative attitude or distractibility and assess the degree of disorientation.

Memory impairment. Immediate recall beyond three words or more is impaired in patients with DAT or ADHD. ADHD patients often need repetition to recall four words. In the delirious patient, immediate memory fluctuates with the severity of the disorder.

Table III–3. Deficits in the early stages of disorders with cognitive dysfunctions—intelligence

	Intellectual ability			
Disorder	Problem solving	Knowledge	Arithmetic	Judgment
Attention-deficit/ hyperactivity disorder[a]	–	–	(+)	–
Amnestic disorder	–	–	–	–
Delirium	+	–	+	+
Vascular dementia	+	–	+	+
Dementia due to Pick's disease	–	–	–	+
Dementia of the Alzheimer's type	+	–	+	+
Mental retardation	+	+	+	–
Affective[b] disorder with cognitive impairment	–	–	–	+

Note. – = cognitive impairment usually absent. + = cognitive impairment usually present. (+) = cognitive impairment caused by factors other than system-specific brain lesions.
[a]Attention-deficit/hyperactivity disorder is not listed under cognitive disorders in DSM-IV. However, it is a chronic condition that shares attention deficit, impulsivity, labile affect, and, frequently, disturbances in motor activity, learning, and social judgment with the group of cognitive disorders.
[b]Includes mania and depression.

Recent memory is severely disturbed in amnestic disorder—which gives the disorder its name—but also in delirium and most forms of dementia, with a notable exception of early Pick's disease, which may be misdiagnosed as a mood disorder. In ADHD, the recent memory disturbance is relative to the number of items proposed in the memory test and to the patient's motivation to remember. Patients with mental retardation fail when given four words intermingled with an abstract word, but may succeed if given three concrete objects meaningful for them.

Remote memory is most often affected in amnestic states and becomes progressively impaired with chronic progressive dementia.

Pseudomemory impairment.   The severity of the affective disorder determines the degree to which recent memory is disrupted. Patients with major depression especially complain about failing memory when, in fact, the deficit is a result of their lack of motivation and interest.

Focal impairment: aphasia, agnosia, and apraxia.   Focal neuropsychiatric impairment depends on the localization of the lesion. Aphasia, agnosia, and apraxia may become prominent in patients with vascular dementia and DAT. DAT patients show problems with agraphia before the aphasia emerges. Under time pressure, they have difficulties generating word lists (e.g., of animals, of words starting with the same letter).

Patients with Pick's disease seem to be affected at a later point in the disease. In the earlier stages of the disease, they are more likely to show difficulties with shifting sets and thus show perseveration and pathological reflexes, secondary to the primary atrophy of the frontal lobe. Patients with mental retardation may have no apraxia if the task given is concrete and simple enough for the patient to understand.

Pathological reflexes and responses.   Depending on the type of the disorder, cognitive disorders may be associated with three types of pathological reflexes:

1. Frontal releasing signs (snout, rooting, palmomental, glabellar), observed in advanced frontal lobe disorders such as Pick's disease, severe alcohol dementia, or vascular and neoplastic disorders
2. Positive Babinski reflex, observed in subcortical vascular dementia, lacunar type
3. Lateral nystagmus, sometimes observed in ADHD

Intellectual impairment. To gauge patients' intelligence, you have to compare their problem-solving and arithmetic capabilities with their fund of knowledge. Because ADHD in children also is associated with specific learning disabilities, patients may show intelligence deficits that parallel their circumscribed learning disability. Thus, you can expect poor performance on the Rapid Approximate Intelligence Test (Wilson 1967) in those patients who have a learning disability that affects their mathematical ability.

Problem solving is primarily affected in patients with DAT and vascular dementia, whereas knowledge is relatively spared in early atrophy. If they can be focused, patients in an early stage of Pick's disease can still solve problems. In patients with mental retardation, the intellectual impairment is uniform. Problem solving, knowledge, and arithmetic ability show comparable and equally low performance.

Pseudointellectual impairment. Major depression slows thinking, and mania speeds it up and makes it erratic. The depressed patient has a tendency to respond to problem-solving tasks with "I don't know" or "I can't do it." The patient with mania may offer a guessed solution rather than a computed one. If you encourage and focus the patient, problem solving is possible. However, speed slows down in depression and the error rate increases in mania.

Impairment of judgment. Several DSM-IV Axis I disorders affect social judgment. Most cognitive disorders cause deficits in judgment. This deficit in judgment corresponds to the other cognitive deficits. In Pick's disease, deterioration of social judgment is an early leading symptom.

In bipolar disorder, manic, impairment in judgment corresponds to elation in mood. Risk-taking behavior is increased and frequently leads to painful consequences. Substance abuse often presents with impairment in social judgment.

Impairment of executive cognitive functions. Executive cognitive functioning is defined in DSM-IV as planning, organizing, sequencing, and abstracting. More specifically, these functions include anticipation, goal selection, self-monitoring, and the use of feedback. These functions are based on three frontal subcortical circuits: a medial-frontal, which controls spontaneity versus apathy; an orbitofrontal, which provides inhibition versus disinhibition; and a dorsolateral prefrontal, which regulates go/no-go paradigms versus perseveration (Cummings, in press). These functions complement the posterior cortical functions of memory, comprehension, and recognition. A bedside test, the Executive Interview (EXIT) (Royall et al. 1992), measures a patient's executive functions and provides a sensitive indicator for early dementia of various etiology. The test can also verify decline in functions caused by Parkinson's disease, subcortical strokes, and so-called pseudodementia in major depression and schizophrenia, especially with negative symptoms (see p. 274 and Appendix).

If the testing of impaired cognitive functions leads to inconsistent results, such as disorientation one day followed by orientation the next, test more extensively with the Screening Test for the Luria-Nebraska Neuropsychological Battery (Golden 1987), the full Luria-Nebraska Neuropsychological Battery (Golden et al. 1991; Luria 1966), or the Halstead-Reitan Neuropsychological Test Battery (Reitan and Wolfson 1985). Alternatively, you may proceed with a somatic workup including a magnetic resonance imaging scan, computed axial tomography scan, electroencephalogram, brain mapping, single photon emission computed tomography, positron-emission tomography, examination of the spinal fluid, and determination of serum levels of heavy metals, vitamin B_{12}, and folic acid.

Interpretation of Cognitive Examination

To arrive at a correct diagnosis, interpret cognitive impairment in relation to the patient's educational background, premorbid intelligence, motivation, and severity of illness as well as the possible presence of Axis I disorders that can mimic cognitive impairment and present as cognitive pseudo-dysfunctions.

Educational background.   Patients with a strong educational background may present with an appearance, a demeanor, and language use that can mislead you diagnostically. For example, a person who is mentally retarded may use a sophisticated vocabulary, although incorrectly. You uncover the retardation by testing whether the patient comprehends the meaning of the words he is using (see Bleuler 1972; Othmer and Othmer 1994). Do not rely solely on an assessment of vocabulary to determine the patient's level of intelligence, because bright people with little education may show poor vocabulary but good reasoning power and a high score in the problem questions of the Kent Test (Kent 1946).

Level of premorbid intelligence.   A patient's level of premorbid intelligence frequently determines whether a test examines her capacity to think or her ability to remember or concentrate. For example, the inability to perform serial 3s backward fluently and without error represents an attention deficit for a high school graduate with at least average intelligence, but is not indicative of an attention deficit for a patient with mental retardation. For the latter, the failure to subtract reflects her low intelligence, not her lack of concentration. Thus, you test concentration in a patient with mental retardation by letting her count backward from 20 or recite the days of the week backward. If she passes, she can concentrate relative to her intellectual functioning. In contrast, you may consider the high school graduate inattentive if she can only perform on the level of a patient with mental retardation, and is slow and makes multiple errors—uncorrected and self-corrected—while asked to do serial 7s or 3s backward.

Motivation.   Uncooperative patients, such as those who want to express their disregard for your examination or the stupidity of the tests, or who malinger, may produce results that disguise their true ability. A classic example is the prison inmate who displays the so-called Ganser's syndrome. He is consistent in giving nearly correct yet implausible answers, such as 8 + 8= 15, a triangle has four corners, the American flag has 12 or 14 stripes, and so on. Obviously, such answers are not evidence of a cognitive dysfunction.

Severity of illness.   Take into account the severity of the illness when you interpret a patient's performance. Patients with severe dementia, for example, fail on virtually all tests. In Tables III–1, III–2, and III–3, the beginning stage of the patient's disorder, when the impairment is not uniform but affects cognitive functions differentially, is presented. At this beginning stage, you can use the profile of the dysfunction to make a tentative diagnosis of the underlying illness process (e.g., vascular versus Pick's versus Alzheimer's dementia).

Cognitive pseudodysfunctions.   Affective and anxiety disorders can mimic cognitive dysfunctions as a result of motivational factors rather than a patient's primary inability. For example, a severely depressed patient may be slow in his thought processes and unmotivated to answer the test questions. A manic patient may be distracted and drawn to respond to other stimuli rather than pursue the one presented by you. Severe anxiety can suffocate a patient's ability to give an appropriate response to tasks. Low self-confidence and the wish to escape the test situation may signify a patient's anxiety level rather than his level of cognitive ability. A patient's failure may represent his general inability to focus on a response rather than a circumscribed deficit due to a localized brain lesion.

We recommend not limiting the testing of cognitive impairment to just patients who show evidence of distractibility, forgetfulness, clouding of consciousness, and concrete thinking. Consider testing cognition as an integral part of all psychological and psychiatric evaluations. You may test for three reasons:

1. *Detection of unsuspected cognitive impairment.* Some patients may have only a very mild impairment that they have learned to compensate for in a skillful manner. A standard examination will alert you to the presence of this impairment. With further tests you can identify its extent.
2. *Baseline assessment.* Cognitive impairment can develop at any time after your initial evaluation as a result of substance abuse, trauma, cardiovascular accidents, tumors, infections, and degenerative brain disorders. Therefore, it is imperative to establish a baseline that allows you to time the onset of the impairment and to estimate its progression.
3. *Standards of care for participation in the Medicare program.* The Health Care Financing Administration of the U.S. Department of Health and Human Resources demands that a specific standard of care be given by hospitals that participate in the Medicare program. Medicare requires two conditions for participation: adequate staffing and adequate medical records. For medical records, standard (b)(6) of the section "Psychiatric Evaluation" [Paragraph 482.61(b)(6)] reads, "Estimate intellectual functioning, memory functioning, and orientation" (Health Care Financing Administration 1989).

A failure to do so in a significant number of records may lead a hospital to fail HCFA standard 482.61(b)(6). In conjunction with other deficiencies, such a failure could lead to focused review and corrective action, which could have been avoided if the standard had been adhered to in the first place.

In summary, adequate evaluation of cognitive functions is not a luxury but a clinical, medical, legal, and regulatory necessity.

Which cognitive functions should be examined in every patient? We recommend testing the following (see also Tables III–1, III–2, and III–3):

- Attention
- Orientation
- Memory

- Problem solving
- Arithmetic

This recommendation coincides with HCFA guidelines.

The five chapters in Part III progress from the disturbance of relatively isolated cognitive functions (i.e., attention) to memory and learning functions to complex interaction of cognitive functions. You see disturbances of the latter in delirium, dementia, and mental retardation. This order is at variance with the order in DSM-IV, which starts with disorders usually diagnosed in infancy (i.e., mental retardation and ADHD), followed by delirium, dementia, and amnestic disorders.

CHAPTER 7

INATTENTION AND HYPERACTIVITY

Summary

Inattention and hyperactivity are signs that are part of attention-deficit/hyperactivity disorder (ADHD) and other psychiatric disorders, especially cognitive disorders. Inattention and hyperactivity are prominent in delirium but also in bipolar disorder, manic state. In this chapter, we show how to recognize and test inattention and hyperactivity, and we discuss the differential diagnosis of these signs.

◆ ◆ ◆ ◆ ◆

They are ill discoverers that think there is no land, when they can see nothing but sea.

Sir Francis Bacon
The Advancement of Learning (1605)

◆ ◆ ◆ ◆ ◆

227

1. What Are Inattention and Hyperactivity?

Inattention and hyperactivity are explicitly addressed in DSM-IV (American Psychiatric Association 1994) within the discussion of ADHD and its subtypes (predominantly inattentive type, predominantly hyperactive-impulsive type, and combined type).

Inattention

Inattention is the inability to sustain concentration. The patient cannot be focused or remain focused. *Attention* is the ability to recognize a stream of stimuli; *concentration* is the ability to attend to and complete a task. According to DSM-IV, inattention is diagnosed by nine criteria, from which at least six should have been persistent for at least 6 months to a degree that is maladaptive and inconsistent with developmental level.

The person with healthy cognitive functioning is alert and aware of both her environment and her internal processes, including her thoughts and feelings. She attends to her environment by filtering out noise, retaining meaningful signals, paying attention, and attending to tasks.

Attention results from a finely tuned interplay of the reticular ascending activating formation and the descending inhibitory system. A subcortical structure—the ascending activating reticular formation—fine-tunes this alertness and awareness. This system originates from brain cells found in the medulla, pons, and midbrain. The pontine nucleus coeruleus feeds into this ascending system using norepinephrine as its main neurotransmitter. This system stimulates the thalamus, limbic system, and cortex, keeping the person alert.

Descending fibers and the ascending reticular inhibiting system work reciprocally to the ascending activating system and direct the person's attention. Serotonergic fibers originating from the upper pontine dorsal raphe nuclei innervate this system. This system activates the inferior parietal lobule consisting of the supramarginal gyrus (Brodmann area 40) and angular gyrus (Brodmann area 39). This third-level association cortex, in which tactile, visual, and auditory stimuli are integrated, is the seat of consciousness. Its activation allows the person to focus on both her environment and her internal sphere (i.e., thoughts and feelings). If this inhibiting system reciprocal to the activating system is disturbed, inattention, lack of concentration, and distractibility result.

Evidence has been presented that inattention without hyperactivity may result from sensory selective inattention (Barkley et al. 1992; Cohen et al. 1993).

Hyperactivity-Impulsivity

Diagnostic criteria for hyperactivity-impulsivity according to DSM-IV include

- Fidgeting
- Inability to stay seated
- Inappropriate running or climbing, or feelings of restlessness
- Difficulty quietly engaging in leisure activities
- Being "on the go" or acting driven
- Excessive talking
- Blurting out of answers before questions are completed
- Inability to wait turn
- Interrupting others

The inattention seen in ADHD may result from impaired response intention and impaired executive functions of the frontal lobe (Barkley et al. 1992; Cohen et al. 1993).

2. Inattention and Hyperactivity in the Mental Status

Inattention

During an interview, you can observe in the patient's mental status three of the criterion characteristics: difficulty in 1) sustaining attention, 2) listening when you speak, and 3) ignoring and suppressing extraneous stimuli. Some patients may report daydreaming. Often the patient loses eye contact with the interviewer; he looks to the side or through you. His eye blink rate may slow down. His facial expression does not reflect an affect that fits the topic of the conversation. At times, his facial muscles may lose their tone and his mouth may open slightly. His reactive movements are initially suppressed when you address him, then are replaced with a startle response when he recognizes that he has been inattentive.

During daydreaming, grooming movements are suppressed or occur in a slow rhythm. Usually daydreaming has a sudden onset and occurs during listening and not talking. When you ask the patient what happened, he may try to cover up and say, "I thought about the things you were talking about"; he may give you an answer that fits a previously discussed topic, not the present one; or he may admit that he was "spacing out." After addressing his tuning out, he may sit up straight, increasing his muscular tension. This shows that he has difficulties paying attention and needs a tense body position to keep himself attentive.

Hyperactivity

The hyperactive person shows an increase in grooming and reactive movements. Grooming movements are frequent and repetitive: stretching and bending of the neck, shrugging of one shoulder, whipping of a leg, rubbing one leg against the other—what most people call *fidgeting*. The hallmark of hyperactivity is goal-directed movements that are interrupted by a rapid change in goals. In younger children, the goal-directed movements are investigative. The youngster climbs on chairs to have a closer look at the phone, starts dialing, then detects a clock, tries out the buttons, sees a pen and doodles with it, and so on. The longer the session, the larger the area of exploration. The adult female patient may open and close her purse and, if uninhibited, use her lipstick, work on her makeup, or take out a cigarette then put it away as she reminds herself that you don't allow smoking in your office. Facial movements sometimes become awkward to the point of repetitive grimacing—pursing the lips, wrinkling the forehead, closing the eyes, and flashing a grin. Repetition shows up in the voice, too (e.g., kids grunt, snort, clear their throat), a tendency that may last into adulthood. Gestures are also repetitive, large, and edgy. Hyperactivity is more common in boys and daydreaming more common in females with attention deficit.

The observed hyperactivity is partly due to the showing of purposeless movements, increased grooming behavior, and the inability to postpone and control the expression of emerging impulses, such as untimely and inappropriate explorative behavior. Screening of responses to incoming stimuli is also impaired. Thus, the patient is often described as impulsive. DSM-IV (American Psychiatric Association 1994) lists three behaviors as indicative of impulsivity:

1. Answering a question before it has been completed
2. Talking out of turn
3. Interrupting and intruding on others

Verbal Characteristics

Verbal strategies show perseveration of affective statements:

Boy, I'm really mad. I'm really mad. You have to do something about it. [Pounding his right fist into his left hand, cracking his knuckles, grimacing] Boy, that really gets me.

The patient has a difficult time staying with one topic and developing details in a logical manner. Instead, he jumps around within the topic or leaves it. Reminders of an emotion will trigger him to follow that affect-laden new topic.

In history taking, ask the patient—child or adult—about school performance, such as being too "hyper" before age 12 years and being often reprimanded because of talking, blurting out answers, interrupting, disturbing others, and daydreaming.

3. Techniques: Testing for Attention Span, Vigilance, and Concentration

The concepts of attention, vigilance, and concentration overlap. *Attention* often refers to the recognition of outside stimuli, *vigilance* to the discriminate recognition of stimuli coupled with a specific response, and *concentration* to the internal manipulation of the stimuli. Yet all three concepts have in common a stimulus recognition task such as recognition of a set of numbers; a required, preset, and preagreed manipulation of the stimulus such as reversing the order of the numbers; and a preset response such as reciting the numbers in a certain order. We selected three groups of tasks that assess these functions.

Tests for Attention Span

- *Digit span test.* Ask the patient to repeat three digits: 7, 4, 9. Then ask him to do it backward. Then use 5, 3, 1, 8. Then 6, 4, 9, 1, 5. Then 9, 2, 5, 3, 6, 8. You can use your own numbers. If a patient fails, give him a second trial. The more digits a patient can remember, the less likely it is that he has an attention deficit. Patients who can repeat seven digits forward and five digits backward probably do not have a clinically significant attention deficit.
- *Digit Span, Digit Symbol, and Arithmetic Subtests of the Wechsler Intelligence Scale for Children—Revised* (Wechsler 1974). These subtests are sensitive to attentional deficits (Kaufman 1979).
- *Spelling words backward.* Ask the patient to spell five- to nine-letter words forward and backward, such as world, flower, trumpet, prome-

nade. If the patient misspells the word in forward mode, ask him to spell it again. If he misspells it consistently, you have two options: expect the same error when spelling backward, or correct the patient and then expect correct spelling backward.

Tests for Vigilance

- *Continuous Performance Test* (Rosvold et al. 1956). Ask the patient to tap on the desk whenever she hears an A or an A preceded by an X among a series of spoken random letters such as K, D, A, M, X, T, X A, F, O, K, L, E, N, A. . . . The number of errors will show her ability to sustain attention. Hyperactive children make increasingly more errors of omission and commission than nonpsychiatric control subjects (Sykes et al. 1973).
- *Go/No-Go Test* (Mesulam 1985). Ask the patient to raise her index finger briefly if she hears one tap ("go") but not when she hears two taps ("no go"). Patients with inattention without hyperactivity show more errors of commission than those with inattention and hyperactivity, but they improve in subsequent trials, whereas inattentive hyperactive patients do not improve (Table 7–1). Patients with hyperactivity show errors of omission but patients without hyperactivity rarely do (Trommer et al. 1988).

Tests for Concentration—Serial 7s, 3s, and 1s

Ask the patient,

Is it easy for you to pay attention and to concentrate?

Table 7–1. Performance on the Go/No-Go Test and the Rey-Osterreith Figure Test by patients with inattention with and without hyperactivity

Type of error	With hyperactivity	Without hyperactivity
Errors of commission	–	+
Improvement of errors of commission	–	+
Errors of omission	+	–
Impairment in copying the Rey-Osterreith figure	–	+

Note. + = increased in comparison to scores of other subtype. – = decreased in comparison to scores of other subtype.

No matter what the patient's answer is, continue:

> May I examine you? Please take 7 away from 100 and after you have the result, take 7 away again, and so on. Try to do it as fast as you can without making any mistake.

The correct answers are 100, 93, 86, 79, 72, 65, 58, 51, 44, 37, 30, and so on.

> Now you have reached 30. Do you think you made a mistake?

The correct answer is,

> No, because $10 \times 7 = 70$ and $100 - 70 = 30$.

Such an answer shows at least average intelligence.

For a patient with lower intelligence, or for a child, use the same test starting at 30 and subtracting 3, or have him count backward from 20.

4. Five Steps to Identify Inattention

Step 1: Listen. Children and adolescents with inattention, impulsivity, or disruptive behavior are often sent to you by their teacher. Adults will come to you and complain about their lack of attention. You may also see patients because of secondary depression, substance addiction, antisocial behavior, bipolar disorder, continuous job problems, marital conflicts, or impulse control.

Step 2: Tag. After you suspect inattention, obtain the patient's school and work history. If you are correct, the report will reflect chronic problems.

Step 3: Confront. Directly address the area of concern. Discuss with the patient your diagnostic impression that he has been experiencing inattention. Very often, the patient will provide more corroborating evidence and be relieved that you have pinpointed a lifelong problem that has caused so many repercussions in his work and social life.

Step 4: Solve. Usually the patient is grateful that you were able to identify his problems and cooperates with the specific mental status testing (i.e., digit span, vigilance testing, serial 7s backward, and backward spelling of long and complicated words).

Step 5: Approve. Share your findings with the patient. Tell him the treatment options and point out what results he can expect with successful treatment.

5. Interview: Mania Versus Hyperactivity-Impulsivity of Attention-Deficit/Hyperactivity Disorder

A colleague asks for a second opinion. She describes the psychiatric history of a patient who has been treated for bipolar disorder by two different psychiatrists. The patient's manic symptoms have not responded to lithium, valproic sodium (Depakote), carbamazepine (Tegretol), and combinations thereof. Now the patient is depressed. She is taking fluoxetine (Prozac) rather than a tricyclic antidepressant to avoid a possible induction of rapid cycling, but there has been no improvement.

In the interview, in Steps 1 and 2 (not recounted here), the patient, Ms. B., asks to be addressed by her first name. She squirms in her chair, stands up and sits down several times, fiddles with her purse, and jumps from topic to topic. She interrupts the interviewer several times.

She denies substance abuse or use. She discloses intermittent and terminal insomnia, reduced appetite, loss of interest in her work, forgetfulness, and an inability to concentrate and complete daily tasks. Her affect appears depressed and she reports depressed mood and lack of energy. She shows no evidence of delusions and denies hallucinations or a suicidal plan. She has insight into the morbid nature of her depressive symptoms and her judgment appears good. She feels she has to get herself together if she wants to have a worthwhile life. (I = interviewer; P = patient)

Step 3: Confront

1. I: I notice that you are restless. Do you have a hard time sitting still?
   P: I do? Really? I'm down.
2. I: Do you feel uncomfortable talking to me?
   P: No, not really. I've talked to a bunch of psychiatrists.
3. I: You've been playing with your purse during the entire interview.
   P: I have? If you say so.

Step 4: Solve

4. I: So you are used to your restlessness?
   P: [Frowns] I don't know. I've been hyper.

5. I: During your depression?
   P: No. I'm slowed down when I'm low like I'm now.
6. I: What are you like when you're not depressed?
   P: Hyper. I move around a lot. I have no patience. I'm always doing something, but I don't get things done.
7. I: And how is your mood when you are not depressed?
   P: Things are closing in on me. I always forget things I have to do. I feel like moving all the time.
8. I: Do you ever get really high in your mood?
   P: [Puzzled] What? Like feel good? No. I feel good if something good happens.
9. I: Do you feel at times that you can do about anything you want to?
   P: Me? [Shakes her head] I wish. I never get things done.
10. I: Do you go on shopping sprees?
    P: Like Christmas? No. I'm usually tight.
11. I: Do you ever get really high strung and full of drive?
    P: No. What did you say? [Interviewer repeats question] My mother says I'm on the go all the time but I feel worn out.
12. I: You mean your mother noticed this? When?
    P: As a child. I could never sit still, she says. I would always talk. Disturb the other kids. Hmmm. [Grunts] The teachers called my mother all the time. My mother says I even kicked her constantly when she was pregnant with me.
13. I: I'm sorry to hear this. You really got a lot of criticism for behavior that is difficult to control. Has it gotten any better?
    P: [Shrugs her shoulders] I'm not sure. In high school I was still very talkative—that's what the teachers wrote. Never had patience.
14. I: What kind of grades did you get?
    P: Average. I could have done better. I could not sit still. I always got up from my work. Took me forever to finish.
15. I: Could you concentrate in high school and listen to the teacher?
    P: My mind would wander off . . . daydreaming.
16. I: How is your attention now?
    P: Awful. I still can't finish a book. I'm trying to take some classes. It's hard. I just look at the words. I just don't get it.
17. I: Do you have children?
    P: Two.
18. I: How are you doing with them?
    P: My son has attention-deficit/hyperactivity disorder (ADHD). He's on Ritalin. I scream and yell at him all the time. My husband can't stand it.
19. I: Let's test your attention.
    P: Good luck. [Laughs nervously]
20. I: Take 7 away from 100 and keep doing it.
    P: 93, 93, 93—is that right?
21. I: I'm sorry. I want you to take 7 away from the remainder. So take 7 away from 93 and keep going.
    P: 89, no it's 87. Sorry. Let me start again. 100, 93, 93 take away 7 is 86, take away 7 is 89, no what am I saying? 79, 72, 65, 50. Where was I?
22. I: 65.

     P: What did you want me to take away?
23. I: 7. 65 take away 7.
     P: 65 take away 7—58, 51. I can't do that.
24. I: Maybe we can start with 30 and you can do the same thing except you take
         away 3.
     P: Oh, that's easy. 30, 30. 27, 24, 21, 19—is that right? 30, 27, 24, 21, 21 take
         away 3 is 18, 15, 12, 9, 6, 3.
25. I: Let's do something else. I'll give you a few numbers and I want you to repeat
         them. And then repeat them backward.
     P: Oh, I was never that good in math.
26. I: You won't get any grades here. We are doing this to get an idea how your
         concentration is working. Let's start. 4, 7, 2.
     P: 4, 7, 2.
27. I: And now backward.
     P: 4, 7, 2. Hmmm. 2, 7, 4.
28. I: That's right. 3, 9, 5, 1.
     P: 3, 9, 5, 1.
29. I: And backward?
     P: 3, 9, 5, 1. 1, 5, 3, 9. No, 9, 3.
30. I: Okay. Let's keep going. 3, 8, 2, 1, 6.
     P: 3, 9, 1, 2, 6.
31. I: Let me give you the numbers again. 3, 8, 2, 1, 6.
     P: 3, 8, 2, 1, 6.
32. I: And backward?
     P: Oh, that's right. What were the numbers?
33. I: Can you remember?
     P: That's really hard. 3, 1, 6, 2. I don't know.
34. I: 3, 8, 2, 1, 6.
     P: [Fast] 3, 8, 2, 1, 6—3, 8, 2, 1, 6—3, 8, 2, 1, 6—3, 8, 2, 1, 6—3, 8, 2, 1, 6—3,
         8, 2, 1, 6.
35. I: And backward?
     P: 3, 8, 2, 1, 6—3, 8, 2, 1, 6—6—3, 8, 2, 1, 6—6, 1—hmmm—3, 8, 2, 1, 6—3,
         8, 2, 1, 6—6, 1 , 8, 1, 3.
36. I: Okay. That's fine. Did you think about something else when you tried to do
         the numbers?
     P: No. It's like somebody wipes off the blackboard where the numbers are.
         [The patient can multiply 2×96 and answer the four problem questions of
         the Kent Test (Kent 1946; see Chapter 11, "Mental Retardation"). She has
         difficulty repeating four words immediately. She remembers two of them
         after 10 minutes and recognizes the other two from multiple choice.]

     The interviewer noticed the distraction in the patient's answer (A. 3) and
therefore targeted her inattentiveness (A. 4), history of impulsivity and
fidgetiness, and present mental status. He distinguished these from her
elation (Q. 8), which could be related to flight of ideas with distractibility
and surplus of energy.

The patient answered all questions but in an abrupt and choppy manner. She appeared inattentive (A. 9). Her constant movements were distracting. When the interviewer expressed empathy (Q. 13), she responded by shrugging her shoulders (A. 13).

Increased spontaneous motor activity is typical of an attention deficit, disorder, whereas mania shows an increase in expressive, reactive, and goal-directed movements. Fragmented sentences are also typical of an attention deficit, whereas mania would show circumstantiality with flight of ideas. This patient's affect appeared restricted. She reported problems with her husband and children (A. 18) and depressed mood (A. 5). She showed a short attention span by having difficulties with serial 7s and 3s and recalling four objects. She made errors when asked to recall more than five digits forward and backward. Her impairment was most likely attributable to attention-deficit rather than low intelligence as the correct answers to the problem questions in the Kent Test place her in the average range or above.

Step 5: Approve

The interviewer explains to the patient her family history (i.e., her son having ADHD [A. 18]). He points out that her restlessness between depressive episodes possibly is not a sign of mania but a residual of ADHD. He discontinues her lithium and carbamazepine and starts desipramine, which may help her depression and her inattention. He explains to the patient that he may add methylphenidate (Ritalin) later if there is not sufficient improvement.

Diagnosis

1. The patient gave a convincing history of major depression in Steps 1 and 2. Her depression was characterized by intermittent and terminal insomnia, reduced appetite, and loss of interest in her work. She reported depressed mood and showed depressive affect.
2. It is still conceivable that the patient has a bipolar disorder and has been treatment resistant. However, she denied elation in mood, increased energy, shopping sprees, or grandiosity. Her restlessness and lack of concentration and patience appeared to be a result of her inability to focus rather than a result of distraction by external stimuli, as would be observed in mania. She also did not report experiencing an elated mood when she was most distractible.

3. ADHD, combined type, adult residual.
4. The patient's inattention could also be a result of substance intoxication or withdrawal. However, the patient denied substance use.

The patient had been referred because the treatments she had received had failed; however, her attention deficit, impulsivity, and persisting hyperactivity when she was not depressed had been misdiagnosed as manic distractibility and increased energy. She experienced no elation in mood, no shopping sprees, and no expansive or grandiose thoughts. Because patients during a depression frequently forget that they were manic earlier, the interviewer questioned Ms. B.'s family members, including her mother, father, and husband, who confirmed the absence of elation and money squandering. She did have a family history of ADHD (A. 18).

Misdiagnosis of patients like Ms. B. is common because psychiatrists specializing in adults may not be sufficiently familiar with ADHD (Bellak and Black 1992; Denckla 1991; Hechtman 1991; Shekim et al. 1990). Furthermore, a female's hyperactivity persisting into adulthood is atypical; usually, hyperactivity is more pronounced in males, whereas females show more problems with daydreaming. Ms. B.'s prolonged depressive episodes contrasted with her restless hyperactivity when she was not depressed. The misdiagnosis would explain the patient's lack of responsiveness to mood stabilizing medications.

6. Inattention and Hyperactivity in Psychiatric Disorders

The differential diagnosis of inattention and hyperactivity hinges on the symptoms and signs associated with them. If inattention and hyperactivity are associated with impulsivity, distractibility, daydreaming, or a learning disorder, the diagnosis of an attention deficit with or without hyperactivity and with or without a learning disability can be made.

Follow-up studies of patients who have childhood ADHD show that these patients may be prone to impulsivity, drug and alcohol abuse, conduct disturbances, and even antisocial personality disorder as an adult. Thus, substance abuse preceded by a history or persistence of attention deficit during drug-free intervals warrants the additional diagnosis of attention-deficit/hyperactivity disorder, adult residual type. The same is true for antisocial personality disorder associated with a history of ADHD.

Bipolar disorder may be complicated by ADHD. If a history of inattention and hyperactivity preceded the occurrence of a manic or depressive episode, and the inattention and hyperactivity persist when the patient is in remission from his affective disorder, make the additional diagnosis of an attention-deficit disorder. If the distractibility is limited to the manic state of a bipolar disorder, consider it a sign of mania rather than of an independently existing disorder.

If inattention and hyperactivity are associated with disorientation, a fluctuating level of alertness, and perceptual disturbances, especially visual and haptic hallucinations, consider them part of a delirium.

Inattention and hyperactivity also occur in states of mild to moderate substance intoxication or substance withdrawal. Usually, distractibility is not a leading sign of dementia or amnesia but may occur in moderate to severe forms of these disorders.

CHAPTER 8

AMNESIA

Summary

In this chapter, we demonstrate how to test for amnesia and how to induce confabulation. The differential diagnosis of amnesia is also discussed. Anterograde amnesia is a key sign of all cognitive disorders. Amnesia can also occur in affective disorders, but here it reflects more a lack of concentration and motivation in storing and retrieving information rather than a true inability to store. Retrograde amnesia without anterograde amnesia may occur in dissociative disorders, such as dissociative amnesia and dissociative fugue.

◆ ◆ ◆ ◆ ◆

To know one's ignorance is the best part of knowledge.

Lao-Tzu (sixth century B.C.)
The Simple Way

◆ ◆ ◆ ◆ ◆

1. What Is Amnesia?

Amnesia is the inability to recall events. According to the definition in DSM-IV (American Psychiatric Association 1994), a cognitive disorder that is mainly characterized by a memory impairment in the absence of other significant cognitive impairment and that is due either to the direct physiological effects of a general medical condition or to the persisting effects of a substance is called an *amnestic disorder.* Individuals with amnestic disorder are "impaired in their ability to learn new information or are unable to recall previously learned information or past events" (p. 156).

When describing memory dysfunctions, clinicians use a brain trauma as a reference point. If the patient cannot recall what happened prior to the insult, it is called *retrograde amnesia.* Retrograde amnesia leads to disturbances of remote memory, which can wipe out a patient's identity. If a patient cannot recall what followed the insult, it is called *anterograde amnesia.* Anterograde amnesia affects recent and immediate recall. A disturbance of recent memory disrupts orientation and learning. If the amnesia is part of a delirium or dementia, it is not classified as an amnestic disorder.

The amnestic disorders are subclassified according to presumed etiology: related to a general medical condition, induced by a substance, or not otherwise specified. Dissociative amnesia (see Chapter 2, "Dissociation") is distinct from an amnestic disorder. Patients with dissociative amnesia can learn and recall new information but are unable to recall previous memories, usually of a traumatic or stressful nature. Furthermore, they do not show an association with a preceding general medical condition or substance use. Amnesia that occurs only during substance intoxication—"blackouts"—or withdrawal is diagnosed as such and not as amnestic disorder.

Orientation

The human brain consistently monitors the coordinates of its position—in time, geographic and social location, and personal identity. Cortical and subcortical areas responsible for recent memory (see below) serve this orienting function. If this tracking is disturbed, the patient becomes disoriented and confused.

Learning

The association areas of the cortex that surround the primary sensory areas register and interpret inside and outside stimuli. These brain areas enable the person to recall stimuli within a few seconds (immediate memory).

Significant stimuli are sorted out and stored with the assistance of hippocampal cholinergic neurons. The association areas of the cortex retrieve these memory imprints with the help of the mammillary bodies and the dorsal medial nuclei of the thalamus (recent memory) and enable a person to learn new information. If any of the brain areas involved in the storage and retrieval process are disrupted, learning cannot take place and anterograde amnesia results.

Subcortical Amnesia

Amnestic disorder, as defined in DSM-IV, represents a subcortical amnesia (also called *axial amnesia* [Karp 1992]) in which bilateral lesions of the dorsal medial nuclei of the thalamus, the mammillary bodies, the fornix, and the hippocampi occur (Young and McGlone 1992). Thiamine deficiency leading to an amnestic confabulatory syndrome (Korsakoff's psychosis), as seen in patients who have chronically abused alcohol, is a frequent cause. Other causes of amnestic disorder include closed head trauma, penetrating missile wounds, surgical intervention, hypoxia, infarction of the territory of the posterior cerebral artery, and herpes simplex encephalitis. These lesions prevent both storage and retrieval of recently acquired memory engrams. Patients with subcortical amnesia retain their ability to repeat words immediately but cannot remember them 5–10 minutes later. At an early stage of the disorder, patients frequently make up words (confabulate) when exposed to the memory task.

As noted in DSM-IV, transient global amnesia is associated with disease of the vascular vertebrobasilar system or with episodic physiological or metabolic disorders, including seizures. Unilateral left temporal lobe lesions produce deficits in the acquisition, storage, retrieval, and recognition of verbal information. A unilateral right temporal lobe lesion leads to storage, retrieval, and recognition problems of geometric figures and melodies (Young and McGlone 1992).

The amnestic syndrome affects mainly the representational memory system. A second memory system involving the cortex with the striatum and associated structures within the extrapyramidal system and cerebellum may stay intact. Therefore, the amnestic patient retains his motor skills and can still acquire some new motor skills (Young and McGlone 1992).

Cortical Amnesia

Cortical amnesia is associated with syndromes involving agnosia, as seen in dementia of the Alzheimer's type. Such patients may often have a loss of immediate memory but may be able to recall words after a few minutes or a few hours if repeated several times (Karp 1992).

2. Amnesia in the Mental Status

For the amnestic patient, the world renews itself from minute to minute. People she met only minutes earlier become new acquaintances when she meets them again a few minutes later. The patient becomes so used to this process that she may no longer greet you with signs of unfamiliarity but will hail you like an old friend; alternatively, she may greet you as a stranger after you have just left her. In conversation, the patient may either rehearse old stories or stay with the here and now, expressing simple needs, such as hunger or needing to use the rest room. Usually, the patient does not complain about amnesia. Often, she gives a rationalization why she is not interested in the news any longer, or why she does not need to know the date. She may become jovial and try to talk you out of insisting on an answer to a probing question.

　　If the onset of the amnesia is relatively acute, such as in substance-induced (i.e., alcohol) persisting amnestic disorder (also referred to as Korsakoff's psychosis), the patient may at least initially fill in the memory gaps with confabulation. Another patient may perseverate on a theme, saying, for example, "I want to go back to my 4 acres," referring to her home. Although the patient forgets all other elements of the conversation, she returns with regularity to such favored topics.

3. Techniques: Testing for Orientation,
Four-Word Memory, and
Induction of Confabulation

Orientation test. Assess orientation by asking the patient how well he keeps track of time. Then test it. Do not excuse yourself by apologizing that you have to ask a "stupid" question. Let the patient know you are concerned about his health and that you would like to ask him a few questions. If your question is truly stupid, don't ask it.

Memory test. Assess three different memory systems: immediate, recent, and remote. For immediate and recent memory, use four words, one being abstract. For example, use 34th Street, honesty, tulip, and eyedropper. The four-word test helps you to identify milder memory disturbances. Have the patient repeat the four words.

With regard to recent memory, if the patient cannot recall the four words 10 minutes later, give her a multiple choice for the missed word; for example, if the word "honesty" was missed, ask, "Was it equality, honesty, justice, or righteousness?" If the patient can recognize the right word, she has shown that she can still lay down memory traces but has a problem with retrieval.

With regard to remote memory, select questions for which you can obtain verification either from the patient's record or informants.

Confabulation. Patients who confabulate are very suggestible. When pressed for information, they invent it. However, they may not confabulate spontaneously. Confabulated stories are false but not fixed in content. The patient will change them if you offer new details. Try to induce confabulation by asking the patient about things that you know about.

- Have we met before?
- (If you know the patient was in the hospital sleeping) What did you do yesterday night?
- Do you remember what we did together?

The patient with dementia and amnesia will often admit that he does not remember meeting you before, whereas the patient with amnestic syndrome can be prompted to produce a colorful story.

4. Five Steps to Identify Amnesia

The five steps—listen, tag, confront, solve, and approve—may often be brief, because the interviewer may turn to outside informants or may immediately conduct a mental status examination (Step 4), as soon as he detects a more severe cognitive disorder. As soon as you suspect amnesia, address the problem (Step 4—solve) using questions such as,

How well do you recall what you did on [fill in time period]?

Be sure to ask the patient about a time period when you know what she did. If you suspect confabulation, induce her to confabulate on the spot. Step 5 may often only consist of one reassuring sentence designed to calm the patient down and indicate the end of the interview to him.

5. Interview: Delusion Versus Confabulation in an Amnestic State

Mr. D., a 43-year old, white, divorced male, is brought to a Veteran's Administration Hospital emergency room by his brother, who reports the following:

> My brother is embarrassing us. He has gone downhill since his wife left him. Last time he was in the hospital, he was just out of it. Now he claims that his boss forces him to have sex with the boss's wife and some other nonsense like that. He has a violent temper and drinks too much, but he hasn't had a drink for the last month since he's been living with us.

A first year resident admitted the patient. The next morning, he presents him to the staff with the following explanation:

> Mr. D. drinks a lot, but everybody here does. He has not been drinking lately. The nurses' log shows that he slept well last night. His vital signs are normal. He showed no tremor yesterday or this morning. So I believe that his brother is right that Mr. D. has not been drinking lately, not even secretly. But I'm not so sure that the brother is right in not believing what the patient says about him having been forced to have sex with the boss's wife. Where I come from, we joke about what goes on in the mountain part of the state. I certainly don't think the patient has an affective disorder because his affect is bright and he relates warmly to me. Also, his memory seems to be fine, because he greeted me in a very friendly way after I came back from lunch to complete his workup. So he remembered me.

The resident brings in the patient, who is smiling broadly, nodding at all residents, and greeting them with "Hi there," and "How are you today?" (I = interviewer; P = patient; R1 = presenting resident; R2 = second resident)

Step 1: Listen

1. I: Hi, Mr. D. Your resident doctor told us a little bit about you.
   P: Call me Ray.

Step 2: Tag

2. I: He told us that you have some problems with your boss.
   P: Boy, oh boy. My boss is a pervert.

Step 3: Confront

3. I: It seems that your brother doesn't believe you.
   P: Oh boy. My brother is a pervert.
4. I: How's that?
   P: My brother forces me to do pervert things.
5. I: With whom?
   P: With my grandmother.
6. I: Ray, would you mind if I ask the residents what they think about your problem?
   P: [With a smile] They all need to hear what's going on.
7. I: [To the presenting resident] What do you think now about Ray's experience?
   R1: I admit Ray's experience is extreme, isn't it, Ray? [Ray nods.] But I still think Ray is a victim. Maybe we should ask Ray some questions from the Kent Test. Some patients who have problems with these questions may be prone to become victims. [To Ray] You wouldn't mind if we asked you to figure out some problems? [Ray grins.]
   R2: Come on. Ray clearly has some unchangeable beliefs that we won't be able to verify.
8. I: [To second resident] Really? Let's see. Let's ask Ray.

Step 4: Solve

9. I: [To Ray] Ray, you spent last night here?
   P: (Boisterous) Did I ever.
10. I: Can you tell the residents how the nurses treated you here last evening?
    P: It was nighttime. The supervisor—I guess—took me into the examination room and forced me to have sex with the nurses.
    R2: [To the presenting resident] Now that will even convince you that Ray has problems with delusions.
11. I: [To the patient] What about me? What did I do?
    P: When you came, it was all over. They let go of me by then. Or maybe you broke it off.
    R1: [To interviewer] But you were at the residents' party last night. How could you be in two places at the same time?
12. I: [To presenting resident] Ask Ray. In Ray's mind I can. Ray can make me appear and disappear. [Looking over at Ray who is chatting with one of the residents not paying attention] We call that confabulation.

        [To all residents] When a patient tells you about an experience that is extreme, examine the patient about a time interval and location familiar to you. If he or she reports experiences like Ray just did, you know where to direct your diagnostic evaluations. Let's do that now. Ray, I would like you to remember the following words that I will ask you to repeat back to me: honesty, tulip, eyedropper, and yellow. Okay, now can you repeat them?
    P: Yellow, eyedropper.
13. I: Fine. What words did I mention first? One was a flower.

P: Rose.
14. I: No. Honesty and tulip.
P: Honesty and tulip.
15. I: Let's say them together. Honesty, tulip, eyedropper, and yellow.
P: [Together with the interviewer] Honesty, tulip, eyedropper, and yellow.
16. I: I will ask you those words again. Remember them! [The interviewer asks the patient to demonstrate how to hang a picture, which he can do, and to write down why he is in the hospital. He writes "I'm here because of my boss. What he made me do." The patient knows that Monday comes before Wednesday and he answers all questions on the Kent Test (Kent 1946) correctly except he does not know how many stripes the American flag has and that one can make glass out of sand. He can multiply 2 × 96. He is not oriented to day, date, or month. He is off in the year by one year. His reflexes are normal.]
17. I: I asked you to remember four words. Do you remember them?
P: Yes.
18. I: What were they?
P: Glasses. . . . [Laughing] That's stupid. You said glasses and [looking at the pen on the table] I think it was pen . . . chair and table.

Step 5: Approve

19. I: Ray, your mind is filled up with all kinds of experiences. I hope you can find some peace here. We will do our best to make you feel comfortable.
P: Thank you. You're nice.

From the beginning, the patient showed familiarity with all people in the room. Throughout the interview, he related in a friendly manner with the interviewer, never contradicting him. The patient showed jovial affect and behaved as if he knew everybody. Such displayed familiarity instead of perplexity helped him to cover up his uncertainty about whether he knew the interviewers or not. When looking only superficially, one could believe there was good rapport between the patient and the doctors.

When the interviewer used the patient's brother's statement to express doubt about the patient's story, the patient made the brother part of his sex perversion story. This was the clue for confabulation. To test it, the interviewer tempted the patient to confabulate about the night nurses and himself.

The patient had slight difficulties in registering the four words. After 10 minutes he confabulated them. He seemed unconcerned about his memory problems. In contrast, he performed well on the Kent Test. Most but not all patients with Korsakoff's psychosis, however, are disoriented and show evidence of impairment of orientation and of recent memory, as did this patient.

Confabulation differs from a delusion. A delusional patient is fixated on a certain false thought content that cannot be changed by verbal suggestions. In this case, the second resident erroneously interpreted the patient's tendency to confabulate as a delusion. A confabulation is false but not fixed. Even though this patient perseverated on a sexual theme, the content of the story changed readily and could be modified by questions. Perseveration on a theme can make a confabulation sound like a delusion.

Diagnosis

Axis I

1. Alcohol-induced persisting amnestic disorder
2. Chronic alcohol abuse by history

Axis II. None.

Axis III. Presumable avitaminosis of B_1.

Axis IV. None known.

Axis V. Global Assessment of Functioning (GAF) Scale score = 30.

Alcohol abuse and dependence are common; so is the alcoholic acute amnestic state—the blackout state—listed in DSM-IV. This example shows the most severe form—the relatively rare Korsakoff's psychosis. Milder forms of memory disturbance secondary to vitamin B_1 deficiency may remain undetected because they may be attributed to some transient phenomenon or atypical withdrawal symptoms.

This patient's dramatic case will sensitize you to memory failures stemming from alcohol abuse. Patients who complain about or display memory disturbances should be thoroughly tested, especially if you suspect a nutritional deficit. The amnesia of these patients is anterograde and retrograde, and the retrograde amnesia may indeed have an impact on their remote memory.

This case demonstrates how one can misdiagnose a cognitive disorder as a delusional disorder or as major depression with psychosis. Confabulation as a result of alcohol-induced persisting amnestic disorder is mainly present at the acute onset of the disorder, during the first weeks or months of the amnesia (Strub and Black 1988). This phase passes and gives way to apathy and withdrawal. Confabulation vanishes during the chronic stage of the disorder, although induced confabulations appear to outlast the spontaneous ones. The addiction to alcohol also disappears during the chronic phase (Strub and Black 1988). Confabulation usually cannot be induced in patients with vascular dementia, dementia of the Alzheimer's type, or dementia due to Pick's disease.

Alcohol abuse may lead to

- Alcohol-induced persisting amnestic disorder
- Alcohol-induced persisting dementia
- Alcohol intoxication delirium
- Alcohol withdrawal delirium
- Alcohol-induced psychotic disorder

Besides severe chronic alcohol abuse, the abuse of other psychoactive drugs may also lead to substance-induced cognitive impairment, such as

- Amphetamine- (or cannabis-, cocaine-, hallucinogen-, inhalant-, opioid-, phencyclidine-, sedative-, hypnotic,- anxiolytic-, or other [or unknown] substance-) induced psychotic disorder with delusions (Chronic abuse of stimulant drugs in a high dosage may lead to a delusional disorder characterized by persecutory ideas.)
- Substance intoxication delirium
- Hallucinogen persisting perception disorder
- Inhalant-induced persisting psychotic disorder with delusions
- Inhalant-induced persisting dementia
- Sedative-, hypnotic-, or anxiolytic-induced persisting dementia
- Sedative-, hypnotic-, anxiolytic-induced persisting amnestic disorder and psychotic disorder with delusions

6. Amnesia in Psychiatric Disorders

Different forms of amnesia occur in several groups of psychiatric disorders. Most cognitive disorders show anterograde amnesia. In progressive dementia, retrograde amnesia also emerges.

Trauma to the brain shows both retrograde and anterograde amnesia. One special trauma is electroconvulsive therapy: the retrograde amnesia is partially reversible, but the anterograde amnesia is permanent.

During intoxication, substance-related disorders may lead to reversible anterograde amnesia, such as in acute alcoholic blackout. More permanent amnesia occurs in amnestic disorder. Delirium is also associated with anterograde amnesia.

Schizophrenia, other psychotic disorders, and mood disorders may lead to pseudoamnesia because the patient does not register certain stimuli, is distracted, or is unmotivated to retrieve the previously stored information. Correct answers to multiple-choice questions and to prodding differentiate this form of amnesia from anterograde amnesia. This pseudoamnesia may also be seen in subcortical dementia, as assessed with the Qualitative Evaluation of Dementia (QED; see Appendix).

Patients with a dissociative disorder, especially dissociative fugue and dissociative amnesia, show exclusive, massive retrograde amnesia. However, their ability to learn new things and their orientation is intact.

CHAPTER 9

DELIRIUM

Summary

In this chapter we discuss how to examine a patient with delirium. Such a patient shows deficiencies in selected tests of cognitive functions. Impaired cognitive functions occur in all cognitive disorders, but hourly fluctuating scores characterize delirium.

◆ ◆ ◆ ◆ ◆

Frons est animi janua.
The forehead is the gate of the mind.

Marcus Tullius Cicero (106–43 B.C.)
De Provinciis Consularibus

◆ ◆ ◆ ◆ ◆

1. What Is Delirium?

In DSM-IV (American Psychiatric Association 1994, p. 129), delirium is defined as

1. Disturbance of consciousness . . . with reduced ability to focus, sustain, or shift attention.
2. A change in cognition (such as memory deficit, disorientation, language disturbance) or the development of a perceptual disturbance that is not better accounted for by a preexisting, established, or evolving dementia.
3. The disturbance develops over a short period of time . . . and tends to fluctuate during the course of the day.
4. There is evidence from the history, physical examination, or laboratory findings that the disturbance is caused by the direct physiological consequences of a general medical condition, substance intoxication, or substance withdrawal.

In a delirium (from the Latin *de-lira,* "off the track or furrow") hypervigilance with motor hyperactivity may turn into somnolence with psychomotor retardation or restlessness. Recent recall may turn into disorientation, and acute awareness of the surroundings into visual and haptic illusionary and hallucinatory perceptions.

The individual with intact cognitive functioning is alert and aware of both his environment and his internal processes, including his thoughts and feelings. A subcortical structure—the interconnected ascending activating and descending inhibiting reticular formation—tones this alertness and awareness. The descending part of the system originates from brain cells found in the medulla, pons, and midbrain. The pontine nucleus coeruleus feeds into this ascending system using norepinephrine as its main neurotransmitter. This system stimulates the thalamus, limbic system, and cortex, keeping the person alert.

When the activating part of the cognitive system is disturbed, the patient shows decreased response to his surroundings, and will become gradually lethargic, somnolent, obtuse, stuporous, and, finally, comatose. If the entire system is overinhibited or overstimulated in an unbalanced manner, the patient shows fluctuations in consciousness ranging from lethargy to hyperalertness, and the result is an acute confusional state (one example is the alcohol withdrawal delirium called *delirium tremens*).

Predisposing factors for a delirium include age over 60 years, brain injury or brain disease, a prior cardiotomy, extensive burns, substance intoxication or withdrawal, and acquired immunodeficiency syndrome (AIDS). Facilitating factors include psychosocial stress, sleep deprivation, sensory deprivation or overload, or immobilization (Lipowski 1990; Wise and Brandt 1992).

Causes of delirium differ depending on the patient's age. During childhood, fever-producing infections, poisoning, epilepsy, tumors, or trauma may lead to a delirium. In adolescence, we still look for infections and head trauma, including subdural hematoma. Other possibilities include intoxication or withdrawal from street drugs such as phencyclidine, alcohol, barbiturates, meprobamate, and benzodiazepines. During middle age, metabolic and endocrine disorders or neoplasms can cause delirium. In advanced age, organ failure becomes a predominant physical problem, resulting in hepatic, uremic, pulmonary, and cardiac causes of delirium (for more detail, see Horvath et al. 1989).

In DSM-IV, the causes of delirium are subclassified into four broad categories:

1. Delirium due to a general medical condition
2. Substance-induced delirium (including during the intoxication and withdrawal phases)
3. Delirium due to multiple etiologies
4. Delirium not otherwise specified

The majority of patients with a delirium recover. A subgroup of patients with delirium end in a demented state. According to Wise and Brandt (1992), 25% die within 6 months after they receive the diagnosis of delirium from a consultation psychiatrist.

To reach an appropriate diagnosis of the cognitive dysfunction, the interviewer needs to correctly identify and interpret symptoms and signs of possible disturbances. These symptoms may be mistakenly interpreted as part of an affective or anxiety disorder if not carefully evaluated.

2. Delirium in the Mental Status

When you *observe* the delirious patient, she may stand in a perplexed state or walk around restlessly. The lack of purpose behind her actions becomes obvious. Another patient may doze off and appear lethargic during the day but be hyperalert and agitated at night. If the delirium is more severe, you may see the patient manipulating invisible objects such as bugs on her skin or small animals on the floor. She may talk back to a dark corner of her room, obviously seeing things obscured to you.

When you engage her in a *conversation,* she gives inappropriate answers, cannot grasp the meaning of your questions, and cannot follow your train of thought. *Exploration,* such as for a chief complaint, produces meaningless answers. Usually, her affect is labile and fluctuating in intensity and quality, reflecting anxiety, anger, depression, apathy, or euphoria. Usually, you quickly get an indication of a coarse disturbance of brain functions so that you can assess orientation and recent memory. You will find the patient confused and amnestic. Her inattentiveness and hallucinations round off the diagnosis of a delirium.

3. Techniques: Repeated Examination of Orientation, Four-Word Memory, Digit Span, Word Spelling, and Serial 7s or 3s

Assessment of attention and concentration are the key techniques in delirium. You will observe dramatic fluctuations in the patient's performance from hour to hour. These fluctuations set delirium apart from dementia and an amnestic syndrome. As tests for determining delirium, perform the following:

- Assess the patient's orientation.
- Assess the patient's memory (give patient four words to repeat immediately and after a 10-minute delay; see Chapter 8, "Amnesia").
- Examine attention (digit span [repetition of 7 digits forward and 5 digits backward] and word spelling), vigilance, and concentration (serial 7s and 3s [serial subtractions by either 7 or 3]) (see Chapter 7, "Inattention and Hyperactivity") in addition to orientation and recent memory.
- Observe the patient's psychomotor activity (this can vary from withdrawal to pacing) and emotional outlets.
- Explore the presence of haptic and visual hallucinations.
- Determine the patient's level of consciousness. Talk to the patient frequently over the span of a day if you suspect clouding of consciousness.

Fluctuating error rates in these tests together with lethargy and sleepiness or marked distractibility indicate clouding of consciousness.

4. Five Steps to Identify Delirium

Usually, the first three steps (listen, tag, confront) are passed over and you move onto Step 4 (solve), in which you examine the severity of the impairment. Your examination may agitate the delirious patient. Be prepared to take him to a quiet room, sit down with him, and talk to him in a reassuring way (Step 5—approve).

5. Interview: Mania Versus Delirium in Human Immunodeficiency Virus (HIV) Infection

Mr. G., a 25-year-old, white, unmarried, homosexual male, is admitted to the hospital because of a recurrent depression which in the past was successfully treated with nortriptyline (Pamelor). Because at least one of these episodes was preceded by reduced sleep, increased energy, laughing, joking, and being teased about being a drug abuser (i.e., because of the change in his behavior), even though he was not, he receives the admission diagnosis of bipolar II disorder, depressed. His psychiatric family history is negative. He does not abuse drugs, alcohol, or nicotine, confirmed by a negative urine screen on admission. His dexamethasone suppression test shows escape with a cortisol level of 8 ng/ml.

Mr. G. reports that he practices safer sex with his homosexual, HIV-positive partner. Two months ago, Mr. G.'s screening test for HIV antibodies was negative.

Mr. G. is started on lithium and fluoxetine (Prozac). Several days after admission, a nurse calls the interviewer and tells her that Mr. G. has suddenly switched into mania. He is talking a lot, pacing, behaving as if in a trance, and entering other patients' rooms. She feels that his lithium dose needs to be increased because his level from the previous day is only 0.4 mEq/L.

When the interviewer enters the ward, the patient is standing in the middle of the lounge gazing around and looking perplexed. (I = interviewer; P = patient)

Step 3: Confront

1. I: Mr. G., you look lost. How are things going?
   P: What? [Picking on his chest and arms, looking down on his body] Going where? Who are you? Need to get out. Feel great. [Smiles, appears elated] What's that?

2. I: What is on your chest and arms?
   P: I chased them away now.
3. I: What did you chase away?
   P: Don't ask. . . . See? Away they run.
4. I: Mr. G., the nurse tells me you are wandering into other patients' rooms.
   P: Rooms? Wandering yeah and nay. All these faces. Where are we? What's going on?

Step 4: Solve

5. I: Where's your room?
   P: [Looks perplexed and points down one side and then the other side of the L-shaped ward] There or there—who cares?
6. I: Let's go to your room.
   P: [Goes back and forth, then walks down one wing and looks in all the patients' rooms] See, all these faces on the wall here? [Points into other patients' rooms]
7. I: Do you know what date it is today?
   P: [Does not know the date or recognize the interviewer. When asked to repeat three objects after 5 minutes, Mr. G. fails. Mr. G. also fails the easiest of the four-problem questions of the Kent Test (Kent 1946): "When the flag points to the south, where does the wind come from?" When failing a question, he is unconcerned and laughs.]
8. I: Everything's all right.
   P: [Breathes heavily and starts crying] What's happening? [Whispering] I'm scared.
9. I: [To the nurse] I'm glad that you called me. I will sedate Mr. G. with some chlorpromazine (Thorazine). More than mania may be causing his trouble.

Step 5: Approve

10. I: Mr. G., I will give you some medication that will calm your nerves and give you some rest.

The patient's perplexed staring around gave the interviewer the first clue that Mr. G. was disoriented. The interviewer could not establish interactive rapport (A. 1–5). Disorientation is unusual for mania. Even a severely excited, manic patient is usually oriented to person, relates well, and often infects people with his elation and puns. Mr. G. appeared lost and struggling to orient himself. Therefore, the interviewer acted as an ally who physically assisted him in finding his room. At the same time, she is testing his cognitive functioning.

The initially observed perplexity (reduced clarity of awareness) prompted the interviewer to immediately test cognitive impairment. She avoided stressful questions that would irritate and frustrate the patient and push him beyond the marginal control that he still was able to maintain.

Mr. G. looked lost and inattentive. His awareness of his environment seemed limited. His motor activity was increased. Observation (A. 1) guided the interviewer to explore tactile hallucinations (A. 1–3) and orientation. The patient showed rapid speech, and short, unconnected, fragmented sentences (A. 1, 4) with rhyming (A. 5). He had labile affect, ranging from perplexity to laughter and from elation to crying and fear. He had visual hallucinations (A. 6). He was disoriented to place (A. 4–6), person (A. 1), and time (A. 7) and could not solve the problem questions of the Kent Test that he could on admission. Because the patient was inattentive and could not focus, the interviewer did not test for apraxia, agnosia, and aphasia. The patient had no insight (A. 1, 4), and his actions reflected impaired judgment.

Diagnosis

Axis I

1. *Delirium of unknown causes.* However, HIV infection is suspected because the patient reports having an intimate relationship with his HIV-infected friend. The patient fulfills the following DSM-IV criteria for delirium:
   a. Impaired environmental awareness and reduced ability to focus
   b. Changes in cognition, the inability to grasp the meaning of simple questions, visual and tactile hallucinations in the absence of auditory hallucinations and delusions, disorientation, deficits in recent memory and simple problem solving, signaling agnosia
   c. Emergence or worsening of possibly previously undetected cognitive deficits over a short time period
   d. Suspicion from history of a nonpsychiatric medical condition, namely HIV infection

   Because the interviewer suspected an activation of a dementia complex of HIV in the form of a delirium, she ordered another screening test for HIV antibodies—the ELISA (enzyme-linked immunosorbent assay) test. The patient's parents were asked to give permission to run the test (they were aware that their son was homosexual and had an HIV-positive lover) because the patient's ability to fully consent appeared to be impaired. The test was positive as was the confirming Western Blot Test.

2. *Bipolar disorder, manic*. This diagnosis is obscured by the patient's present delirium, yet the patient appeared elated in his affect and mood, which was a dramatic switch from the depressed affect observed at admission. Visual hallucinations occur in severe mania, yet tactile hallucinations are rare. They fit better into changes of cognition observed in delirium. On the surface, acutely manic patients may appear disoriented. However, if you give them enough time and encouragement, they prove to be surprisingly well oriented and their recent memory—if you can prompt them to focus long enough—is intact. Their symptoms rarely fulfill the diagnostic criteria for a delirium.

Axis II. None.

Axis III. Suspected HIV infection (proven after the test results were received).

Axis IV. None.

Axis V. Global Assessment of Functioning (GAF) Scale score = 20–30.

Cognitive impairment associated with HIV infection may precede the manifestation of AIDS (Maj 1990). However, so far only one cognitive impairment typical for serum-positive HIV infection has been identified—slowing of psychomotor speed as measured by the Trail Making Test B and Digit Symbol or Symbol Digit Tests (Van Gorp et al. 1993). Most other damage to the central nervous system by the neurotropic retrovirus is highly variable, including dementia (Navia et al. 1986) and psychosis; at times, no cognitive impairment is apparent. In Halstead et al.'s (1988) study of 2,200 patients with HIV infection, only 5 (.2%) presented with such a psychosis. These 5 patients had neither a personal nor a family history of psychiatric disorder in their first-degree relatives. (A similar finding was made by Buhrich et al. 1988.) Other psychiatric syndromes, including mania without cognitive impairment, have been reported in connection with HIV infection (Dilley et al. 1985; Gabel et al. 1986; Perry and Tross 1984; Schmidt and Miller 1988; Wolcott et al. 1985). Therefore, one can repeat for HIV what has been said about the spirochete bacteria that can cause neurosyphilis—it is a great imitator of mental disorders.

In the above example, the cognitive impairment took the form of a delirium, which appears to be rare in a patient who is otherwise free of psychiatric disorders. Mr. G.'s switch into mania may have precipitated the delirium. Because early treatment with zidovudine (Retrovir, formerly called azidothymidine [AZT]) seems to halt or reverse a development of AIDS-related dementia, early detection in high-risk patients can be beneficial for the patient's quality of life (Egan 1992; Forstein 1992). Such patients may come to treatment because of increasing social or work-related problems related to impaired brain functions. The Neuropsychiatric AIDS Rating Scale (Boccellari and Dilley 1992), which classifies HIV-related cognitive impairment along a six-stage continuum, may help to quantify this impairment.

The above interview demonstrates how important it is to conduct an interview targeted at cognitive dysfunctions with patients who have already been diagnosed with a psychiatric disorder. When these patients present with an unusual clinical picture, it should be accepted as atypical only after alternative explanations have been excluded. Cognitive impairment as a complication of HIV-related infection will be a common problem for physicians worldwide (Pajeau and Roman 1992).

6. Delirium in Psychiatric Disorders

Delirium may be due to a substance or a general medical condition. Its presentation varies.

- About 20% of all cases show psychotic features, as occurred in Mr. G. (Horvath et al. 1989). This presentation may lead to misdiagnosis of mania with psychosis, depression with psychotic features, schizophrenia, or brief reactive psychosis.
- Another 20% show depressive, anxious, labile, or irritable mood together with fatigue, subjective weakness, vivid dreaming, and hypersensitivity to stimuli. These symptoms may be misdiagnosed as major depression or generalized anxiety disorder, or both.
- Another 20% show behavioral disturbances, such as irascibility, demanding behavior, uncooperativeness, and, in the case of inpatients, the demand to leave the hospital against medical advice. Such behaviors may lead to an Axis II personality disorder diagnosis.
- About 30% of patients with psychotic features present with dominant cognitive impairment, directing the interviewer to the correct diagnosis of a delirium.
- The remaining 10% show mixed features.

Besides the mental status examination, the electroencephalogram is the single most helpful test because it shows slowing and disorganization of alpha frequency and onset of sporadic theta waves. With increasing severity of the delirium, bilaterally synchronous delta waves emerge.

Both the toxic effects of substances of abuse or withdrawal from such substances may lead to a delirium. Phencyclidine intoxication or sedative withdrawal syndromes (including alcohol) are classic examples of delirium. Furthermore, medications used to treat psychiatric disorders, especially those with strong anticholinergic action such as amitriptyline and protriptyline, may lead to a delirium, especially in elderly individuals. High dosages of these medications or problems with elimination lead to drug accumulation and make the patient susceptible to a delirium. High serum levels of lithium can lead to toxic effects that can cause a delirium. Rarely, lithium may suppress thyroid functions, leading to hypothyroidism, the possible cause of a delirium.

An Axis I psychiatric disorder, such as a bipolar disorder or schizophrenia, may accentuate a preexisting cognitive dysfunction and lead to a delirium-like presentation.

Acute depersonalization or derealization can be mistaken for a delirium. However, the absence of a metabolic disturbance and the presence of a history of dissociative symptoms may guide the interviewer to the correct diagnosis.

Special forms of bipolar disorder can be associated with disorientation and memory impairment. Furthermore, visual hallucinations and rapid change in occurrence of manic and depressive symptoms may lead to a delirium-like presentation. Leonhard (1979) considered this disorder as a special form of cycloid psychosis called *confusional psychosis.*

CHAPTER 10

DEMENTIA

Summary

In this chapter, we show how to establish the diagnosis of three kinds of dementia, two of which are common forms—vascular dementia and dementia of the Alzheimer's type (DAT)—and one of which is a rare form—dementia due to Pick's disease. Besides a general decline in intelligence and recent memory, patients with any of these types of dementia show poor judgment and insight, as well as agnosia, aphasia, apraxia, and decline in executive functions. Pathological reflexes may emerge.

◆ ◆ ◆ ◆ ◆

Animi labes nec diuturnitate evanescere nec amnibus ullis elui potest.
A mental stain can neither be blotted out by the passage of time nor washed away by any waters.

Marcus Tullius Cicero (106–43 B.C.)
De Legibus

◆ ◆ ◆ ◆ ◆

1. What Is Dementia?

Dementia is a simultaneous decline in memory (amnesia); focal cortical cognitive functions, such as language (aphasia), recognition (agnosia), and execution of motor activities (apraxia); and executive functioning from a previous level of functioning. Dementia is used to describe decline that occurs during adulthood, whereas a deficit of these functions during the developmental years is called *mental retardation* (see Chapter 11, "Mental Retardation"). In this chapter, we will describe amnesia, cognitive focal functions, insight, and judgment (for memory functions, see Chapter 8, "Amnesia").

In DSM-IV, eight types of dementia that result from a general medical condition are listed along with their criteria; the types are differentiated based on their etiology. Several other medical causes are also listed, but no criteria are provided for these (Table 10–1).

Amnesia

Cortical and subcortical damage of memory circuits prevents registration of new stimuli and the laying down of memory traces (retention). Thus, words cannot be immediately repeated (impairment of immediate memory), or, if some are repeated, cannot be retrieved (recalled) after several minutes. They also cannot be recognized from a list of words because they have not been stored. Thus, the patient cannot recall events that happened days, hours, or minutes earlier (recent memory).

The association cortex stores patterns of stimuli for long-term reference. The retrieval of these stimuli occurs without the help of the hippocampus, the mammillary bodies, and dorsal medial nuclei of the thalamus. Thus, if profound widespread neuronal cortical damage occurs (as happens in the later stages of DAT), remote memory will be lost.

Table 10–1. Types of dementia listed in DSM-IV

- Dementias resulting from a general medical condition
  Dementia of the Alzheimer's type
  Vascular dementia
  Dementia due to HIV disease
  Dementia due to head trauma
  Dementia due to Parkinson's disease
  Dementia due to Huntington's disease
  Dementia due to Pick's disease
  Dementia due to Jakob-Creutzfeldt disease
- Dementias caused by other medical conditions (no criteria given for these in DSM-IV)
  Brain tumors
  Subdural hematoma
  "Normal pressure" hydrocephalus
  Hypothyroidism
  Hypercalcemia
  Hypoglycemia
  Deficiencies in thiamine, niacin, or vitamin B_{12}
  Neurosyphilis
  Cryptococcosis
  Multiple sclerosis
  Renal and hepatic dysfunction
- Substance-induced dementias
  Alcohol-induced persisting dementia
  Inhalant-induced persisting dementia
  Sedative-, hypnotic-, or anxiolytic-induced persisting dementia
  Other (or unknown) substance-induced persisting dementia
- Dementias resulting from multiple etiologies
- Dementias not otherwise specified

Focal Cortical Cognitive Functions

The brain perceives the environment by its sensory organs, interprets events (integrating them with the present need state and with past experiences), and then responds to the stimuli in the here and now. The patient with focal, multifocal, and generalized cortical damage misinterprets his environment and produces inappropriate responses. For example, he fails to

- Recognize familiar objects—e.g., naming his own fingers or pointing to them or to the interviewer's fingers (agnosia), a deficit seen most frequently in patients with localized lesions of the dominant parieto-occipital areas
- Understand spoken language (sensory aphasia), a deficit that results from the destruction of Wernicke's area of the left upper temporal gyrus (Brodmann area 22)
- Produce meaningful sentences (expressive aphasia), a deficit that results from the destruction of Broca's area in the prefrontal gyrus (Brodmann area 44)
- Perform simple actions, such as using a hammer with the right hand (ideomotor apraxia), a deficit that occurs with damage to any of the cortical areas that control the action of that hand, as listed below:
  - Brodmann area 22 (for comprehension of the task)
  - Brodmann areas 1, 2, 3, 39, and 40 (for activation of kinesthetic memories in the supramarginal gyrus and post-Rolandic parietal cortex)
  - The association fibers that lead to the premotor areas
  - The premotor areas themselves, which order the task
  - The pyramidal neurons, which perform the final action
- Operate familiar machinery (ideational apraxia), a deficit that most frequently occurs with bilateral destruction of the parietal lobe (for more details, see Young and McGlone 1992; Strub and Black 1977, 1988)
- Carry out executive functions, such as "anticipation, goal establishment, planning, response trials, monitoring of results, and the use of feedback" (Young and McGlone 1992, p. 55). In DSM-IV (American Psychiatric Association 1994), these functions are defined as planning, organizing, sequencing, and abstracting. Damage to the frontal lobe of the brain significantly impairs these functions.

You want to recognize agnosia, aphasia, apraxia, and disturbance of executive functions so that you can diagnose dementias (see "3. Techniques" below; also Othmer and Othmer 1994).

Insight

A healthy person has some appreciation of her strengths and weaknesses. She can understand criticism of her shortcomings and she can criticize herself. The nondominant parietal lobe participates in these functions. Destruction of this parietal lobe leads to a loss of insight and to a neglect of the left side of the body and of stimuli arising in the left visual field, which is controlled by the right side of the brain (Strub and Black 1977).

To arrive at the correct diagnosis, the interviewer must be able to separate a lack of insight caused by cortical brain lesions from a lack of insight caused by other noncognitive Axis I psychiatric disorders or psychological defenses.

Judgment

Individuals integrate their hierarchy of needs with their physical and social environment. Relative success in this task makes the person appear wise or foolish. Several brain functions participate in this task. Subcortical structures signal to the cortex basic needs such as hunger, thirst, sleep, sexual desires, personal safety, and social recognition. Unlearned, instinctual behaviors become activated. The hypothalamus and the limbic system are the sources for the emotionally charged experiences that influence judgment by evoking feelings such as pain, anxiety, or lust. Cortical functions, including the frontal lobe, integrate these internal needs and motifs with past experiences and environmental cues. They control these needs by suppressing, delaying, or satisfying them in a socially acceptable manner. If these control functions are disturbed, a patient may blurt out his needs in a demanding, coarse, indiscreet, and socially unacceptable way, showing poor judgment.

Poor judgment can be the result of physiological or psychological processes; the interviewer needs to examine all possible etiologies to arrive at an accurate diagnosis.

2. Dementia in the Mental Status

A patient with beginning dementia who is free of hallucinations, neurological focal signs, and depressive symptoms, may appear normal in expression of affect and psychomotor behavior. Superficial conversation may not reveal the beginning dementia either. To determine if the patient has dementia, focus on recent events, decision making, or problem solving that may prompt the patient to use rationalization. Words she cannot find remain on the tip of her tongue and become replaced by circumscriptions. The timing of recent events becomes unimportant; she may explain she is retired. Dates lose their meaning. Decisions are of no consequences. The patient appears to have adjusted to a lower level of intellectual and executive functioning without regretting the loss.

An examination of cognitive functions yields deficits in memory, use of language, performance of a series of meaningful actions, and recognition of formerly familiar objects.

3. Techniques: Testing for Aphasia, Agnosia, Apraxia, Executive Functions, Pathological Reflexes, Judgment, and Insight

Focal Neuropsychiatric Signs

Aphasia. To identify and classify different types of aphasias, use four tasks summarized in the mnemonic "WRITE, REPEAT, and COMPREHEND FLU-ENTLY."

WRITE. To screen for any aphasia, ask the patient,

> Please write down in one sentence what problems brought you here to see me.

If the patient can write down a meaningful sentence using correct grammar, a moderate to severe form of aphasia is unlikely.

REPEAT. Ask the patient to repeat "Mississippi River." If he can do it, have him repeat, "The tall, young janitor cleaned the floors upstairs." Ask the educated patient to repeat, "Every aspect of the problem needs more detailed discussion."

COMPREHEND. Ask the patient the following questions:

> Do women wear athletic supporters?
> Do you harvest potatoes in Iowa in December?

Missing the questions on the Kent Test (Kent 1946) that measure problem solving (see Table 11–1) may also indicate a problem in comprehension.

FLUENTLY. Generally, a lack of fluency is immediately apparent in the interview. However, whether the patient is fluent or not, if the content of his speech is agrammatical, he is suspect for having an aphasia.

Agnosia. Screen for agnosias with two types of questions:

- Ask the patient to identify fingers (finger agnosia), faces from photographs (prosopagnosia), and right-left locations of body parts (right-left agnosia) and to find locations on a map (geographic agnosia). A combined right-left and finger agnosia is called *Gerstmann's syndrome.*
- Have the patient name different objects that you point to (actual visual agnosia), describe their color (actual color agnosia), and name other objects after you have described their use (associated visual agnosia). Have the patient list different colors (associative color agnosia). (For more details and a decision tree, see Othmer and Othmer 1994.)

Apraxia. While testing for apraxia, make sure that a possible deficit is not due to a paralysis or paresis.

Ideomotor apraxia

- *Limb apraxia.* Ask the patient to show you how she brushes her teeth, would hammer in a nail, or would flip a coin.
- *Buccofacial apraxia.* Ask the patient to show you how she would blow out a match or drink through a straw.
- *Whole body apraxia.* Ask the patient to show you how she bends her knees or would swing a golf club.

Ideational apraxia

- *General.* Ask the patient to show you how she would sign a letter, fold it, put it in an envelope, seal it, address it, and put a stamp on it.
- *Dressing.* Ask the patient to show you how she would put on one sock, then put on one shoe, lace it, and tie it.
- *Constructional.* Ask the patient to draw a diamond and a cube and outline a cross. Then have her take three matches and form a triangle, and then take six matches and form a pyramid. Then have her draw a clock that shows the current time. All these tasks are more difficult for the patient to do if she has to perform them on request only, without having a model to copy from.

Executive Functioning

Test the patient's executive functioning by having him tell you similarities, count to 10, recite the alphabet, subtract serial 7s or 3s, name as many animals as possible in 1 minute, draw a line with continuous m's and n's, and use shifting sets. To test shifting sets, ask the patient:

> When I say A1, B2, C3, how do you continue?

The correct answer would be "D4, E5, F6," and so on. A patient with frontal lobe damage may perseverate (e.g., say "D4, D5, D6, D7" or "D4, E4, F4, G4") (Othmer and Othmer 1994).

Clinically relevant bedside assessment techniques have recently been developed, including the Executive Interview (EXIT; Royall et al. 1992) and the Qualitative Evaluation of Dementia (QED; Royall et al. 1993). (Both are reprinted with permission in the Appendix.)

The EXIT is a standardized and validated instrument that assesses impairment of executive functions. It contains 25 tasks scored as 0, 1, or 2 (0 = normal; 1 = partially impaired; 2 = impaired). The authors recommend a cutoff point of 15—scores above 15 indicate impairment. However, community studies are in progress that, in the opinion of Royall et al., may lead to a lowering of the cutoff point to 10.

The QED is a brief, 15-item checklist that differentiates cortical from subcortical dementia. A score of 0 indicates pure subcortical dementia characterized by apathy, and a score of 30 indicates pure cortical dementia characterized by disinhibition. A score of 15 indicates normal function (see Appendix). Blinded raters show an 80% accuracy in their assessment with this instrument.

Pathological Reflexes

- *Snout reflex.* Tap the patient's upper lip with your finger or a reflex hammer. A snoutlike movement (called a *snout reflex) is a positive response.*
- *Rooting.* Scratch below one angle of the patient's mouth. A pulling down of the ipsilateral angle of the mouth is a positive response.
- *Palmomental reflex.* Scratch across the patient's palm with a key. A pulling down of the ipsilateral angle of the mouth is a positive response.
- *Grasp reflex.* Scratch the patient's palm longitudinally with your fingers. The patient's grasping your fingers is a positive response.

- *Sucking reflex.* Lightly stroke the patient's upper lip. A sucking movement is a positive response.
- *Glabella reflex.* Tap the patient's forehead above the bridge of the nose. The eyes cease to blink after a few taps. The test is positive if no extinction occurs (perseverative glabella reflex).
- *Babinski reflex.* Scratch the outside margin of the sole of the patient's foot longside. An upward motion of the patient's great toe is pathological.

Judgment

Clinicians often test judgment in two ways:

- *Social judgment.* One commonly used example is to ask the patient,

  If you find an addressed, stamped letter, what do you do?

  The correct answer is,

  You put it in a mailbox.

  An inappropriate response would be,

  Take the stamp off and use it.

- *Personal planning.* Examples (for more details, see Othmer and Othmer 1994):

  - What are your plans for the future?
  - What are your chances of making a new start in life?
  - Do you think you can make a major invention?

Insight

A patient possesses insight when she is aware of her deficit and recognizes it as part of a psychiatric disorder, rather than as the result of external or magical forces, or denies them categorically. Such a denial is typical for dementia.

The standard question to assess insight is:

Do you think you have a problem?

If the patient answers yes, then ask

> Is it part of a disorder? Do you need help for it?

4. Five Steps to Identify Dementia

A five-step approach will yield the information necessary for an understanding of the patient's degree of cognitive dysfunction.

Step 1: Listen. Often the problem comes to your attention through the patient's friends or relatives. Such intervention by a third party should alert you to three diagnostic possibilities: 1) the patient is psychotic, 2) he lacks insight, or 3) he is anxious or dependent. Sometimes the police intervene if the patient acted socially inappropriately, such as running naked in the street, or acted in a dangerous manner.

Step 2: Tag. Repeat the patient's problem to the patient or informant or both. Separate the factual occurrences from the patient's and the informant's interpretation. The patient and informant often share the need to minimize to you the patient's intellectual limitations and to maximize conflicts and environmental stressors, thus obscuring the patient's real loss of cognitive functioning.

Step 3: Confront. Focus the patient and the informant clearly on the cognitive failure, suggesting alternative reasons for the problem than their interpretations and the need to explore this possibility with the patient. Then tell the patient that you can help him understand his problem better if he agrees to answer some specific test questions.

Step 4: Solve. First, test the patient's attention and concentration, then his orientation and memory. Second, test praxis, speech, and reflexes. Finally, test the patient's intelligence and judgment. Compare the patient's knowledge with his ability to think. Knowledge represents past cognitive functioning frozen into remote memory traces; thinking represents present ability to solve a problem.

At its onset, dementia impairs the current thinking process more than remote memory. Select tests targeted at the early detection of the suspected cognitive dysfunction. Apply the mental status battery described below. Apply this systematic testing to suspected psychosis and cognitive dysfunction. The battery will confirm impairment in the cognitive disorders but will exclude them in schizophrenia and schizophreniform, schizoaffective, delusional, brief psychotic, and shared psychotic disorders as well as in the mood disorders.

Step 5: Approve. Summarize your findings for the patient and his family. If you detect cognitive impairment, tell all involved how important it is to 1) verify your impression, and 2) identify the underlying cause in order to develop a management and treatment plan.

In the following section, we present three patients with different types of dementia: vascular dementia, dementia due to Pick's disease, and DAT. With our present knowledge, we may be able to slow down the progression of vascular dementia by agents that in vivo prevent vascular coagulation. Therefore, the recognition of vascular dementia has therapeutic implications. DAT is the prototype of senile dementia. Yet, symptoms typical for this form of dementia are not found in the early stages of Pick's dementia. Thus, Pick's dementia may be treated as an atypical bipolar disorder. Such a diagnostic miss may be costly and may prevent the family from taking appropriate steps for the future care of such a patient.

5. Interview A: Retarded Depression Versus Apraxia in Vascular Dementia

The nurse from the emergency room at a hospital phones the interviewer about a 76-year-old farmer, Mr. M., who was referred by his internist, Dr. I., for possible admission because of a suicidal gesture. The patient's wife had found her husband handling shotgun cartridges.

Dr. I. had earlier reported to the interviewer the following items: Mr. M. has been healthy except for hypertension; his psychiatrist, Dr. P., is retiring; and Mr. M. needs help with his bipolar disorder. Dr. I. added that now when Mr. M. gets depressed, he appears to become more confused. The wife feels she cannot manage him at home. The patient refuses admission.

The interviewer asks the nurse to give the phone to Mr. M. (I = interviewer; P = patient; W = wife)

I: [On the phone with the patient] Hi, Mr. M. I'm Dr. O. I was expecting you. I'm glad that you arrived. Dr. I. asked me to check you out. Dr. I. is a friend of mine. So I better do what he asked me to do. I'll look you over as soon as I come to the hospital. Is that okay with you?

P: Sure, doc.

I: If you want me to do what Dr. I. says, you have to sign the paper. And I want the nurse to help you with that. I will tell her to help you. Please hand her the phone. [To the nurse on the phone] Give Mr. M. a pen now so he can sign in. Tell him I will be in later. [With surprise, the nurse reports to the interviewer that Mr. M. is signing in.]

Step 1: Listen

When the interviewer arrives at the hospital, he shakes hands with Mr. M., asking him at the same time if he is right-handed, which Mr. M. and his wife confirm.

1. I: What seems to be the problem?

   W: For 20 years my husband has had bipolar disorder. He's been on 300 mg lithium at night. His blood level is 0.7. But lately, he's been acting up again, and Dr. P. gave him 200 mg of Mellaril [thioridazine] at night to calm him down because he's had spells of crying and laughter and walks with stiff legs. He's still not right and Dr. P. is retiring.

2. I: Can you give me an example of his "acting up again"?

   W: He suddenly became so depressed that he couldn't do anything. Our furnace broke down the other day and he tried to fix it. When he did not come back from the basement, I followed him. He stood in front of the furnace with two shotgun cartridges in his hand trying to light them. He's been suicidal before. So I called our son over for help. But then my husband told him exactly how to fix the furnace but could not do it himself. The next day, my husband was in the furnace room again. This time he had one hand in a bucket with ice water and with the other hand he pushed against the fuse switch, saying he wanted to keep the furnace running. You see, my husband is so depressed he doesn't know what he's doing.

   P: [While the wife talks, Mr. M. is sitting in his chair looking at the interviewer. When the interviewer tries to include him in the conversation, he smiles and nods but does not make any effort to disagree with his wife. Therefore, the interviewer summarizes his impression for Mr. M.]

3. I: It seems, Mr. M., that you have had some problems that both your psychiatrist, Dr. P., and your internist, Dr. I., have recognized. They trust me with this and I will do my best to work along with them. With your help, we'll find out what may have caused your problems.

   The interviewer initiated rapport with the patient over the telephone, as evidenced by the patient's compliance. Because the interviewer was told by Dr. I. that the patient was depressed and confused, the interviewer told the patient why he had to sign in, thereby assisting the wife who stated that she was unable to handle the patient. Such an approach—to tell the patient what to do—worked for two reasons: first, it did not activate the ambivalence typical of depression by asking the patient to make a decision; second, it avoided challenging the patient's failing intellectual powers. To confront him would provoke him to become stubborn and unable to reason. Many patients with suspected cognitive impairment try to appear competent. Thus, they agree with rather than oppose an esteemed authority figure. They follow familiar environmental cues. Because Mr. M.'s remote memory was still intact, he could understand the reference to his former caregiver.

The interviewer allowed the wife to answer because the patient might not have been able to.

The patient is right-handed. He appeared impaired and socially dependent. His affect was unchanging; he kept a rigid smile even when his cognitive failures were discussed in his presence. This observation alerted the interviewer to search for the cause of this passive behavior, such as the presence of a cognitive dysfunction, psychomotor retardation, or dependent personality as seen in a subcortical form of dementia (see the QED in the Appendix).

As to diagnosis, the wife's report of Mr. M.'s knowing how to light the furnace (as evidenced by his directions to his son) but not being able to do so himself would suggest sudden onset of apraxia; the cartridge handling may have been a sign of confusion and not a suicidal gesture, which was the wife's interpretation. Because the patient could instruct his son how to fix the furnace, his posterior cortical areas storing his remote memory appeared to function. His not being able to fix the furnace himself would indicate that certain cortical functions of the dominant parietal lobe areas, the interconnections of parietal to prefrontal areas, or the prefrontal areas themselves might be impaired and hinder execution of these actions by the patient himself. This interpretation was supported by the wife's report that Mr. M. was walking with stiff legs, which could point to a lacunar stroke and an impairment of the pyramidal cortical spinal tracts. In this context, crying and laughter could be a sign of pseudobulbar palsy supporting the presence of a lacunar stroke and presence of vascular dementia.

Step 2: Tag

4. I: You are telling me that your husband knows what he wants to do, he can explain to your son what to do, but can't do it himself.
   W: That's right.
5. I: Mr. M., do you remember that you tried to light the cartridges? [When the wife tries to answer again, the interviewer signals with a gesture that he wants Mr. M. to answer.]

P: [With a smile and normal rate of speech] Well, I had the cartridges out because the hunting season is starting.

6. I: What about having your hand in the bucket with ice water?

P: I guess I was trying to clean up the furnace room.

Step 3: Confront

7. I: Do you mean that your wife really didn't understand what you were trying to do?

P: Yeah, that's right. She worries a lot and she looks out for me.

8. I: Do you feel she needs to look out for you?

P: [Without answering the question] You see, I have over 2,000 acres of land and my annual payments are due at the end of the year and I'm always worried about it.

9. I: Well, Mr. M., it sounds like your wife describes something more than worrying. It sounds like you get confused.

P: I guess I get confused when I worry.

The interviewer shifted his attention to Mr. M. (Q. 5) who cooperated. His responses were inappropriate; they reflected a routine response prompted by familiar cues and appeared to be a manifestation of impaired brain function rather than resulting from motivational factors, such as a wish to mislead (A. 5, 6, 8). The interviewer did not confront the patient with the inappropriateness of the answers but accepted them in order not to annoy Mr. M.

Mr. M.'s reason for lighting the cartridges was poor, as it had no logical connection to the hunting season. The ice water justification was equally inappropriate. Mr. M.'s explanations did not have the quality of rationalization. The logic lacking in his answers pointed to his decreased reasoning power (A. 5–8).

As to diagnosis, Mr. M.'s poor reasoning power and sudden onset of apraxia would support the diagnosis of vascular dementia in addition to the known bipolar disorder. The coexistence of DAT is not excluded.

Step 4: Solve

10. I: Mr. M., I think I would like to ask you a few questions that will tell me how well you can track things.

P: Oh, go right ahead.

11. I: Well, can you keep track of time?

P: [Cheerfully] I think so.

12. I: Do you know what date it is?

P: Oh sure, it's 1992. Matter of fact it's December. [Answers correctly]

13. I: Do you know the day?

P: It's Wednesday. [It is Friday.]
14. I: Do you know the date?
P: Oh, it's the sixth or the seventh. [It is the eleventh.]
15. I: Can you repeat four words for me: honesty, yellow, eyedropper, and tulip?
P: Yes.
16. I: Which ones were they?
P: Yellow, tulip. . . . Hmmm, I didn't pay any attention to the others.
17. I: They were honesty, yellow, eyedropper, and tulip. Can you do it now?
P: Eyedropper, tulip, yellow . . . [then, with a triumphant smile] honesty. Yes, that was it.
18. I: Keep them in mind because I will ask for them again. In the meantime, let me ask you a few other questions. At what time of the day is your shadow the shortest?
P: In the morning or in the evening. I guess it's in the evening.
19. I: Why does the moon appear larger than the stars?
P: Because it is larger. God wanted it that way.
20. I: If the flag floats to the south, where does the wind come from?
P: Oh, from the north.
21. I: If your shadow points to the northeast, where is the sun?
P: Oh, in the southeast.
22. I: How many stripes does the American flag have?
P: [With triumph] Thirteen for the original thirteen colonies.
23. I: What metal does a magnet attract?
P: Steel and other ferrous metals, like iron.
24. I: What can you make out of sand?
P: Concrete.
25. I: Anything else?
P: [Laughing] Sandcastles.
26. I: Anything more?
P: [Grinning] Sandpaper.
27. I: If I say A1, B2, C3, how would you have to continue?
P: D4, E5, F6, G7.
28. I: Mr. M., could you show me how you sign a letter, fold it, put it in an envelope, seal it, and stamp it?
P: Okay. [He mimics folding a piece of paper, and then folds it again, and then looks at the interviewer in a befuddled way.]
29. I: That's fine. Now, can you tap your right knee two times with your right hand and then tap your left knee one time with your left hand?
P: Can you say that again?
30. I: [Repeats question]
P: [Starts to tap his right knee with his right hand and keeps doing it]
31. I: What I want you to do is tap your right knee just twice.
P: [Does it] Like that?
32. I: Yes. And tap your left knee just once.
P: [Taps his left knee with his right hand once]
33. I: No. Use your left hand for your left knee.
P: [Taps his left knee with his left hand continuously]

34. I: No, just once.
    P: [Does it once]
35. I: Do you understand? Can you now do it?
    P: [With a confident smile] Sure. [With both hands taps both knees continuously]
36. I: May I test a few reflexes?
    P: Go ahead.
37. I: [Snout, sucking, glabella, and palmomental reflexes are negative; Babinski reflex is positive.]
38. I: Do you still remember the four words that I told you to remember?
    P: What four words?
39. I: The four words I asked you to repeat?
    P: Yeah?
40. I: Do you remember any of them?
    P: [Looks bewildered]
41. I: One was a color. Do you remember the color?
    P: Yellow, wasn't it?
42. I: Yes. And one was a flower.
    P: Was it rose?
43. I: No. I also gave you an abstract word. Can you pick which one it was? Justice, honesty, and equality.
    P: Was it justice?
44. I: [To the wife] Was your husband ever confused before?
    W: Yeah, I think so. Last year, he wanted to run his tractor and didn't know how to. I thought he had worked too much. So we went to my sister's in Minnesota for 2 weeks. I drove the whole way. When we came back, he went right to the tractor and got it started without any problems.
45. I: How was he doing afterward?
    W: Oh, he wasn't high then as he was this time when it started.
46. I: Was he different in any way?
    W: No, I don't think so.
47. I: Was he more forgetful?
    W: No,. that was the first time, the winter before. He got up at 3:30 A.M. and said he had a headache and felt dizzy. And then he looked out of the window and it was snowing. "I better clean the driveway," he said, and went out to the shack. I followed him after a little while and he didn't know what he was looking for. I said, "You wanted to use the snowblower." And he said, "Where is it? What does it look like?" And the blower was just sitting in front of him. Then we went to Florida, and he seemed to be more forgetful. It took him longer to do things. And Dr. P. thought he had a depression and stopped some of his medication.
48. I: Did anything unusual happen this time that did not happen before?
    W: [Hesitates] Like what?
49. I: Well, your husband walked with stiff legs. He lost some control. . . . How was his bladder control?
    W: [Looking at her husband, who smiles] I think the lithium made him drink too much. He had an accident one night.

Step 5: Approve

50. I: Well, I'm glad that you came to see me, Mr. M. This is very important. We
        want to know what's going on.
    P: Okay, I want to go now.
51. I: We really have to find out what is going on this time. [To the wife] Can you
        look out for your husband at home?
    W: Not really. I have to call my son over to help, but he can't always come. And
        if he starts something like with the cartridges, I can't stop him. I can't always
        watch him.
52. I: Well, Mr. M., I think you should stay in the hospital. I want to stop all your
        medication, run a brain map, get a magnetic resonance imaging [MRI] scan
        and a few other tests to see what is going on. I wouldn't want anything to
        happen to you while we stop your medication.
    P: No. I'm going home.
53. I: I talked to Dr. P. before you came here. He told me that you get confused
        at times, usually when you get depressed. I promised him to take good care
        of you as he has done for the last 20 years. I can't go bad on my promise.
    P: [Grunts]
54. I: Mr. M., you are a farmer. You understand what it means living up to a
        promise. And we will do what Dr. P. would have done, run a few tests.
    P: I guess we'll have to go ahead with it.

The patient was friendly and tried to appear healthy. He minimized his
problems (A. 16). He was cooperative and objected only when asked to stay
at the hospital (A. 52). At that juncture, the interviewer again borrowed the
authority of the patient's former psychiatrist and family physician to prevent
the patient from signing out. As we pointed out before, patients with
dementia depend on their remote memory and Drs. I. and P. were both part
of that prior, intact perceptual world with which Mr. M. felt comfortable. Mr.
M. could safely go along with the interviewer because the interviewer
represented an extension of Drs. I. and P., whom the patient trusted.

The centerpiece of the technique used in this interview was the mental
status examination of cognitive and intellectual functions. Besides recent
memory and orientation (A and Q. 12–14), present praxia was examined
(Q. 28–35). The interviewer obtained an outside history of the patient's
confusion and praxia from the wife (Q. 44–49).

To test the patient's cognitive impairment, the interviewer used the
abbreviated Kent Test (Kent 1946). The patient could answer four knowledge questions very well (A. 20, 22–24). He missed only 2 points out of a
possible 13, namely, that one can make glass out of sand (A. 24–26). In
contrast, he failed three out of four questions that involved thinking (A. 18,
19, 21). He passed only the easiest of the four problem-solving questions

(Q. 20). Of 14 possible points for these four questions he received only 3. This means that Mr. M.'s knowledge is proportionately better preserved than his problem-solving ability.

Mr. M. was grossly oriented to time. He showed short-term memory impairment; out of four test words, he could repeat only one after 10 minutes. He could do the shifting set (A. 27). It took the hand-clapping test to reveal his problem with alternating movements (A. 28–35). Perseveration in motor activity is an indicator of frontal lobe impairment.

The patient's recent history demonstrated apraxia—his inability to light the furnace—and agnosia—his inability to recognize the use of shotgun cartridges. In combination with these symptoms, the right positive Babinski reflex was a red flag. It indicated a lacunar stroke and identified Mr. M.'s disorder as vascular dementia, which was affecting most connections to the frontal lobe.

The patient had no insight into his deficits. His recent history and his behavior surrounding his hospitalization showed his lack of judgment.

The customary method for testing cognitive functions (assessing only orientation and asking simple memory questions [recalling three words, such as pencil, car, and watch]) would have failed to identify the patient's cognitive impairment, which was severe enough to possibly cause harm to himself and his property. The more elaborate mental status testing validated the wife's report, which suggested cognitive dysfunction.

Diagnosis

Axis I

1. *Subcortical vascular dementia (lacunar syndrome).* The vascular dementias share diagnostic criteria with other dementias, but are distinct in showing hypertension and focal neurological signs, such as exaggerated deep tendon reflexes, extensor plantar response, pseudobulbar palsy, gait abnormalities, and weakness of an extremity. Multiple vascular lesions of the cerebral cortex and subcortical structures can be diagnosed using computed tomography and MRI, as noted in DSM-IV.

   The present episode of intermittent confusion in Mr. M. appeared to be the result of a vascular problem—infarctions at deeper structures of the brain that acutely but only temporarily interfered with cognitive intellectual functions. This confusion was less likely the result of bipolar disorder, lithium, or thioridazine side effects. Mr. M.'s gait disturbance;

equivocal, right-sided, positive Babinski reflex; intermittent bed-wetting; emotional lability; and lack of motivation confirmed this diagnosis. He seemed to experience mini-infarcts of small vessels of the brain stem caused by hypertensive small vessel disease. This disease causes a progressive lacunar state with a positive Babinski reflex and pseudo-bulbar palsy (Roman 1985).

2. *Cortical vascular dementia.* Mr. M. also could have ischemia of the middle cerebral artery, which would contribute to his transient state of apraxia and intermittent confusion caused by arteriosclerotic or hypertensive disease of large arteries. His Hachinski Ischemic score (Horvath et al. 1989) (Table 10–2) was 15 when the interviewer rated Mr. M.'s history of symptoms and signs.

3. *Rule out dementia of the Alzheimer's type.* At its onset, DAT affects predominantly the hippocampal area and thus interferes most strikingly with orientation to time and recent memory. Mr. M.'s presenting impairment was an intermittent apraxia, intermittent bed-wetting, and possible residual damage to the corticospinal pyramidal tract. Thus, his problems could be better explained by a vascular dementia than by DAT.

4. *Bipolar disorder (by history).* Mr. M.'s wife and Dr. P. both chalked up the patient's episode as one of his usual periods of excitement or retarded

Table 10–2. Hachinski ischemic score for patient in interview A

Feature	Score
Abrupt onset	2
Stepwise orientation	1
Fluctuating course	2
Nocturnal confusion	1
Relative preservation of personality	1
Depression	1
Somatic complaints	0
Emotional incontinence	1
History of hypertension	2
History of strokes	0
Evidence of associated arteriosclerosis	0
Focal neurological symptoms	2
Focal neurological signs (excluding aphasis and apraxia)	2
Total score	**15**

depression during which he needed medication adjustment. Only a thorough cognitive evaluation and investigation of the history led to the correct diagnosis.

Axis II. None.

Axis III. Hypertension.

Axis IV. Mild to moderate.

Axis V. Global Assessment of Functioning (GAF) Scale score = 30; highest level of functioning during the last year = 60.

Follow-Up

Mr. M.'s MRI was within normal limits. No atrophy of the lobes, enlarged ventricles, or evidence of infarction was found. These results excluded cortical vascular but not subcortical vascular dementia, as infarctions may be small and nondetectable.

   Brain mapping suggested mild vascular problems. The Mini-Mental State Exam (Folstein et al. 1975) and the Screening Test for the Luria-Nebraska Neuropsychological Battery (Golden 1987) were abnormal. However, the patient improved dramatically within a 1-month follow-up period during which he was continued on lithium and started on aspirin and dipyridamole (Persantine). This course would support the diagnosis of a vascular dementia, in which an improvement of functioning occurs after the initial edema surrounding the mini-infarcts has been reabsorbed. The continuous control of the bipolar disorder with lithium prevented interference by this disorder, which otherwise could have complicated the course.

5. Interview B: Mania Versus Frontal Lobe Inhibition in Pick's Disease

Ms. R. is a 38-year-old, white, married production line worker who is brought to a university clinic by her husband for psychiatric consultation. The husband reports, "She's on the go all the time."

   While the patient waits in the lounge, her husband gives a short account. Her supervisor had called from work to ask her to stay home and see a doctor because she had shut down the production line a number of times. She took her colleagues' food impulsively and, when reprimanded, just smiled and said, "okay," and continued with her behavior.

Her husband continues,

> She is in constant motion during the day, but in good spirits. At night she is exhausted and sleeps soundly for 6–8 hours. When she gets up, she is in motion again.

Somewhat embarrassed, he adds,

> She often makes sexual remarks.

Ms. R. drinks neither alcohol nor coffee, but she craves chocolate milk. She puts a lot of cigarettes into her mouth, takes a few puffs without inhaling, and throws them away. She has not abused any drugs and has only tried marijuana once or twice. Her family history is negative for psychiatric disorders.

The family physician has recommended consulting a psychiatrist. "Your wife has a classic case of bipolar disorder," he told the husband.

The interviewer asks the husband to bring Ms. R. in from the lounge. Her hair seems washed but is uncombed. (I = interviewer; P = patient; H = husband)

Step 1: Listen

1. I: Ms. R., your husband told me that you move around a lot. Do you notice that yourself?
   P: [With a mechanical smile] Yes.
2. I: By the way, what would you like me to call you?
   P: [Rapidly] Linda.
3. I: Linda, that must feel awful when you can't stop moving.
   P: Let's go.
4. I: Linda, could you sit still if you wanted to?
   P: Yes. [Stands up and says to her husband] Let's go now.
   H: Sit down, Linda, and let's talk to the doctor.
   P: [Pressed and rapidly] I have to go to the bathroom.
   H: Just wait a minute.
   P: I have to go pee-pee. [Leaves the office]
   H: [After the patient has left] That's how she is at home now all the time.
5. I: Linda uses baby language—"having to go pee-pee"—is that new?
   H: She started that a few months ago. She does that even in public.
6. I: How did this all start? When is the first time you remember her acting strange?

H: Maybe 8 months ago, she started to repeat herself. She was telling me the same story about what happened at work that day several times in one evening. [Patient comes back.]

P: You're good looking, Dr. X. [Grinning]

H: Linda, sit down now.

Step 2: Tag

7. I: Linda, your husband just told me you go to the bathroom often.

   P: [Rapidly] Yes.

8. I: Do you have to urinate a lot?

   P: No, not much. I just have to go.

9. I: What's on your mind when you go to the bathroom?

   P: Can I go and have a cigarette?

10. I: I would like to talk to you first.

   P: Okay. You're good looking, Dr. X. [Smiles again]

11. I: Are you a heavy smoker?

   P: No, I don't inhale. I just take a few puffs. Can I go outside and have a cigarette now?

12. I: What did I just ask you to do, Linda?

   P: [Rapidly] To sit and talk to you.

13. I: And do you remember what you answered me?

   P: I said okay.

14. I: So let's try to do that.

   P: I want a cigarette now. [Getting up]

   H: Linda, sit down and wait a little bit.

   P: I'll have a cigarette now. [Smiles at the interviewer and leaves the room]

15. I: [To the husband] So Linda notices that she is restless? She agrees to sit down but then does not do it?

   H: [Nodding] That's exactly what she does.

16. I: I guess we'll wait until Linda comes back.

   H: That usually does not take very long. She wanders away just to come back.

17. I: Has she ever gotten lost?

   H: No, not really, she finds her way around, and she hasn't taken off yet. [Patient comes back in.]

Step 3: Confront

18. I: Linda, you could have hardly lit up a cigarette, let alone smoked it.

   P: [Mechanically smiling] I don't smoke. I just puff.

19. I: Whenever you walk away, it is because you want to smoke or because you want to go to the bathroom . . .

   H: Or she wants to drink chocolate milk.

   P: [Smiling]

20. I: Linda, all your actions involve some basic need.

   P: [To her husband] Can we go now?

H: [To Linda] Just a moment. [To the interviewer] Yes, and that also includes sex. She talks about it more than she used to and then she won't do it.

21. I: Does she cut all her actions short?

H: Yes, except for sleeping. She hardly gets up during the night.

Step 4: Solve

22. I: [Asks patient to repeat four words, which she does] Linda, I'd like you to write down why you are here.

P: I want to go now.

H: Linda, write down what the doctor asks you to do. And then we'll go.

P: [Takes a pencil and writes, "I here."]

23. I: Can you sign it?

P: [Signs her first name]

24. I: Can you tap your right knee twice with your right hand and your left knee once with your left hand?

P: Yes.

25. I: Please do it! [Demonstrates how to do it]

P: [Slaps the desk with her right hand continuously]

26. I: Linda, do you know what date it is and where we are?

P: [Gives the correct date and place]

27. I: Okay, Linda, when I say A1, B2, C3, what would be next?

P: [Getting up] A1, A2, A3, 4, 5, 6, 7.

28. I: Okay, stop. Let me do a simple test, Linda. I will tap your upper lip with this reflex hammer. Is that okay with you?

P: Fine, but I want to go.

29. I: [Walks over to the patient and taps her upper lip. She shows a snout reflex. Then he scratches the palm of her right and left hand with the handle of the hammer. The angles of her mouth pull down slightly. He asks her to repeat the four words. She needs only help with one word.] [To the husband] We need to do a thorough workup of Linda's brain functions, and we have to make appointments for that.

H: That will be difficult. I can't handle her at home any more.

Step 5: Approve

30. I: Well, we can admit Linda to the hospital and I will arrange for a neurological consult.

H: That's fine.

31. I: Linda, your husband will take you over to the hospital and I will see what I can do about your restlessness. [To the husband] Your wife may not be a classic case of bipolar disorder but may have a brain disease.

The patient answered the questions about her hypermotility to the point. However, her answers were mechanical and lacked an emotional engagement with the interviewer (A. 1, 2, 4, 7, 8, 11–13, 18, 19, 22–24). She ignored the empathy the interviewer expressed for her hypermotility (Q. 3) and the request to sit still. She could not be directed. Instead, she repeated her demand to go (A. 3, 4, 20, 22, 28), use the bathroom (A. 4) or smoke (A. 9, 11, 14). Several of her answers appeared inappropriate: baby language (A. 4) and complimenting the interviewer about his looks (A. 6, 10). The interviewer did not become an ally, an expert, or an authority; he remained a casual acquaintance. She was too preoccupied with her activities to talk to him. Instead, rapport developed with the husband. The husband's answers contributed more than the patient's responses.

The techniques that yielded the most information about the patient were not *conversation* and *exploration* but *observation* and *testing* (Q. 22–29).

As to her mental status, Linda was alert. Her hygiene was fair. She noticed her own behavior but gave no indication that it caused her any suffering (A. 3). She had a short attention span. Her concentration was decreased not because of outside stimuli but because of her internal need to move. Her motor behavior was stereotyped—it did not serve any meaningful purpose. The driving force for her actions was her need for increased motor activity, not actual goals. She hardly modified her motor behavior when asked to sit still, even though she had agreed to do so (A. 10). Her motoric actions constituted perseveration. Her perseverations were not related to her forgetting that she had already smoked, used the bathroom, or promised to sit still, but to a primary impulse to repeat. According to her husband, verbal repetition had signaled the onset of her disorder (A. 6). Because her short-term memory was intact at the time of the interview (A. 12, 13, 22) and probably was at the onset of the disorder, the verbal repetitions were an early sign of perseveration.

The patient answered questions in a telegrammatic style that—in the context of this mental status examination—bordered on a nonfluent expressive aphasia. Her brief, agrammatical written note (A. 22) would support this notion. Her answers were truthful and accurate, but her motor perseveration disrupted communication.

Linda's affect was restricted and mildly inappropriate. She showed mechanical smiling (A. 1, 6, 10, 18, 19). The interviewer did not assess her mood himself but accepted the husband's statement that she felt good.

The patient was oriented (A. 26). She failed alternate tapping of her knees (A. 25) and performing shifting sets (A. 27), which confirmed her tendency for perseveration, a localized defect of the frontal lobe. This was supported by the positive snout and palmomental reflexes (Q. 29).

The patient showed deteriorating judgment by increased use of baby language (A. 4), by complimenting the interviewer (A. 6, 10) and by being sexually indiscreet (A. 20).

Diagnosis

Axis I. Dementia due to a neurological condition, most likely Pick's disease.

Patients in the early stages of Pick's disease show changes in personality, deterioration of social skills, emotional blunting, disinhibition, expressive language abnormalities, decline of executive functions, and appearance of prominent primitive reflexes. Apathy and agitation occur. Amnesia, apraxia, and disorientation occur at a later stage. Brain imaging reveals either frontal or temporal atrophy or both, as well as hypometabolism. A brain biopsy or autopsy reveals characteristic intraneuronal argentophilic Pick inclusion bodies (DSM-IV, p. 150). This triad (frontal and/or temporal atrophy, hypometabolism, and intraneuronal argentophilic inclusion bodies) differentiates Pick's disease from other frontotemporal dementias (Baldwin and Förstl 1993).

At the onset of Pick's disease, a sudden deterioration in the judgment of a patient who shows no clear increase in energy, push of speech, or decreased need for sleep may alert you to the presence of the disease. For example, a male teacher started to exercise in the nude on his front balcony while his students walked by on their way to school. He had no insight into his inappropriate behavior. Poor judgment, sexual and social disinhibition, and frontal lobe signs are characteristic of dementia caused by Pick's disease rather than of DAT, the early stage of which is characterized by disorientation and recent memory impairment. At a later stage of dementia of both etiologies, these distinguishing features merge because all cognitive functions become affected.

Many of Linda's behaviors were similar to those of a manic patient, yet they differed in fundamental ways. Her hypermotor activity was driven by perseveration, not by its opposite—involvement in multiple activities. She showed rapid speech, but her sentences were very brief, without circumstantiality or flight of ideas. In fact, she showed the opposite of flight of ideas; she perseverated on a fixed set of subjects. Her affect was bright, but her smile was rigid and her affect not engaging like that of a manic patient.

We selected Pick's disease, which affects mainly middle-aged females, for this chapter because of its rarity and symptom profile. Pick's disease may be misdiagnosed as a mood disorder such as mania and lead to costly treatment attempts before its general medical nature is detected (Baldwin and Förstl 1993). Such treatment may even occur while you suspect a neurological condition because our diagnostic certainty based on clinical criteria is less than 100%. Even a brain biopsy may not be conclusive.

A second reason to include Pick's disease here was to present a patient who presumably had frontal lobe damage. These patients show poor social judgment, motivation, foresight, and planning, all indicative of frontal lobe damage. They are moody, forgetful, and show slow and concrete thinking. They score low on the Halstead Categories Test (Horvath et al. 1989). To quantify the progressive impairment on a serial basis, use the Executive Interview (EXIT; see Appendix), which includes similar tests as applied in A. 22–29.

5. Interview C: Marital Conflict Versus Amnesia in Dementia of the Alzheimer's Type

The interviewer receives a telephone call from an English professor at a northeastern university requesting a second opinion on her husband's worsening psychiatric problems. Her husband is a history professor and has been in psychiatric treatment for the previous year. The interviewer agrees to meet with the couple.

The patient is in his mid-50s. At the interview, he is meticulously dressed in a blue blazer and gray pants. His gray hair is combed neatly back, and he sports a thin gray mustache. He wears a silk scarf with a white shirt. He is accompanied by his wife who wears a gray suit, flat shoes, and horn-rimmed glasses, giving her a professorial look. (I = interviewer; P = patient; W = wife)

Step 1: Listen

1. I: [To the patient] Did you have a good flight?
   P: Thank you for asking.
2. I: Your wife called me and told me that you both would like to have a second opinion about your problem. I'm glad to help if I can.
   P: [With a thin smile] Yes, Louise seems to worry.
3. I: What seems to be the problem?
   P: Hmmm . . . well. . . . [Shrugs his shoulders and looks over to his wife with an inviting gesture] Well, . . . Louise?
   W: Don't you want to tell him what the problem is?
   P: You seem to be so much better in putting it all together.

W: But Dr. C. has told you and me several times I should not be so controlling and domineering. He seems to think that's one of your problems. So why don't you tell him.

4. I: So Dr. C. felt that you [gesturing toward the patient] are too dependent on your wife?

W: Yes. He felt that, because we have no children, I care for Dave as if he's my son and not my husband. And he felt that this has interfered with our sexual relationship. But that is so much better now.

5. I: What got you to see Dr. C. in the first place?

W: I'll let Dave tell you that.

P: [Looks at his wife, bewildered, then at the interviewer. Smiles, spreads out his arms] Well . . . here we are.

6. I: [To the patient] What would you like me to call you?

P: Dave is fine.

7. I: Well, Dave, what kind of problems brought you to Dr. C.?

P: [Putting up his hands] It seems to be a long story. I guess, Louise will do much better with it.

8. I: [Looking back and forth between the couple] Well? . . .

W: You see, doctor, this is just it. This is what Dr. C. does not seem to understand. For some time now, Dave leaves most things up to me. And I kind of feel compelled to jump in.

9. I: Okay. Maybe you give me your version first, and then Dave can fill in.

W: Well, what really got us to see Dr. C. was when Dave lost his train of thought in a lecture to his students and just ran out of the classroom. I had noticed for some months that he had not finished preparing for his lectures and that he seemed to have lost interest in his work. He did not seem to pay any attention to me either. So I was worried about this, and then we decided to make the appointment with Dr. C.

10. I: Hmmm.

W: Dr. C. pointed out to us that I'm taking over too much and I've tried to change that. But we don't seem to make any headway. The day I called you, Dave didn't come back from Dr. C.'s session. The police called me. He had driven over to the next state and had stopped a police car and told the officer that he was lost.

11. I: So what did you do?

W: I drove over and had Dave follow me home. And when I informed Dr. C. about it, he told me that this was Dave's way of protesting my dominance. He said sometimes things have to get worse before they get better. I have difficulties with that explanation.

12. I: So how did you get to me?

W: One of the teachers, Dr. K., from our psychiatry department knows you. He later told me that you have a different approach to psychiatry than Dr. C. and that I should give you a call. And that got us here.

The patient was meticulously groomed and was able to handle social formalities (A. 1, 2, 5, 6). He left the history telling to his wife, dodging all attempts by the interviewer to encourage him to tell his own story. This behavior contrasted with the patient's educational and social level. His affect was euthymic, but depressive mood could be considered because the patient had lost interest in his work and in his wife. Most remarkable was that 1) the patient could not continue his lecture; he ran out rather than handling the situation; 2) he got lost driving home from the session with the psychiatrist; and 3) his wife felt she had to play an increasingly larger role in managing her husband's behavior.

Differential Diagnosis

1. Dementia
2. Amnestic disorder
3. Major depression
4. Dissociative disorder

Step 2: Tag

13. I: [To the patient] It is significant that you lost your train of thought in a lecture. Has that happened again lately?
    P: Oh, I haven't lectured lately.
    W: Dave asked to be relieved from the lecturing until such a time that his problems could be resolved.
14. I: Dave, did you get lost again since the time you got lost after you left Dr. C.'s office?
    P: I must have had a lot of things on my mind.
    W: That's right, Dr. C. told us that he was not surprised that Dave got lost because they had had a very traumatic session. And Dave has always been an absent-minded professor.
    P: [Smiles]

Step 3: Confront

15. I: It seems that your memory is not working right and that you get lost at times. Dave, do you feel that you have problems with your memory?
    P: [Mildly annoyed] My memory is fine. I just don't care that much.
16. I: Have you been smoking more or drinking more?
    P: I don't smoke.
    W: [Nods, approving and confirming] He drinks maybe once or twice a year at a Christmas or New Year's Eve party.
17. I: Have you been more depressed?
    P: No, I feel fine.

W: He seems to have lost interest in all his work. He says he wants to go back full time, but he doesn't read any journals in his field.

The interviewer tagged the memory disturbance and the disorientation by the history given. He distinguished these cognitive impairments from the couple's interpretations of being overworked. The interviewer's confronting the patient about his memory disturbance and disorientation prompted the patient to deny them (A. 15). He remained emotionally and intellectually uninvolved in the interview but maintained a socially acceptable demeanor, which contrasted with the poverty of his speech. Without any increase in latency of response or decrease in fluency, he answered with only one-liners. His affect was euthymic. He smiled appropriately and used appropriate gestures. He denied depressed mood. He had no insight into the severity of his memory disturbance and denied it. He did not contribute to the history of his problems. He showed no concern about his problems.

Differential Diagnosis

1. Drug and alcohol abuse appear unlikely.
2. The patient's lack of interest in his work is compatible with depression, but his affect and mood appear nondepressed.
3. This leaves dementia and, more remotely, a dissociative state as diagnostic possibilities.

Step 4: Solve

18. I: Let me just ask you how your memory is working now.
    P: Oh, my memory is fine.
19. I: How well can you track time? Do you know, for example, what today's date is?
    P: [Smiles, shrugs his shoulders, looks at his wife] I don't pay any attention to that. But then. . . . [Starts to look at his watch]
    W: Don't forget, doctor, he is not working now. He does not have to keep track.
20. I: [Raising his hand] Please, don't look at your watch. Can you tell me without looking at it what date it is?
    P: Oh, what is it? Wednesday? Or is it still Tuesday? [It is Friday]
21. I: Maybe I'll just ask you for the year.
    P: I don't really see why I should answer that.
22. I: It would help me to help you.
    P: Thank you.
23. I: So can you tell me what the year is?
    P: I have more important things to worry about.
24. I: Guess! [Patient does not answer.] What year is it?

P: It ought to be 1968. [It is 1976]
W: Oh my God. [To the patient] Dave, you know what year it is.
P: Of course I do.
25. I: Well, that's all right.
W: [Begging] Dave, say it!
P: What do you want me to say?

The interviewer completes the mental status examination.[1] The patient cannot repeat five digits backward. He shows agraphia. He has ideomotor apraxia. He bangs the desk with his fist when asked how to hammer a nail into the wall. After two attempts, he repeats the words pencil, car, and watch accurately and touches his watch when he says the word watch. The only word he can remember after 5 minutes is watch. On the Kent Test (Kent 1946), he answers that the sun is in the west when the shadow points to the northeast, and he repeats east, west. He says the wind comes from the south when flag floats to the south. He appears to be proud that he can answer the questions, even though the answers are wrong.

26. I: [To the wife] Was there anybody in Dave's family who had problems with memory?
W: Yes, Dave's mother is in a nursing home. She has Alzheimer's, but she is 86 years old.

Step 5: Approve

27. I: I'm very glad that you came and gave me a chance to examine you. At this time, we will run a brain scan, an electroencephalogram, and a few blood tests. [To the wife] Is Dave taking any prescription drugs?
W: No.
28. I: Does he have any medical illnesses?
W: No, but that is how Dave's mother was until she lost her mind.
29. I: I will order these tests that we have discussed now and then we will see how I can help.

Throughout the interview, rapport existed mainly with the wife. The interviewer included the patient, even against his mild resistance (A. 15), to determine to what extent rapport was possible. Even though the interviewer signaled to the wife not to answer, she had a difficult time staying out of the

---

[1] You should proceed with the mental status examination despite a patient's insistence that his memory is fine. Frequently, a well-dressed and well-educated patient has a mildly intimidating effect on an interviewer, who may feel embarrassed to ask simple questions, such as date, time, or place. Such an omission can be detrimental for the patient. Therefore, if you do not want to be distressed later, never skip the examination of cognitive functions.

interview process (A. 13, 14, 17). It appeared that some denial on her part dictated her assisting behavior (A. 25).

The patient showed contrasting behaviors throughout the interview: emotionally, he remained attentive and tuned in; intellectually, he appeared to lose the thread of the examination. He moved in and out of responding to the context (A. 22, 24, 25). His answers were short and limited to the immediately preceding question without grasping the context. It seemed that his train of thought was not continuous, which would point to a short-term memory impairment. His inability to follow the conversation was a significant indication of his cognitive deficiency. The existence of this deficit was further born out by the fact that the patient was grossly disoriented to time. Because orientation to time is a recent memory function, the interviewer tested the patient's other cognitive functions and found symptoms and signs indicative of agraphia, aphasia, apraxia, and decline of problem-solving ability in the Kent Test (Kent 1946).

A patient with a progressive dementing disorder is dependent on a support person. Therefore, it is important to help the support person (in the above case, Dave's wife) to understand the disorder.

Diagnosis

Axis I

1. *Dementia of the Alzheimer's type, pending further studies.* This diagnosis is supported by the mental status examination and by the patient's family history.
2. *Major depression.* At the onset of the disorder, the patient may have had a depression, which obscured the then-mild cognitive deficit. During psychotherapy, the therapist focused on interpersonal conflicts and failed to periodically examine the client's cognitive competence.
3. *Dissociative disorder.* This diagnosis is ruled out because of the patient's mental status. Patients with psychogenic amnesia are usually oriented to time and place, but often not to person, and have intact short-term memory. Only their remote memory is not accessible.

Axis II.   None.

Axis III.   Not assessed.

Axis IV.   None obvious.

Axis V.   Global Assessment of Functioning (GAF) Scale score = 20.

Follow-Up

Dave's brain scan showed signs of ventricular enlargement and cortical atrophy. There was no evidence of a normal pressure hydrocephalus or deep structure scars, like those seen in multi-infarct dementia.

DAT is age related. The increasing population of elderly individuals will lead to an increase of this disorder (Jorm 1990). Sometimes, the family covers up the deficits or tries to explain them away. For example, the president of an insurance company was asked by his board to get a health clearance from a psychiatrist. He showed severe cognitive defects and had to retire, but his wife resisted the diagnosis because his demeanor was still authoritative. Another patient's cognitive deficits became prominent when the family traveled to Las Vegas, where he walked into mirrored doors. The family believed that the stress of the trip and the overstimulation in Las Vegas were responsible. Occasionally, a patient may have visual or haptic hallucinations. For example, one patient in the beginning stages of DAT reported that multiple tongues with tubes underneath them popped up in his mouth and caused continuous salivation.

If the cognitive defects are not assessed or misinterpreted, patients may be misdiagnosed as having a psychotic disorder without appreciation of the associated dementia. To quantify the progressive impairment, use for serial follow-up—besides the EXIT (see Appendix)—the Mini-Mental State Exam (Folstein et al. 1975; also Othmer and Othmer 1994).

6. Dementia in Psychiatric Disorders

Dementia is a process independent of any psychiatric disorder. However, it can occur in conjunction with any of the disorders and aggravate them. Dual diagnoses of dementia and affective disorder, substance-related abuse, or schizophrenia may even prevent the detection of the dementing process, because the symptoms and signs of dementia may be attributed to the coexisting psychiatric disorder. Furthermore, special forms of dementia— those that affect orientation and memory in a later stage, such as dementia due to Pick's disease—may be mistaken for a noncognitive psychiatric disorder rather than recognized as a primary degenerative cognitive disorder.

CHAPTER 11

MENTAL RETARDATION

Summary

In this chapter, we show how to test quickly for signs of mental retardation and how to distinguish these signs from dementia.

◆ ◆ ◆ ◆ ◆

Vivere est cogitare.
To live is to think.

Tusculanarum Disputationum,
Book V, Chapter 38, Section III
Marcus Tullius Cicero (106–43 B.C.)

◆ ◆ ◆ ◆ ◆

1. What Is Mental Retardation?

The following diagnostic criteria for mental retardation are listed in DSM-IV (American Psychiatric Association 1994, p. 46):

1. Significantly subaverage intellectual functioning: an IQ of approximately 70 or below on an individually administered IQ test.
2. Concurrent deficits or impairments in present adaptive functioning . . . in at least two of the following areas: communication, self-care, home living, social-interpersonal skills, use of community resources, self-direction, functional academic skills, work, leisure, health, and safety.
3. The onset is before age 18 years.

Mental retardation is coded on Axis II.

The normally functioning brain can understand and solve a variety of problems in a timely and economical fashion. It can access its fund of knowledge, retrieve old solutions, and find new ones and express them in language and action. Diffuse, widespread damage or lack of development of cortical brain areas interferes with problem solving and causes mental deficiencies. These deficiencies affect interpersonal communication, self-care, home living, social skills, use of community resources, self-direction, functional academic skills, work, leisure, and safety. If these disturbances occur during development before age 18 years, they are called *mental retardation*. If they have an onset during late adolescence and adulthood, they are called *dementia*.

In adult patients, mental retardation can interfere with the accuracy of your diagnosis because you may mistake mental retardation that occurs with psychosis as dementia with psychosis or as delirium, rather than as a dual diagnosis of mental retardation with schizophrenia, schizophreniform disorder, major depression, or bipolar disorder with psychotic features. Some patients develop suspiciousness, dependency or anxieties, or phobic behaviors as a result of their low mental functioning. You may misdiagnose a patient with mental retardation as having a delusional disorder or paranoid personality disorder; dependent personality disorder; or avoidant personality disorder.

2. Mental Retardation in the Mental Status

Indicators of mental retardation during the mental status examination depend on the severity of the mental retardation and the stress the patient experiences. Patients who have mild mental retardation and good social support and who are functioning can appear well adjusted. However, certain behavioral patterns may tip you off to the existence of mental retardation, such as social dependency, suspiciousness, pseudointellectualism, concreteness in thinking, and trivial social conflicts.

Social dependency. The adult mentally retarded patient has a minimum-wage job, still lives with her parents, and refers to her parents in a reverential way, using terms like "mommy" and "daddy." This pattern of dependency may carry over into the interview situation where the patient tries to be on friendly terms with you, thus inviting your support rather than showing autonomy.

Suspiciousness. The patient may have experienced teasing, rejection, and failure in reaching personal goals. In response, he may have developed a suspicious, cautious pattern of behavior that becomes evident in your examination.

Pseudointellectualism. A patient who comes from an educated family may have developed behavior patterns and a vocabulary disproportionate to her intellectual capacity. Such a patient uses abstract and elaborate words incorrectly.

Concreteness in thinking. The patient may reveal his disorder by giving concrete answers. For example: You discuss drug therapy and psychotherapy for the treatment of his depression with the patient. You then ask him how he would like to be treated. He responds, "Nicely." If you ask him what that means, he may tell you he likes to have doughnuts every afternoon.

Trivial social conflicts. Patients with borderline intelligence may present with interpersonal conflicts that appear trivial when you analyze them. Rather than looking for a complicated answer, you may first want to resort to examining their intelligence.

3. Technique: Intelligence Testing

Intelligence testing is the key technique to establishing below-average intelligence. The Wechsler Adult Intelligence Scale—Revised (WAIS-R; Wechsler 1981) and the Wechsler Intelligence Scale for Children—Revised

(WISC-R; Wechsler 1974) are examples of comprehensive tests. Digit span and similarities, which are two parts of a subtest of these instruments, are often used for bedside testing. To test a patient's concept of similarities, ask

What do an apple and an orange have in common?

The patient gets the highest score if she answers,

They are both fruit.

A person who can think in abstract categories is usually not mentally retarded. The same is true for the abstract interpretation of proverbs. As an example, ask the patient,

Can you tell me what the proverb, "A stitch in time saves nine" means?

The correct answer would be,

If you tend to a problem early on, it may save a lot of work later.

Such evaluations do not require computation. A procedure that can be done at bedside and that will give you a more differentiated idea of a patient's intelligence is the combined use of the Kent Test (Kent 1946) and the Rapid Approximate Intelligence Test (Wilson 1967). Both are easy to remember.

We have reorganized the Kent Test into four problem-solving questions and six knowledge questions (Table 11–1). A patient who can solve the four problems correctly has at least average intelligence. We give such a patient credit for the first three knowledge questions because of their simplicity. Therefore, such a patient has the following score:

12 points credit for the simple knowledge questions
14 points credit for the problem-solving questions

The bright, normal person or the person with superior intelligence can also correctly answer the last three knowledge questions. A patient who fails to correctly solve the four problem questions is then evaluated with the three simple knowledge questions. If she fails to answer these, her brain functioning falls clearly in the defective range and may be diagnosed as mental retardation if her school record also shows poor performance. Thus, you need only four problem-solving questions and one multiplication task from the Rapid Approximate Intelligence Test (i.e., 2×48) to exclude or establish the presence of subnormal intelligence.

Scores of both types of questions may be added up and used to estimate

Table 11–1. Kent Test

Question	Maximal score
Problem solving	
If the flag floats to the south, from which direction is the wind?	
Answer: North	3
At what time of the day is your shadow the shortest?	
Answer: Noon	3
Why does the moon look larger than the stars?	
Answers:	
Lower down (2 points)	
Nearer (3 points)	
Nearer objects appear larger	4
If your shadow points to the northeast, where is the sun?	
Answer: Southwest	4
Knowledge	
What are houses made of?	
Answer: 1 point for each material, up to 4 points	4
Tell me the name of some fish.	
Answer: 1 point for each fish, up to 4 points	4
Give me the names of some large cities.	
(Small hometowns are excluded.)	
Answer: 1 point for each city, up to 4 points	4
What is sand used for?	
Answers:	
Playing (1 point)	
Constructive use (2 points)	
Making glass	4
What metal is attracted by a magnet?	
Answers:	
Steel (2 points)	
Iron	4
How many stripes are in the United States flag?	
Answer: 13	2
Maximal score	**36**

Source. Reprinted from Kent GH: *E-G-Y Scales.* New York, Williams & Wilkins, 1946. Used with kind permission from The Psychological Corporation, 555 Academic Court, San Antonio, Texas.

the patient's intelligence. In Table 11–2, Kent Test scores and the IQ levels indicated by them are matched with the most difficult multiplication problem from the Wilson Test that a patient at that level could answer.

4. Five Steps to Identify Mental Retardation

Use the five-step approach (i.e., listen, tag, confront, solve, and approve) in an abbreviated fashion. When you suspect mental deficiency, you should politely but immediately ask the patient how easy it is for him to figure out problems. His reply may prompt you to ask about whether or not he required special education in school. Then ask him how easy it is now for him to do math. This will lead directly into Step 4 (solve). In Step 5 (approve), you may give the patient positive feedback about the tasks he was able to solve and emphasize some other strength or asset he has shown.

5. Interview: Dementia With Hallucinations Versus Bipolar Disorder With Psychosis in Mental Retardation

Mr. L. is a 34-year-old, white, single man. As a teenager, he was adopted by the owner of a nursery and he has worked there ever since. The first-year psychiatric resident reports:

Table 11–2.　Approximate IQ levels indicated by performance on Kent and Wilson Tests

Intellectual abilities	Approximate IQ	Score on Kent Test	Level reached on Wilson Test[a]
Defective	<70	0–18	2×12
Borderline	70–80	19–20	2×24
Dull normal	80–90	21–23	2×48
Average	90–110	24–31	2×96
Bright normal	110–120	32–33	2×192
Superior	120–130	34–35	2×384
Very superior	>130	36	$2 \times ?$

[a]Rapid Approximate Intelligence Test (Wilson 1967) should be implemented as a series of progressive multiplications: 2×3, 2×6, 2×12, 2×24, and so on.

Mr. L. was brought in by his father with his chief complaint being, "I want to stab myself. I need help." He has heard voices for at least 5 years and has taken thioridazine (Mellaril) in the past. Now, the voices are back. They tell him to stab himself. Mr. L. also has visual hallucinations; he sees the killer knife in the kitchen sink. He denies being depressed but is angry, disagreeable, and argumentative with his adoptive father. The hallucinations keep him from sleeping but his appetite is fine. As for the mental status examination, Mr. L.'s affect is flat. He is disoriented to the day of the month. Even with help, he can remember only one of four words. He also has difficulties in problem solving; he does not know where the sun is when a shadow points to the northeast. He has poor judgment. He has no insight because he feels he has to obey the voices. On the screening test for the Luria-Nebraska Neuropsychological Test Battery (Golden 1987), his score is 24; the cutoff point is 8. Thus, he shows neuropsychological impairment. I conclude that he has dementia with hallucinations. Maybe he was exposed to some toxins that they use as pest control or as herbicides in the nursery.

The interviewer asks the patient into his office. (I = interviewer; P = patient)

Step 1: Listen

1. I: Hi, Mr. L. You have problems with voices, your resident told me?
 P: [Without a change in facial expression, staring at the interviewer's forehead] Yes.
2. I: Tell me about these voices.
 P: [After a pause] Stab myself.
3. I: Can you tell who they are?
 P: [Looks puzzled, after a pause] Don't know.
4. I: Is your own voice among them?
 P: [Stares at the interviewer's forehead, hesitates] Doesn't sound like it. Sometimes like my father's.
5. I: Where are they coming from?
 P: [Keeps staring at the interviewer's forehead] Right here. [Points at his own head]
6. I: Right from your head?
 P: Yes.
7. I: What are they all saying?
 P: Stab myself.
8. I: What else are they saying?
 P: Stab myself . . . cut myself.
9. I: Did they ever tell you anything else?
 P: [Closes his eyes; replies after 3 seconds] Nope.
10. I: Do you hear them all the time?
 P: [Frowns and pauses] Nope.
11. I: How do you feel when you hear the voices?
 P: [Stares at the interviewer for a while] Awful, mixed up . . . I can't sleep.

Step 2: Tag

12. I: I'm sorry that you feel so bad. Let me make sure that I understand you correctly. You hear a voice that comes from inside your head? And you feel awful and mixed up? And you can't sleep?
    P: Yes.
13. I: [Waiting for a more explicit answer] Do you cry?
    P: [Looking down on his knees] I cry.
14. I: And that voice tells you to stab and cut yourself and nothing more?
    P: Yes.

Step 3: Confront

15. I: How do you feel now?
    P: Mixed up. I wish I'm dead.
16. I: [Raises his eyebrows as if he does not understand]
    P: Upset. The voice upsets me.
17. I: Do you hear the voice now?
    P: [Looks frightened, leans forward, looks the interviewer in the eyes and whispers] Yeah.
18. I: How long have you felt upset and mixed up?
    P: [Gazing around as if looking for an answer] I don't know. For a while.

As to rapport, Mr. L. answered the interviewer's questions with yes (A. 1, 6, 12, 14, 17), no (A. 9, 10), and short, fragmented sentences void of elaboration (A. 2, 4, 5, 7, 8). Before several answers, the patient stared at the interviewer without making eye contact (A. 1, 4, 5). Mr. L. did not pick up on the interviewer's expression of empathy (Q. 12). Thus, rapport remained restricted.

The patient was alert and paid attention. He comprehended the questions. His answers seemed fragmented and agrammatical—he left out part of the infinitive (A. 2, 7, 8), *from* (A. 5), the subject (A. 3, 4), and the verb (A. 4). He showed prolonged latency of response (A. 1–5, 9–11, 18). His affect was restricted. He described his mood as mixed up (A. 12, 15). His insight was good because he had told his father that he needed help.

The interviewer's open-ended questions did not yield elaborations (Q. 2, 3, 5, 7, 8, 11, 15). The interviewer confronted the patient with questions to persuade him to confirm what the patient was experiencing at the time of the interview (A. 9, 15–18).

Differential Diagnosis

Axis I

1. *Dementia with hallucinations due to unknown etiology.* The patient's telegraph style with grammatical errors is possibly indicative of an expressive aphasia. So far, the interviewer has only confirmed auditory but not visual hallucinations. He has not tested cognitive functions. Therefore, this diagnosis is open for revision or confirmation.
2. *Major depression with psychosis.* The patient showed prolonged latency of response, poverty of speech, restricted affect, depressed mood, and auditory hallucinations.

Axes II through V. Not assessed.

Step 4: Solve

Orientation

19. I: You say you feel mixed up. Can you tell me what day it is today?
    P: Tuesday. [Correct]
20. I: And what month?
    P: November. [Correct]
21. I: Do you know which date it is?
    P: Tuesday.
22. I: No, Mr. L., which day of the month is it?
    P: Don't know.
23. I: Do you know the year?
    P: 92. [Correct]

Intelligence

24. I: Can you name all the months of the year? Please start with January.
    P: January . . . [pause], February, March, April.
25. I: What comes after April?
    P: Don't know.
26. I: Take a guess.
    P: August.
27. I: And after that?
    P: September.
28. I: And then?
    P: Don't know.
29. I: Guess.
    P: November.

Immediate memory

30. I: So it's hard for you to remember these things. Let's see if you can remember three things: pencil, car, and watch. Can you say them?
    P: Now?
31. I: [Nods]
    P: Pencil, car, and watch.
32. I: I want you to remember pencil, car, and watch because I want you tell me them again later on.
    P: Okay.

Kent Test

    I: [Interviewer gives the Kent Test (Table 11–2).]
33. I: Mr. L., let me ask you some other things. Tell me when is your shadow the shortest?
    P: At night.
34. I: Can you tell me the name of some fish?
    P: Catfish.
35. I: [Nods]
    P: Croppie.
36. I: Yes. Tell me some more.
    P: Don't know.
37. I: Just try. I bet you know some more fish.
    P: [Frowning, then with a broad smile] Bass.
38. I: And one more!
    P: Goldfish.

When asked to name major cities in the United States, the patient says Chicago, Florida, and New York. With prodding, he continues, naming Los Angeles, Dallas, and Kansas City (where he lives). He names wood, two-by-fours, and a hammer as building materials for houses; with prodding, he adds concrete and nails. He knows that the wind comes from the north when the flag points to the south, but fails all other questions of the Kent Test. He can multiply 2×3 and 2×6, but does not know 2×12. When the interviewer explains that this is the same as $12 + 12$, Mr. L., with some hesitation, answers 14.

Gnosia. The patient knows that Monday comes before Wednesday.

Praxis. Mr. L. can correctly demonstrate how to sow lettuce seeds.

Aphasia. He can write "Stab myself." Reflexes are normal.

Recent memory. The patient can recall pencil, car, and watch after 10 minutes.

39. I: How are you feeling now?
    P: Down. I want to stab myself.
40. I: Down? Have you ever felt up?
    P: Yes.
41. I: How do you sleep when you feel up?
    P: Don't. Two hours. That's all.
42. I: Have you always heard the voice?
    P: Nope.
43. I: Do you also see things?
    P: The knife in the sink.
44. I: Was the knife really in the sink?
    P: Yes. It was there. Then I heard the voice. I was so scared. I told my Mom. She put it away.
45. I: Have you ever seen other things?
    P: No.
46. I: When did you first hear the voices?
    P: About 4 or 5 years ago.
47. I: What happened 4 or 5 years ago?
    P: I got all upset and excited. I felt good, really.
48. I: Anything happened?
    P: I walked around a lot. Didn't need sleep.
49. I: And then?
    P: I talked. My Daddy said shut up. Didn't shut up. [Laughs] The voice started and I got frightened. I cried a lot. Couldn't eat. I wanted to die. And my father put me into [names a state hospital].
50. I: You say the voice started. How many did you hear?
    P: Just one. I hear just one voice.
51. I: How were you doing in school?
    P: Slow. I was in special ed.
52. I: Did you hear voices then?
    P: No.
53. I: How does your medication, the Mellaril, help you now?
    P: I don't take it. I feel so tired from it. I sleep a lot when I'm on it. But the voice stops.

Step 5: Approve

54. I: I'm glad that you are here. I want you to come to the hospital.
    P: I want to go back home.
55. I: You will go home after you feel better and after the voice has stopped. I don't want you to hurt yourself. We can watch out for you better in the hospital. We have nurses here to help you.
    P: Okay.
56. I: I hope we can find a medication on which you don't sleep so much.

When the interviewer realized that the patient was mentally slow, he himself began to use short questions to help the patient comprehend them. To ask simple questions is a prerequisite for the development of trust. Also, the interviewer made sure that he understood Mr. L. correctly. He picked up on the patient's statement that "the voice" started (Q. 50) and learned that the patient only heard one voice, even though he had never corrected the interviewer who assumed from the resident's presentation that the patient heard several voices (Q. 46). With a mentally retarded patient, it is helpful to cross-check your understanding of his statements because he often feels inferior and will not contradict you.

The patient continued to be attentive. He replied to the point when he knew an answer. He recalled three out of three objects immediately. Therefore, the interviewer skipped counting backward from 20, which would have been a test appropriate for a patient with Mr. L.'s suspected IQ. His remote memory was intact. He could give a correct history, the details of which were confirmed by his father later.

Mr. L. was oriented to year, month, and day of the week, but not to the date, which was in keeping with his suspected IQ. His Kent Test score was 14, which would correspond to an IQ below 70, in the defective range. Mr. L. had no evidence of aphasia, agnosia, or apraxia when tested on his intelligence level.

The resident had reported that the patient also had visual hallucinations. However, this was most likely a misinterpretation of what the patient had said. Mr. L. happened to see a real knife in the sink when he heard the voice tell him to stab himself, or the sight of the knife may have triggered the auditory hallucination (Q. 43, 44).

Diagnosis

Axis I. Bipolar I disorder, most recent episode depressed, with psychotic symptoms with mood-congruent features.

Axis II. Mental retardation, mild.

The giveaway for this disorder came from the patient's longitudinal history—mental retardation clearly existed before the onset of the second psychiatric disorder—and from the profile of his cognitive dysfunctions, which showed his main deficit to be low intelligence. The parents confirmed that the patient was mentally retarded with an IQ of 69, but that the hallucination had started when the patient was only age 29 years. After the low IQ was taken into account, the patient had no deficits in attention, concentration, or memory. He showed absence of apraxia, agnosia, aphasia, pathological reflexes, and problems with shifting sets.

From the mental status examination alone it may at times be difficult to differentiate a cognitive disorder with psychosis from a dual diagnosis of mental retardation with major depression and psychosis or bipolar disorder with psychosis. In the German literature the word *Pfropfpsychose* (from the German *Pfropf,* meaning a plug or a graft) is used to refer to a functional psychosis grafted onto mental retardation (Bumke 1948).

Epilogue

This patient was started on lithium because of his manic episode (A. 47–49) and because of the relapse. When he became depressed, he experienced a command hallucination. He responded to an antidepressant with the addition of a low dosage of a nonsedating neuroleptic—perphenazine (Trilafon).

6. Mental Retardation in Psychiatric Disorders

Mental retardation does not protect a patient from developing any other psychiatric disorder. The frequency with which a psychiatric disorder is found in conjunction with mental retardation approximates the frequency of psychiatric disorders in the general population, but this dual diagnosis is often difficult to recognize. In the example, Mr. L. indeed did show some symptoms of a cognitive disorder. He could not solve problems well, his arithmetic abilities were poor, and he seemed to have difficulty naming the date. His recent memory appeared relatively impaired if one did not take into account his preexisting mental retardation. If such a patient develops major depression or bipolar disorder with psychosis, he may be diagnosed as having an affective disorder due to a general medical condition or substance induced and receive chronic treatment with neuroleptics rather than with mood stabilizers.

Mental retardation may worsen the treatment outcome of an Axis I or other Axis II disorder. Moderate or severe mental retardation may lead to the diagnosis of schizophrenia, a cognitive disorder, or an intermittent explosive disorder, rather than to the dual diagnosis of bipolar disorder with mental retardation.

In the next section, Part IV, "Self-Protective and Deceptive Behavior," we return to the management of psychological factors in the interview.

PART IV

SELF-PROTECTIVE AND DECEPTIVE BEHAVIOR

SELF-PROTECTIVE AND DECEPTIVE BEHAVIOR

◆ ◆ ◆ ◆ ◆

Si operam medicantis expectas, oportet vulnus detegas.
If you expect to be cured, you must uncover your wound.

Anicus Manlius Severinus Boethius
De Consolatione Philosophiae (524 A.D.)

◆ ◆ ◆ ◆ ◆

Some difficulties with patients are easy to suspect but hard to accept. Health professionals are trained to be understanding, nonjudgmental, and empathic toward their patients' pathology. Therefore, they may experience a personal difficulty when interviewing patients who minimize, hide, falsify, lie, falsely accuse others, produce factitious symptoms, and deny their obvious patterns of abuse. They may have a hard time recognizing the sadistic, paraphiliac, or pedophiliac patient, sometimes a respected teacher in the community.

The prevalence figures in DSM-IV (American Psychiatric Association 1994) show that categories that depict socially scorned behavior are used the least, despite increasing numbers of reported cases of physical and sexual child abuse, substance abuse, suicides, homicides, and other violent crimes. Health practitioners are members of society and, as such, are

311

exposed to all of its problems. Therefore, they must learn to recognize their own tendency to deny hostility, destructiveness, and sadism in their patients. They must learn to face up to these patients and familiarize themselves with interviewing techniques that may combine empathy and the wish to help with a hard-nosed toughness and willingness to identify and to detect. This means they may have to consider adopting legal techniques into modern psychiatry (see Chapter 13, "Falsifying and Lying," and Chapter 14, "Factitious Behavior").

The following four chapters (12–15) address self-protective and deceptive behaviors as they are manifested in the psychiatric interview. Such behaviors can mislead the interviewer and stall the interview. They erect a wall between the interviewer and the patient and limit rapport by casting the interviewer as an adversary. The patient pretends to want help, yet sabotages that alliance.

In DSM-IV, deceptive behavior is recognized on three levels:

1. *Directly, as a direct symptom or sign of a disorder and therefore as a criterion for such a disorder.* For example, in DSM-IV, criterion A11 of conduct disorder states that the individual "often lies to obtain goods or favors or to avoid obligations (i.e., 'cons' others)" (p. 90). Criterion C2 of antisocial personality disorder states that the individual practices "deceitfulness, as indicated by repeated lying, use of aliases, or conning others for personal profit or pleasure" (p. 650). Criterion A of factitious disorder describes "intentional production or feigning of physical or psychological signs or symptoms" (p. 474), whereas malingering is described as "the intentional production of false or grossly exaggerated physical or psychological symptoms" (p. 683).

2. *As an associated feature of a disorder that is not included in the diagnostic criteria.* For example, in the discussion of substance-related disorders in DSM-IV (p. 189), it is stated that individuals "incorrectly assure themselves that they will have no problem regulating substance use." Within the discussion of bulimia nervosa in DSM-IV, it is stated that "individuals with bulimia nervosa are typically ashamed of their eating problems and attempt to conceal their symptoms" (p. 546).

3. *Indirectly, as a mediating behavior in the service of a personality trait.* For example, in pedophilia, some individuals "threaten the child to prevent disclosure" (DSM-IV, p. 528). Patients with borderline personality disorder may use deceptive behavior if they fear abandonment. In DSM-IV, criterion 1 for borderline personality disorder states that they may make "frantic efforts to avoid real or imagined abandonment" (p. 654).

All these behaviors have common denominators: first, the patient is conscious and aware of her self-protective and deceptive behavior; second, the behavior is volitional and ego-syntonic; third, it is intentional—that is, the behavior serves a purpose. Nevertheless, this self-protective and deceptive behavior is part of the patient's pathology and therefore requires our understanding and empathy rather than moralistic and legalistic rejection.

On the basis of the patient's intent, we can observe four forms of deceptive behavior: concealment, falsifying and lying, fabrication in factitious behavior, and self-deception. A chapter is devoted to each of these because each reflects a unique type of psychopathology that can be associated with a different group of psychiatric disorders or personality disorders.

You meet the guilt-ridden deceiver in Chapter 12, in which concealing is explored. *Concealing* occurs when patients hide information, feelings, or activities, such as substance abuse, bulimia, or suicidal thoughts. These patients do not feed you false information nor do they feign feelings. They suppress evidence to protect themselves and to cover up their own weakness.

In Chapter 13, we describe the falsifying and lying patient. In *falsification,* a patient not only conceals the truth but invents lies to prevent its detection. He wants to lead you to wrong conclusions. One such patient, to cause a rift between her father and her stepmother, falsely claimed that her stepbrother was shoplifting. Knowingly, the falsifier produces erroneous evidence. In the process of protecting himself he is willing to actively hurt others.

In Chapter 14, on factitious behavior, you meet the patient who invents symptoms and signs of medical and psychiatric disorders either in herself (Munchausen syndrome) or in a close relative, often children under her care (Munchausen by proxy). Such a patient invests herself in the creation of, preferably, physical evidence to convince you that she or a loved one is seriously ill from a condition that you are unable to identify, thus challenging your expertise.

The patient in Chapter 15, on self-deception, deceives you and himself. Whereas the falsifying and the fabricating patient produces false evidence after the event has happened, the self-deceptive patient slants his very perception to fit the desired image. Finally, he cannot separate the truth from wishful thinking.

All four types of deceit have one thing in common: the patient sends you a double message. This double message consists, first, of a false front that the patient puts up that she wants to have accepted as the truth, and second, of myriad giveaways that tell you that a different set of information is hidden behind the false front. That set of information is often an embarrassing truth. However, you have to be able to evaluate the double message correctly so you do not mistake any hidden or suppressed emotion as an indicator of deceit per se. Therefore, familiarize yourself with the patient's responses to neutral and embarrassing control questions such as,

> Have you ever lied to a person who trusted you?

After you know how she responds to neutral and embarrassing questions, you may try to augment her giveaways. A set of probing questions can magnify them and flush out the truth. Such probing questions include, for example,

> Is this the truth? Are you fooling me or yourself?

After you have identified the patient's type of deceit, implement the specific technique that encourages the patient in various ways to give up deceit. For example, for the patient who conceals information from you, weigh the advantages and disadvantages of concealing with the plus-minus technique. With the patient who falsifies and invents elaborate lies, dissect his lies with the cross-examination technique and make him see the unsustainable contradictions in his story. For the patient who fabricates physical evidence and tries to persuade you to accept it as truth, confront him with the evidence for fabrication obtained through voice-stress or polygraphic analysis and persuade him to be truthful under recording conditions. Point out the negative consequences if he continues fabricating. Redirect a patient who deceives himself without any evidence of delusional thinking. Steer him away from talking to you. Focus on his self-talk instead. For example, ask him

> What do you tell yourself about your drinking?
> How well do you control it?
> What do you tell yourself when you are honest with yourself?

Show him the discrepancy between what the truth seems to be and what he would like to portray.

These specific strategies to give up deceit are discussed in Chapters 12–15. The nature of the double message and the use of control and probing questions are described in the section below, as these topics apply to all four chapters.

1. The Double Message of Deceit

To detect deceit, you need to spot its double message—the truth hidden behind a false front. The false front originates from conscious cortical planning to deceive. The hidden truth is associated with the patient's genuine emotions, which originate from the subcortical limbic system and find expression in spontaneous nonverbal behavior. The knowledge of the truth is also represented in the patient's memory and may become evident, for example, in slips of the tongue and in her speech. It may show through in her affect, as is manifested in autonomic responses, reactive movements, facial expressions, grooming, and tone of voice. In addition, it may show through in her psychomotor movements, which are composed of gestures, symbolic signals, and goal-directed movements. Therefore, when a patient shows deceptive behavior, she displays two affects: the suppressed true one and the emphasized false one.

The memory of the hidden truth competes for expression with the patient-sponsored web of deceit. The true memory emerges spontaneously and can be seen in broken off and incomplete gestures, incomplete hand and facial signals, suppressed goal-directed movements, and slips of the tongue.

If a patient's emotional response differs from what she intentionally plans to communicate, her spontaneous response may contradict her intended response, and a double message emerges. This double message in effect occurs because the patient responds spontaneously (fast response) and intentionally (slow response) to a stimulus. The spontaneous response, which is not under voluntary control, floods the autonomic and extrapyramidal motor system of the brain. A genuinely experienced emotion reveals itself before it can be controlled by the slower-working voluntary control centers. For example, a probing surprise question may provoke anxiety of being found out (detection anxiety) in the deceiving person. This anxiety leaks out before the patient can hide it behind faked confidence.

If a patient has a genuine and consciously accepted position toward a topic, her spontaneous response matches her intended response. You receive the impression of a genuine response in which spontaneous and intentional expressions agree.

2. How to Draw Out the Double Message

Experienced deceivers are accustomed to lying, can minimize the double message, and easily present a "natural front." To help draw out the patient's double message, you can use two strategies: provide security or increase awareness of negative consequences.

Providing a secure setting at the beginning of the interview invites a patient to let down his guard. Increasing the patient's awareness of negative consequences intensifies his emotions, which then become more difficult to conceal and falsify. For example, for a patient who has a history of, or who may possibly be, lying, clarify his position as follows:

> If you accuse your stepfather wrongfully of physical abuse, *you* may be kicked out of the family, not him.

If he lies in response to your statement, he may show a tremor in his voice and trembling of his hands while trying to appear relaxed, although more accomplished individuals will often be able to control such signs.

Double messages tell you that the patient is experiencing two opposing emotions, and that he wants you to recognize one and miss the other. Double messages do not automatically signal deceit. For example, a person who is wrongfully accused of lying may appear relaxed and hide his secret anger about the false accusation. Thus, he may send out a double message.

Therefore, double messages have to be interpreted accurately. They have to be evaluated in the context of more than one interchange and possibly in the context of the patient's history. The use of control questions helps you in this interpretation.

3. Control Questions

If you know a patient well, you know how she responds to neutral or sensitive topics or to your suspicion. With a new patient, study her emotional responses to different topics. Control questions for use in detecting deceit are listed in Table IV–1.

When you know the patient's range of responses, you are prepared to correctly interpret her double messages. To further guard against misinterpretation, carefully study similar emotional responses to different types of probing questions. In Table IV–2, reactions to probing questions and statements of a truthful person and a deceitful person are compared.

An alternative way to ascertain the patient's general credibility is to weave into the interview a few questions about an event that you are familiar with but that the patient most likely does not know you are familiar with.

Table IV–1.   Control questions to detect deceit

Topic	Sample question or statement
Neutral	How do you spend a 24-hour day?
Invested	What are your hobbies, your most significant losses, your goals in life?
Sensitive	What are your weaknesses and shortcomings? Did you ever lie to a person who trusted you?
False accusations	I hear that you did not do your homework that you had promised to do.
Intentional falsification	Please assume a false first name and insist to me that it is your true name when I question you about it.
Praise of truthfulness	I believe you. You told me the truth about having done your homework.
Express acceptance of an untruth	I believe you. You told me the truth about never having lied to your mother about your homework (when interviewer knows that the patient did lie).

Table IV–2.   Sample responses of a truthful person and a deceitful person to probing questions and statements

Example of probing	Truthful person's reaction	Deceitful person's reaction
Is this really true? I have doubts that you are truthful.	Frustration at being falsely suspected	Anger at being found out
Are you lying? You are lying!	Anxiety at being disbelieved	Fear of being found out
Please tell me the truth!	Anger at being distrusted	Guilt about deceit
I believe you.	Relief	Contempt, triumph over deception
You finally confessed to me.	Anger over implied lying	Anger at being caught; relief of guilt and anxiety

Note. You have to know a patient well to correctly interpret the meaning of anger and anxiety. It is dangerous to draw conclusions from one single response.

CHAPTER 12

CONCEALING

Summary

Concealing reflects the patient's self-censorship and anxiety, guilt, or ambivalence about hiding and revealing information, feelings, or activities, but also his distrust and suspicion. To help the patient overcome this concealing behavior, the interviewer weighs with the patient the advantages and disadvantages of revealing versus concealing. This plus-minus technique gives the patient the opportunity to reconsider his concealing behavior. The interviewer helps to tip the scale in favor of disclosure and thus alleviates the discommunication. This leveling relieves the patient of his guilt and supports him in dealing with his weakness.

◆ ◆ ◆ ◆ ◆

Sers ton mari comme ton maître,
Et t'en garde comme d'un traître.
Serve your husband as your master,
And beware of him as a traitor.

Michel de Montaigne (1533–1592)
Essays

◆ ◆ ◆ ◆ ◆

1. What Is Concealing?

The concealing patient knowingly and voluntarily suppresses information. She conceals embarrassing symptoms and pathological behaviors to avoid rejection, disrespect, and punishment. Concealment often is used to cover up experiences such as promiscuity, incest, pedophiliac tendencies, rape, substance abuse, suicidal plans, and personal failures. A concealing patient avoids making up lies. As mentioned in the introduction to these four chapters, concealing may be directly associated with substance-related disorders and eating disorders, and indirectly associated with borderline personality disorder and pedophilia.

Concealment occurs in two forms. The patient either admits that she is concealing or conceals her concealment. The patient who admits that she is concealing something often tells you,

> I can't talk about it. I'm sorry. I'm too ashamed about it. I know you would not want me as a patient any more.

If the interviewer goes along with the patient's secretiveness, the patient may initially feel relief. However, later the patient may experience guilt. First, she feels guilty that she is concealing something. Second, she feels guilty about what she is concealing. This double burden may drive her to admit both.

If the patient conceals her concealing, her discomfort is threefold: the guilt of concealing, the anxiety of being caught, and the fear of punishment. Burdened by guilt and anxiety, she realizes that she cannot permanently conceal her deceitful maneuvers. Her guilt is increased by your trust that she feels she does not deserve. Throughout the interview, such a patient struggles with her concealing. She wants to relieve her conscience because her guilt outweighs her fear of punishment.

2. Concealing in the Mental Status

Before we describe signs of concealing, we would like to emphasize that all these signs are best observed and interpreted if the patient serves as his own control. In other words, learn about the patient's mental status when you interview him about neutral and emotionally sensitive subjects as are outlined in Table IV–1, and then when you interview him about subjects in which he may be concealing. Only if you can identify differences in his responses to the two types of subjects have you controlled for the interview situation, personality, and cultural factors.

Like a tightrope artist, the concealing patient balances the need to preserve a secret against the need to confess. If he fears you may reject him, he will remain secretive. If he feels overburdened by guilt, he will admit and accept the fact that he may be punished, but lose the burden. This conflict tinges the mental status during the interview. Concealing forces the patient to experience three emotions that may show up in the mental status.

First, you may see the patient's guilt about concealing flit across his face before he can assemble his false front, because true emotions usually precede verbal output. In contrast, nonverbal expressions of his feigned strength typically follow his concealing lines. Secretly, he may ask himself,

Is it worth concealing for this?
Is there a better way to solve my problem than concealing?
What will happen if I share my guilt? Will I lose face? Will I lose trust?

Second, the patient's anxiety of being caught and shamed may overlay his guilt. Therefore, fragments of anxiety may precede his feigned, self-assured affect.

Third, the patient may fear that detection puts him in jeopardy:

Will I be placed in a group home?
Will I lose my job?
Will my wife divorce me?
Will I lose custody of my children?

Although the patient may succeed in suppressing the truth in his verbal productions, he has increased difficulty in suppressing his guilt, anxiety, and fear in his nonverbal behavior. His nonverbal behavior gives you a double message: he presents a false front of self-assurance, straightness, honesty, and confidence, but behind this posture lurks anxiety, guilt, and fear. These feelings show as giveaways before the patient can put up his false front.

Double messages of concealing emerge in affect and in psychomotor movements and speech of the mental status. Ekman (1992), a researcher who investigates deceit, introduced the term *leakage* for behavioral signs that appear outside of the patient's control and point to the hidden truth. These giveaways or leakages of the truth frequently occur immediately after your probing questions address a sensitive, concealed subject. They precede the patient's pretended emotions and his verbal productions.

Double Message in Affect

Genuine emotions, as opposed to pretended emotional expressions, originate from the limbic system. There are five emotions the concealing patient experiences as true: guilt, anger, anxiety, shame, and fear. These emotions emerge out of the patient's dilemma—guilt because she conceals, anger because she feels suspected, anxiety because she may be detected, shame because she may be publicly exposed, and fear because she may be punished. These emotions are displayed in reactions in the autonomic nervous system, such as blushing and blanching. They are expressed by the involuntary extrapyramidal nervous system, which controls reactive movements to new stimuli, facial expressions, grooming movements, and tone of voice. The patient hides these emotions by tensing up, flattening her facial expression, or deliberately relaxing. In general, her affect fluctuates; at times she appears restless and flighty, and at others, emotionally engaged. The ways in which concealment is expressed in affect are summarized in Table 12–1.

Autonomic response.   Your quest for the truth in a concealing patient leads him to have an adrenergic autonomic response. He may show a rapidly pulsating neck artery, wetting of lips, and trembling hands. His pupils may dilate, and he may sweat as if ready for action. The patient may blush and swallow frequently. He may cast his eyes downward. His breathing may become audible, irregular, fast, or shallow; it may stop

Table 12–1.   Manifestations of concealing in affect

Expression	Leakage of anxiety, guilt, fear	False front
Autonomic responses	Dilation of pupils, increased breathing rate, increased heart rate, sweating	Deliberate relaxation
Reactive movements	Startle	Deliberate stretching, suppression of all reactive movements
Facial expressions	Symmetrical, flashed-on affect, repressed affect	Prolonged, flat affect
Grooming behavior	Fast, incomplete, broken-off	Suppressed or absent
Voice	Initially increased or decreased pitch, tremble	Monotone pitch

temporarily or deepen with occasional sighing. The concealing patient tries to suppress these responses and appear relaxed. The more experienced and skillful the concealing patient is, the more he is able to control his autonomic responses by convincing himself that his presentation is the truth.

Reactive movements. A noise or a sudden movement prompts a response that expresses attention. The patient looks up and turns to the stimulus. Similarly, an unexpected question or a change in voice solicits a reactive movement. The concealing patient suppresses reactive movements when she wants to hide surprise. Alternatively, she may increase her reactive movements in the hope that an interruption could rescue her from the uncomfortable interview situation.

Facial expressions. Concealed emotions manifest themselves most clearly in facial expressions. Patients cannot control every spontaneous response and you may see the beginning of one emotional expression that is quickly repressed. The secret emotion flashes on and off (Ekman 1992). In his effort to control his expression, the patient's expressive facial movements may appear wooden. He may wear an artificial smile, which, according to Ekman's (1992) work, appears stronger on the left side than the right side in right-handed patients.

Grooming behavior. Animals and humans alike groom themselves. A scolded dog may turn away and lick his crotch. This grooming behavior may indicate an attempt to regain composure. A human in distress may unknowingly massage her nose or scratch her head or any other part of her anatomy, and, when she realizes what she is doing, break off these movements because they are known giveaways for distress. A male patient may loosen his collar as if it were strangling him. Shoulder shrugging or stretching or nose twitching may emerge.

Voice. The tone of voice reflects the patient's affect. Increased pitch signals excitement, tension, and anxiety, culminating in a loss of voice. Decreased pitch reflects sadness and sorrow. Experimental data seem to support these clinical observations (Ekman 1992). The concealing patient may try to hide his emotions by using a monotonous tone of voice and rhythm. Alternatively, the patient may use rapid speech and enthusiasm to keep the interviewer from interrupting.

Double Message in Psychomotor Movements and Speech

The patient who conceals is aware of the truth. She is cautious toward the person who pressures her to reveal that truth. She screens and filters what she does and what she says. Yet the truth leaks out preceding, intermingled with, or following the patient's concealing responses. You can observe these leakages of truth in the patient's voluntary psychomotor responses—for example, in her gestures, hand and facial signals, goal-directed movements, and pattern of speech (Table 12–2).

Gestures.   In normal communication, gestures simultaneously describe an individual's words. German actors call it *mahlende Bewegungen* (painting movements). Ekman (1992) called these gestures *illustrators*. When a patient wants to move a suspicion away from himself, for example, he makes a pushing movement, or when he wants to show how small something is, he puts his thumb and index finger closely together. When a patient is trying to conceal something, an incomplete gesture may give away a different thought content than the patient is trying to present. Some concealing patients may not use any gestures at all. Leakages of the truth (giveaways) can be expressed by an avoidance of eye contact, a retraction of legs, or a crossing of arms. The adolescent may hold a hand or fingers over his mouth to remind himself to stay quiet. He appears tense and anxious. If he can introduce a story that may distract you from your line of questioning, he may increase the size and number of gestures.

Table 12–2.   Manifestations of concealing in psychomotor movements and speech

Expression	Leakage of truth	False front
Gestures, expressive and illustrative	Decreased	Artificially increased for distraction
Symbolic gestures	Decreased or peripherally and incompletely displayed	Artificially increased for distracting stories
Goal-directed movements	Diminished, tense, or incomplete and interrupted	Relaxed
Speech	Slips of the tongue, interjections, unwarranted pauses, rehearsed quality	Slow, planned, organized

Hand and facial signals. Every culture has signals or symbolic movements that have a specific, precise meaning (Fish 1967). Efron (1972) called
these *emblems,* such as the "A-OK" sign in the American culture, which is
made by forming the thumb and index finger into a circle with the
remaining fingers staying upstretched. These symbols are speech equiva-
lents. They appear to be semiautomatic with gestures accompanying communication. Johnson et al. (1975) counted at least 60 emblems used in the
United States. Ekman (1992) reported that hidden emotions often find their
expression in a symbolic gesture in two ways: first, they can be incompletely
presented, like a shrug of one shoulder rather than a double shrug of
shoulders or raising of eyebrows expressing "I don't know."; second, they
can occur outside the range of the eye field (e.g., a patient may raise the
middle finger communicating an expletive but keeps this obscene sign
buried in his lap).

Goal-directed movements. Goal-directed movements are made to carry
out a task, such as sitting down at the beginning and getting up at the end
of an interview. Secret intentions leak out by the initiation of a goal-directed
movement that is quickly aborted. For example, a patient may whip her foot
as if she is about to walk away. Then she tenses up. The isotonic movement
freezes into an isometric one. After she detects her revealing behavior, she
overcompensates and relaxes her muscles.

Speech. In a concealing person, speech may betray the true intent of his
statement. He may show slips of the tongue (e.g., "I'm slad to see you," with
"slad" being a blend of sad and glad), ehs and ahs, or frequent pauses, all
signs that he has to filter his words. The speech may become faster and
louder. The voice may break—swallowing may interrupt speech. His
thoughts may become jumpy, his speech, circumstantial. His incomplete
sentences express discomfort. The patient may perseverate on a distracting
topic or repeat sentences, words, or partial words. To control his speech, the
concealing patient may slow down and his speech rhythm may become
more deliberated. Again, compare the patient's speech when he is talking
about neutral or sensitive subjects with his speech when talking about
subjects about which you suspect he is concealing.

Verbal Strategies of Concealing

Patients use different strategies to conceal.

Nonhostile concealment.   The patient reduces her communications to elusive statements:

> I don't want to talk about it right now.
> This is not important.

She may be more direct:

> I don't want to cry like a baby.
> Expressing these feelings would be counterproductive.
> Alternatively, she may downplay a problem:

> I don't think much of it.
> It's just something that occurred to me.

She can't talk about it because she fears that she may revive old conflicts or open old wounds, become upset, and embarrass herself in your eyes. She is afraid she will lose your respect, making it impossible for her to continue therapy.

Hostile concealment.   The patient may use both verbal and nonverbal responses at once: refusing to answer questions or elaborate on answers, asking to leave or to use the rest room, or running out of the office.

Distraction.   The patient may avoid your topic and return to a previous one, introduce a new topic, or focus on some irrelevant detail, hoping you will probe only where he shines the light—and not where he hides his problems. He may flatter you and hope you forget your original question. Distraction may be preceded by enthusiasm:

> Do you know that? . . .
> Have you heard? . . .
> Let me tell you. . . .

Distraction can be attempted by the patient's disowning the problem:

> Everybody has that problem.
> Nobody will pin that on me.

Emotional response.   The patient may produce an emotional response, such as crying or expressing anger or shame:

You are hurting my feelings.
You are pushing me.
I've never been treated like this.
You are overstepping your boundaries.
I couldn't look you in the face after I told you.

The patient's emotional responses are designed to arouse your empathy or pity or to encourage you to back off from your questioning. At the same time, the patient may be disappointed if you do not pursue helping her to overcome her resistance. It is important that you pick up the clues of concealing and offer the patient empathy and support before her anxiety and anger cause an emotional outburst.

Amnesia. The patient may claim amnesia about some events.

3. Technique: The Plus-Minus Approach

By using the plus-minus approach, the interviewer challenges the patient's decision to conceal. In so doing, the interviewer asks the patient to weigh the opposing forces of feeling guilt about concealing, anxiety about being detected, and fear of being punished, against the desire to obtain relief by admitting and accepting the consequences of the infraction. The goal is to resolve the conflict through the alliance with the interviewer. The patient may feel that he has more to lose than he can possibly receive. You have to convince him why he should reveal his secret (Fisher and Brown 1988; Fisher and Ury 1991). In the plus-minus approach, you barter with the patient about the advantages and disadvantages of revealing versus concealing, of confiding versus staying secretive. Thus, you start to run a balance sheet with him. What will tip the scale?

The patient fears disclosure for many reasons:

- He feels it would open old wounds.
- He is used to his current way of avoiding his problem.
- He is desperately concerned about the emotional aftermath of revealing his problem.
- He wants to deal with it himself first before talking to you about it.
- He believes that his problems are difficult to understand for an outsider.
- He feels that what he has to say is so embarrassing and shameful that he could not look the interviewer in the eye.

- He is very concerned the interviewer will reject him or pressure him into unwanted therapy.

With the plus-minus technique, identify the patient's concerns and counteract his fears as outlined in the next section under Step 4. First, be sure the patient knows you understand that he is concealing something. When you have evidence of that, convey the message,

> I understand you don't want to talk about _____ [fill in the blank].

Next, point out that you cannot help him if he holds back. If there are any negative consequences of his concealing, you may point them out to him. For example, if, after a severe suicide attempt, a patient evades discussing the value of his life but demands discharge from the hospital or a pass, you can tell him that you cannot grant his request if he is not willing to discuss his suicidal tendencies with you. In contrast, if you can convince the patient that it is in his best interest to admit his concealing behavior and discuss more openly what he is concealing, you have established common ground. Next, elicit in detail the patient's fear that prevents him from leveling with you. Ask him,

> What do you think would happen if you talked to me about it? What would happen to you and how would I respond?

Then, summarize your understanding by reflecting his perspective back to him. Some anxious patients have a narrow perspective about the severity of their misdeed. For such patients you may weave statements such as,

> You haven't exactly robbed the First National Bank.

or

> You haven't exposed yourself in front of the entire track team.

Such exaggerated statements may allow the patient to smile and recognize his unproportionate fear, embarrassment, or guilt. Your statements may serve as ice breakers. They are meant to desensitize the patient to state his own perceived failures.

4. Five Steps to Open Up

How do you overcome the patient's ambivalence about revealing sensitive problems?

Step 1: Listen. Your task is to recognize emotional, verbal, and behavioral signs of concealing. Give the patient the opportunity to talk about her problems. Your openness may uncover her reluctance to share her problems. Ask open-ended questions unless she diverts from the subject. Give her the opportunity to tell her story her way. Encourage her to elaborate on her statements. Make her feel comfortable, express your empathy for her anguish, and praise her accomplishments. If she continues to conceal, she may reveal this behavior best in a double message when you show her understanding and empathy.

The most common signs of concealing are vagueness and discomfort. These behaviors are your cues to ask gently for more details. It is likely the patient will not reveal them early in your interaction. For example, a teenager was suspected by his mother and the police of being involved in a theft. The mother was concerned that her son, who had a history of alcohol abuse but had ceased drinking 7 months earlier, was being influenced by another teenager who had been arrested many times. The interviewer asked the patient about his friend and classmate, John, who was suspected of having broken into a house and stolen a gun. (I = interviewer; P = patient)

1. I: What happened that night?
   P: [Anxiety flashes across his face, then he stretches and yawns.] I don't remember what happened that night. At that time, eh . . . eh . . . I was with a friend, a girl, a girl friend, I think.
2. I: Do you remember her name?
   P: [Has another flash of anxiety; then scratches his neck and chest and wiggles in chair] I just know her first name. Karen. [Then with a broad smile] Some guys even sleep with a girl without knowing her last name.
3. I: Do you know where this girl lives?
   P: [Pushing away motion with his hands] We usually meet at the pizza place. [Leaning forward with emphasis, trying to present certainty] Yes, I enjoy having, having a c-Coke with her. [Broad smile]
4. I: Your mother thinks you were with John last Friday when he and a friend were seen jumping out of the window of a house. Your mother feels you were that other person. It would help if you remembered where you were with your friend at 10:00 P.M. that Friday.
   P: [Has a tortured look, broken up by a smile] Oh, oh, we moved ah . . . around town that night. [Looks at the interviewer, who raises his eyebrows, then makes a waving movement with his body as if driving through curves]

5. I: Do you remember any particular place?

   P: [Deep breath to fill a pause] I . . . I was very tired that night. [Yawns] I really would like to talk to you about something that worries me a lot. My headaches.

This patient's vagueness indicated that he had not prepared his lines. He avoided specific answers. Concealment was indicated in his verbal and nonverbal behavior: ehs, ahs, and repetitions (A. 1, 3, 4); broken-up emotions of anxiety (A. 1, 2, 4), guilt, or surprise preceding the intended artificial emotion (A. 2, 3, 4). These fake emotions, unlike natural emotions, followed the sentence rather than preceded it (A. 2, 3). Abortive, goal-directed movements, symbolic movements, and grooming movements (A. 2) indicated his feelings of helplessness and wish to escape. The patient's gestures died down or appeared in awkward contrast to what he wanted to relate, such as the pushing-away gesture (A. 3), which did not fit the thought content that followed; this indicated that he would like to have the topic pushed aside. A second sign of concealment—the patient's discomfort—increased (A. 2). Finally, the patient employed verbal strategies to escape. He tried distraction by bringing up his headaches (A. 5).

In Step 1, do not indicate that you suspect secretive behavior yet. Ask how you can help.

Step 2: Tag. Tag the patient's sensitivity, vagueness, or discomfort. Tell him that you are unable to understand what really happened. Do not tell him yet that you feel he is concealing the truth. Ask open-ended questions so that the patient has the freedom to tell you more. Tagging can result in three possible outcomes:

1. The patient may tell a coherent detailed history that appears to be true; if so, you no longer need to probe further about that aspect of his story.
2. The patient may make detailed but contradictory statements; then you continue with tactics that deal with contradiction (see Chapter 13, "Falsifying and Lying").
3. The patient may continue to be vague. Ask the patient to write down his story, including the reason why he cannot provide details.

Vagueness may have three sources: The patient may have forgotten part of an event that at one time he could remember better; he may not have paid attention during the event and thus has only a vague impression of it; or he wants to conceal the event. To cover all the possibilities, take the following approach in Step 2:

Was there ever a time when you had a sharper recollection of the event than you have now?

If the patient indicates that he did have a sharper recollection immediately after it happened but then forgot it, offer to help him remember:

Would it help if I tried to refresh your memory? Let me give you some choices.

Another method to tag vagueness is free association. This is particularly effective when the patient has forgotten a name. Cue the patient with words that are similar to what the patient has said:

I: Do you remember the person's name?
P: I really don't have any clue. I know it sounded German—Kindergarten or something.
I: Hmmm.
P: No, it wasn't Kindergarten, it was Klingenfuss. No, Klingenheim.
I: Klingenheim?
P: I think the "Klingen" part is right. But it's more like Klingenburg.
I: So it was Klingenburg.
P: It still doesn't sound right. It was longer. Klingenberger—yeah, Klingenberger.

The patient's anxiety and resistance may prolong this process. Usually, he is aware of his concealing maneuver and will test to see 1) if you notice it, and 2) what you are going to do about it. After several rounds of distraction on the patient's part, and redirection on your part, express your curiosity about his reasons for acting that way. Return to the topic gently but persistently. A patient who habitually distracts the interviewer may smile or make a comment such as, "You caught me." Such a response allows you to respond lightheartedly:

Yes, we went around and around for a while, and I kind of admired you how you could always bring up some new topic. But that is getting old now. I know what you will do, you know what I will do. It becomes a waste of time. We should probably discuss how we can pass this point so that we don't get stuck here.

Your persistence coupled with your offer of alliance may persuade the patient to stay on the topic and finally level with you.

When you tag, it is important that you monitor the patient's emotional response. Emotional discomfort may become more apparent after you tag it.

I think when you get to know me better, you will be able to share with me what you are uncomfortable about. That's the only way I can truly help you. If you feel you have to conceal it, that tells me you don't think you can trust me yet and that your problems are not safe with me. But I hope as we go on you will be able to open up more and more.

Step 3: Confront. At this point, if a patient has still not given up concealment, proceed to confront her with the purpose of her strategy. If you are not sure whether the patient is concealing or whether an Axis I or Axis II disorder (e.g., somatization disorder or histrionic personality disorder) is responsible for her vagueness, you may interject some probing questions (Table IV–1).

Zero in on the tagged areas of the patient's story and confront her. Say in a nonthreatening way,

You give me vague explanations. You try to distract me from asking you about a certain subject and you get upset. I believe you are holding back on me.

Express your regret about this stance:

I'm really sorry that you feel you can't trust me. I think you could use help, but it must be difficult for you to tell me your story so that I can help you.

Ask the patient to consider sharing with you so that you can be an active ally. Make it clear that you can best help her if you know the events as they happened. Ask the patient whether she understands the implications for her future if she withholds any facts. Express your empathy when she shows verbal or nonverbal signs of distress. Switch back to a supportive style of interviewing and accept her defenses.

The patient may show a weakening of her stance by appearing to think about your words, hesitating, or expressing self-doubt. If any of these occur, seize the opportunity to address the change in attitude. Tell her that you notice her conflict about whether or not to tell you. Show understanding:

It must be difficult for you to talk about this.

Show empathy:

I'm sorry that this question upsets you.

Let her discharge and cognitively elaborate on her emotion:

Tell me what makes you so upset.

Step 4: Solve. Step 4 is the centerpiece of your efforts to sway the patient to share her secret with you by implementing the "plus-minus" approach. Help the patient recognize the reality of her situation. It is very important for you to learn exactly what she feels is at risk for her if she opens up to you. Give her vague anxiety a concrete form. Help her by interpreting the emotions she is feeling. Try, for example, to discover the source of her defensive anger or tears. Show empathy for her need to conceal. Often this empathy is enough to encourage the patient to open up, thus freeing her from the burden of concealing. Offer to help her face the consequences of her actions. Equally important, reveal to her how her concealing represents a part of her illness (e.g., a patient with borderline personality disorder conceals the truth to avoid rejection). Tell her that once she begins to get better, her ambivalence about her problem will dissipate.

Finally, the patient may start to admit that she is concealing but bring forth different reasons and fears why she should conceal. Counteract these reasons. In Table 12–3, a patient's arguments for concealment are balanced with an interviewer's arguments for revealing a sensitive problem.

Some concealing patients are accustomed to feeling and thinking in polarities. Therefore, they experience an inherent attraction to an interview approach that plays into their pathology. Because of the associated anxiety, the plus-minus approach works best if it is combined with anxiety-reducing reassurance and empathy in verbal statements and attitude. If you merely make reassuring statements, she may hear you but not believe you. The challenge of using reassurance is not just relaying a reassuring message, but convincing the anxious and suspicious patient of its truth by showing her support in your attitude before offering reassurances in words. Convey the fact that you side with her. Show that you see her problems her way; give your approval from her perspective:

I'm on your side. I'm your ally.

I believe you have a good reason for telling the story as you tell it.

Be sure the patient understands that you are her expert advocate. Express the third vital message of reassurance:

I'm a useful ally because I can help you. *You* are my focus of concern, not your parents, your neighbors, the police, or the IRS.

Suggest specific ways you can protect her interests, such as by speaking to others on her behalf to clarify and negotiate her position. In this way, you

Table 12–3.   Arguments for overcoming concealment

Pro continued concealment	Pro revealing	Element of rapport
● **Not now:** I don't want to deal with it now.	It causes you anxiety and problems. I can help share your pain.	Empathy
I'm used to the status quo.	It causes you discomfort and suffering. I can help relieve these.	Alliance
I don't want to open a floodgate.	I will help you stem the flood.	Expertise
I don't want to have a nervous breakdown.	I'm here to help you sort through things and manage them.	Guidance, healing
● **Desire to do it alone:** This problem is not your [the interviewer's] business.	It's part of your other problems. We should share it all.	Alliance
I can best deal with it alone.	I can be a sounding board to clear up matters. I have worked with similar problems before.	Expertise
Sharing has no bearing on diagnosis or treatment.	Sharing will strengthen our alliance and increase the understanding of your problems.	Alliance
● **Fear of consequences:** No good will come from confiding in you	I can help you face your problem and resolve it.	Empathy, alliance, expertise, guidance
You will not understand.	I understand you. I will help you deal with your problems.	Empathy, guidance, expertise
You will pressure me into therapy.	Together, we will decide about therapy.	Alliance
I will feel shame.	I understand you. We will find out what made you do it. I can help you prevent the problem in the future.	Empathy, expertise
You will abandon me.	I will help you shoulder your problem.	Alliance
I don't want the whole world to know.	Your problems are safe with me.	Confidentiality

transform the misunderstood, lonesome, helpless, and anxious patient into an understood partner who can help to resolve a problem.

Step 5: Approve. A patient often feels embarrassed after he reveals his sensitive problems. Soothe the patient's embarrassment that results from having shared a perceived weakness. Embarrassment breeds more avoidance and resistance. Try to prevent this resistance from reappearing in the next session. Help the patient understand his need to conceal by integrating it into his self-image. In Step 5, you should attempt to make the patient feel good about his choice first to conceal and then to reveal his problem. Summarize for him how confessing his problems serves his needs better than his persistence in concealing them.

Alternative Techniques

What if the plus-minus approach fails? What alternative techniques can you use?

1. Create a vacuum—have a waiting approach. Consider one of the following options: a) Tell the patient the issue is not very important. b) Tell the patient about the waste of time and money that concealing causes. When considering costs, the patient with obsessive-compulsive personality traits, obsessive-compulsive personality disorder, or obsessive-compulsive disorder, who may be usually frugal, especially may reconsider giving up on concealing.
2. Use a dynamic approach. Analyze the patient's defenses. Take this option if concealing is part of the patient's personality style. This would mostly apply to a patient who is secretive, such as one with paranoid personality disorder. Alternatively, acknowledge that the patient has difficulty facing consequences, as in narcissistic personality disorder, or that he has a hard time trusting the interviewer, as in avoidant and paranoid personality disorder.
3. Analyze the patient's relationship to the interviewer, the way he sees you. Tell him he is not trusting you.
4. Consider the cognitive approach for the concealing patient. (See discussion of this technique in Chapter 15, "Self-Deceptive Behavior.")

5. Interview A: Borderline Personality Disorder

Ms. L. is a 38-year-old, white woman who walks with a slight limp. A clinical and structured Psychiatric Diagnostic Interview—Revised (Othmer et al.

1988) supports the diagnosis of bipolar disorder with rapid cycling mood swings. In addition, the clinical interview and the Millon Clinical Multiaxial Inventory—II (Millon 1976) yields a diagnosis of borderline personality disorder. Her father had experienced problems with alcoholism and her mother—an obese woman—had experienced problems with extreme mood swings.

During the interview, Ms. L. reports that she has experienced lifelong rejection by both parents. Her father has constantly teased her about her limp. Her mother has acted as though she hates her daughter, who has tried desperately to win her approval.

In her younger years, Ms. L. was a salesperson in female apparel, insurance, and used cars. In each job, after a short period of success, she would become dysphoric, distrustful, sensitive to rejection and ridicule, and even paranoid. With preemptive strikes, she would ventilate anger, disappointment, and sorrow until she was asked to quit. At those times, she would slash her wrist, overdose on medication, or try to kill herself with exhaust fumes in her garage.

Ms. L. divorced her physically abusive husband. She feels she never loved him. She voices negative feelings, anger, and accusations of others. With full insight, she discusses her mood swings and her unstable, destructive relationships. She readily shares her symptoms with the interviewer. When he asks her about her social history and her present living arrangements, she hesitates. (I = interviewer; P = patient)

Step 1: Listen

1. I: Have you been living alone since your divorce?
   P: [Looks in her lap; face and neck turn red] Kind of.
2. I: Can you explain that to me?
   P: [Closes her eyes and presses her lips together] No, I'd rather not. [Opens her eyes, looks to the side at the floor] That's kind of a sore spot in my life. [Swallows, looks the interviewer in the eye] My family is really down on me for my lifestyle. I don't think you could stomach it either. [Lowers her head as if wanting to knock the interviewer with her forehead]
3. I: So, you feel I would be down on you too if you were to talk about it?
   P: [Looks the interviewer in the eyes] Yes, kind of. I know you are a psychologist and you have heard a lot, but I still feel I can't look you in the eyes any more if you know too much about me—if I feed you all that shit.
4. I: I wonder how I can help you if I don't know your hurts.
   P: There are too many of them. It would make you throw up.
5. I: You mean you are full of them?
   P: That's right.

This patient used orally colored language relating to the digestive tract: "stomach it," "feed you," "throw up" (A. 2–4). Tuning into this idiosyncrasy (Othmer and Othmer 1994), the interviewer used this language himself to create rapport. Still, the patient exempted an area for the interviewer's access, indicating that she feared being rejected by him more than she expected gaining help from him. This constituted an understandable reason to conceal.

Step 2: Tag

This step is omitted because the patient has tagged her concealing herself.

Step 3: Confront

   6. I: [Shrugs his shoulders and looks at the patient]
      P: What?
   7. I: I don't know how I can help you if you just want to talk about your chocolate side.
      P: There isn't that much chocolate. It's more like shit all over. [Flinching and reaching for her weak leg]
   8. I: And you fear that's distasteful to me?
      P: That's right.

The interaction in Step 3 was brief because the patient was aware of her avoidance. The interviewer showed her the consequences of being secretive (Q. 4, 7). The patient countered that she might lose the interviewer as an ally (A. 2, 8). At this point, the interviewer could have assured Ms. L. of his unshakable alliance, but the patient was suspicious of the supportive statements he had previously made (A. 3–5). Therefore, the interviewer opted to reason with the patient using the plus-minus approach.

Step 4: Solve

   9. I: But if you hold it in, I can't help you.
      P: Hmmm. . . . [Bites her lower lip and looks down]
  10. I: If you want to cleanse yourself of it. . . .
      P: [Shakes her head]
  11. I: Well, we were talking about your living arrangements.
      P: Well. . . .
  12. I: What's unusual about them?
      P: [Gets a fold between her eyebrows, looks down and blushes] I live with Carla. [Looks at interviewer from underneath her eyebrows]

13. I: So? What's unusual about it?
    P: [Her eyelids narrow to a slit; defiance enters her voice] Carla is a lesbian.
14. I: So?
    P: Well, my family is down on me for living with a lesbian.
15. I: How do they know?
    P: It's obvious. She's a real butch. She says to everybody she really feels like a man.
16. I: So your family can't stomach her?
    P: [Angry] Damn right. It's really none of their damned business. [Looks away, turns pale]
17. I: Can you stomach her?
    P: [Looks at the interviewer with narrowed eyes, presses her lips together]
18. I: Can you?
    P: [Makes a wiping-away hand movement] Let's just forget it.
19. I: Well, if we do, you are wasting your money and my time . . . just making small talk.
    P: But, you won't get a bitter taste in your mouth when you see me. [Relaxes her shoulders]
20. I: Maybe. But you make me yawn because we are not talking about anything.
    P: So, my choice is to make you nauseated or put you to sleep.
21. I: [Laughs] That's one way to put it. [Shrugs his shoulders and turns his palms up] It's up to you.
    P: [Mocks the interviewer's gesture and his voice] Up to me? [Folds her arms in front of her chest and crosses her legs]
22. I: Up to you! Do you want to impress me? Or do you want to help yourself?
    P: Yeah. [Sighs] It's important to me that you like me.
23. I: To help you, I have to understand what's bothering you. I will accept you anyway.
    P: I can't. [Shaking her head] No. Let's forget it.
24. I: I know it's hard but you'll really win by letting me in on what's bothering you.
    P: [Scratches her head, her face lights up] Okay. . . . [Looks down] It bothers me to be with Carla.
25. I: Why's that?
    P: [Shrugs one shoulder] Because . . . [looking the interviewer in the eyes] I can't really tell her. [Looks frightened] I'll lose her.
26. I: So you're holding back from her too?
    P: I want her to love me.
27. I: And you want me to like you. So you have to hide your true feelings.
    P: Yeah. But you don't understand. Carla loves me like a man does. But, if I wanted a man, I could have stayed with my husband. I'm sorry.
28. I: What are you sorry about?
    P: I don't want to hurt your feelings because you are a man.
29. I: Shall we worry about you or me?
    P: Oh, there we go again.
30. I: Is it more important that I like you or that I help you?
    P: You are playing with my head.

31. I: You stall. You hold back from me and Carla, maybe even from yourself.
    P: Okay, what do you mean?
32. I: Is it more important that you look good to me or that you feel good about yourself?
    P: [Tearful] Okay, I want to be loved. I want Carla to admire me, to look up to me—not to protect me. I'm not sure that I'm a lesbian.
33. I: You want her to be more like a woman. Ms. L., you have to let me know your feelings. It's important that we share. Level with me.
    P: I know myself. As soon as I'm out of here I'll be angry about having told you. I'll feel so bad that I'll want to hurt myself again.
34. I: I understand your feelings. Your feelings flip-flop on you. Trust turns to distrust, like to dislike.
    P: [Interrupting] That's my life story. I can't make up my mind how I feel.
35. I: I'm glad that you talked about your feelings toward Carla.
    P: I'm so screwed up about it. I can't talk to Carla about it.
36. I: Hmmm.
    P: [Mocks him] Hmmm.
37. I: You mock me.
    P: I hate it when you say "hmmm" and don't tell me what you are thinking. I start distrusting you right away and get angry.
38. I: Well, I'm surprised that you don't talk to Carla about your feelings about her.
    P: I don't even dare to think to myself about it.
39. I: Do you know why?
    P: I'm afraid.
40. I: Afraid?
    P: Of losing her. I feel guilty about the way I feel about Carla. I feel if she knows, she'll feel hurt and get angry with me. So, I leave it all unsaid and pretend that everything is okay.
41. I: You trust that little, do you?
    P: I guess.
42. I: I'm glad that you put these feelings into words. I think it may help you in your relationship with Carla.
    P: You think so?
43. I: Well, I hope you will be able to tell Carla about it.
    P: Never! She's so emotional.
44. I: Well, it will help our relationship if you talk to me about it.
    P: I'm surprised that I said what I did.
45. I: Well, if we talk about these feelings again and again, they will become less touchy and easier to put in words.
    P: [Sarcastically] Really?!
46. I: [Ignoring the sarcasm] You may not believe me. I hope we reach a stage where we can bring in Carla and talk about these things.
    P: Let's hold it for now.

From the beginning, Ms. L.'s autonomic responses and her facial expressions showed her double torture of concealing her feelings from the interviewer and her lover (A. 1). The patient had difficulties in accepting her own life-style and projected her rejection of herself onto the interviewer. A psychodynamic interviewer might use this opportunity to make the patient aware of her projection and interpret this as a defense mechanism. In this section of dialogue, the interviewing goals were directed toward the patient's conflict between concealing and being accepted versus revealing and chancing rejection. The patient made only feeble attempts to conceal her lesbian relationship with Carla, even though she feared that her life-style was offensive to the interviewer. What she did hide from the interviewer and Carla was the way she felt about Carla.

The interviewer wanted the patient to give up her concealment. In his plus-minus approach, he offered five reasons for leveling:

1. To be able to receive help (Q. 4, 7, 9, 23, 24, 30)
2. To use time and money wisely (Q. 19)
3. To engage in problem-solving therapy (Q. 20)
4. To help herself rather than impress him (Q. 22)
5. To feel good about herself rather than look good to him (Q. 32)

The most frequently used reason—so that she could receive help—did not work. What weighed in favor of revealing was the prospect that she would feel good about herself after conflict resolution. This observation illustrates a basic principle of the plus-minus approach: depicting the anticipated result, and not the prospect of resolving the problem (as offered in first argument, above), is the most powerful motivation to overcome concealing. This principle is commonly used in marketing, where the consumer is persuaded to decide in favor of a product because it will make him feel clean, good, smart, attractive, and powerful.

Because Ms. L. revealed her feelings about Carla to the interviewer, he tried to encourage her to be more open in her relationship with Carla. Such revealing could resolve her interpersonal conflicts with Carla (Q. 38, 42, 43). However, when Ms. L. expressed her fear of rejection by Carla, the interviewer did not pursue this any further in this session. Thus, he set the stage for future sharing.

Step 5: Approve

47. I: For now. I'm looking forward to our next session. When you go home, I would like you to keep track of your feelings. If you feel guilty or remorseful or angry about what you said today, write it down for next time. And tell yourself that you did the right thing.

P: I better call you when I start to feel sorry about what I told you.
48. I: That's exactly what I want you to do.

Ms. L.'s tendency to conceal her true feelings was indicative of her distrustful, ambivalent relationship with others, which she recognized (A. 34, 37, 44, 45, 47). Therefore, the interviewer anticipated the ambivalent reaction that she might experience on her way home. He invited her to keep track of her feelings and promised to talk to her on the phone about this.

Diagnosis

In addition to bipolar mood swings, this patient presented evidence of borderline personality disorder. She showed frantic efforts to avoid abandonment. She gave a history of unstable, intense interpersonal relationships, identity disturbance, recurrent suicidal behavior, inappropriate intense anger, and paranoid ideation. Patients with this disorder may conceal negative feelings to heighten their acceptance level.

5. Interview B: Incestuous Pedophilia

This patient conceals his secret because he himself rejects his crime and is very remorseful about it. He weighs relief from guilt against rejection by sharing with the interviewer.

Mr. S. is a 6'2", 42-year-old, muscular, white male, recently separated from his wife. The top two buttons of his tight red shirt are open, allowing his dark chest hair to curl out. His brown shorts are wrinkled and stained with food and motor oil. The interviewer shakes the patient's hand, which is damp. Mr. S.'s face is covered with a film of perspiration. Sweat glues his wavy hair to his head. Body odor hangs in the room. When the interviewer invites him to sit down, the patient hesitates. (I = interviewer; P = patient)

Step 1: Listen

1. I: How are you, Mr. S.? How can I be of help to you?
   P: I'm down and worried, can't get any work done. If I don't shape up, I'll lose my job.
2. I: What has happened to you?
   P: Well, my wife just left me. I'm not used to living by myself.
3. I: Hmmm.

     P: Before we got married, I lived with my mom, but she's dead now. And I'm stuck in the trailer all by myself. I can't get things straight.

4. I: Mr. S., what got you separated from your wife?

     P: A whole bunch of things. [Looks down, blushes, and flinches]

5. I: Well, this seems to be rather painful.

     P: Right. [Pauses, looks away out the window, then looks back at the interviewer] What I need now . . . you see . . . I have no pep.

6. I: Hmmm.

     P: I can't get going in the morning. Even when I'm up, I'm just dragging through the day. I can't concentrate on my work.

7. I: Does your dragging get better as the day goes on?

     P: Not really. At night, I sit there and brood.

8. I: And your sleep?

     P: I can't fall asleep.

9. I: Have you had that problem for a long time?

     P: Well, I don't know.

10. I: [Raising his eyebrows] You don't know?

     P: No, I don't.

11. I: I don't think I understand.

     P: Well, you see, I usually had a few drinks in the past. They put me to sleep. But, I'm not doing that anymore.

12. I: You quit drinking?

     P: I guess.

13. I: Did you have a drinking problem before?

     P: I don't know what you call a drinking problem, but I drank.

14. I: Any reason why you stopped?

     P: It caused me lots of problems.

15. I: Problems?

     P: Yeah.

16. I: What kind of problems?

     P: With . . . with . . . [Rings his hands] No, that's over with. [Breathing hard, licks his lips] Let's just talk about what we talked about before—my problems with sleeping.

The patient's discomfort (A. 4), guilt (A. 4, 14, 15), and almost torture (A. 16) showed at the beginning of the interview. But the patient concealed the reason for his distress (A. 4, 5, 14–16). Concealing seemed to be central to the patient's pathology. Therefore, the interviewer decided to forego the assessment of the symptoms of major depression, bipolar disorder, or alcohol abuse to fathom concealment in the five-step approach.

Step 2: Tag

17. I: Okay, let's do that. But I wonder, is that the same reason that you did not want to talk about your separation?

P: [Takes a deep breath] Something like that. But I need help with my sleep now. [Propping himself up to sit straight]

18. I: Okay, you said you can't sleep.

P: Right.

19. I: Any other problems with sleep?

P: Well, I toss and turn, my bed is all messed up in the morning. I sweat. I could wring out the bedsheets. And when I wake up it feels like I have a big headache but I don't really have one.

20. I: Well. . . .

P: And I'm late waking up. I could just sleep forever.

21. I: You have a problem with oversleeping.

P: Yes. Like my mother. She had sleeping problems. She was a manic depressive. She took lithium for 8 years until she died.

22. I: Do you know what that means, manic depressive?

P: Yes, you go down and then some other times, my mother was up all night, yelled at the neighbors, mowed her lawn at 2:00 A.M., and cleaned house all night long.

23. I: Do you get such up periods too? And do some weird things?

P: Like too much cleaning or screaming at the neighbors?

24. I: No, not that, anything weird that may be out of character for you?

P: [Starts to tremble, swallows, looks down, and wipes off a tear] I guess we all do some weird things.

25. I: What weird things did you do?

P: Ah, that's over with.

The interviewer tagged (Q. 17) the patient's evasive answer (A. 16) by linking it to Q. 4 and 5. The patient again avoided talking about the reasons for his separation and his sobriety. The interviewer did not press for the concealed reasons immediately but assessed symptoms for an affective disorder instead (Q. 18–23). However, she returned to the patient's concealed painful problem (Q. 24) and tagged it again (Q. 25).

Step 3: Confront

26. I: You look so miserable. You look so down. And you're fighting off some bad memories.

P: [Suppressing the tears, sits straight up and looks at the interviewer] I'm okay.

27. I: Is it that tough? That hard? You look as if guilt is tearing you apart. I want to help you with that.

P: Do you think lithium would help me like my mother?

28. I: I'm not sure about that. But I'm sure about something else. You are holding things back from me.

P: [Sweat wets his eyebrows, looking down] I'm sorry, but I can't tell you.

29. I: Let's go back to the weird things that you did not want to tell me about. If you want me to help you, I need to know.

P: [Gets up from his chair] I'm sorry, I guess I better leave if you can't help me.

The interviewer's confronting the patient with his attempt to conceal (Q. 26, 28, 29) raised Mr. S.'s anxiety to the point that he wanted to break off the interview.

Step 4: Solve

30. I: That's not what I said. I said I want you to tell me about your weird things so that I can help you. But, I will try to help you any way whether you tell me or not.

    P: But I can't. It's all behind me. I don't want to bring it back. And, if I would, I'm sure you wouldn't want to help me. It's just so low and dirty.

31. I: No matter what you have done, I'll try to help you.

    P: You can't. You'll run. There is no use.

32. I: Well, I'm not here to condemn you or hold judgment over you or punish you. I want to get you out of your mess and help you to work on your future.

    P: There isn't any left.

33. I: A future is there whether you think so or not. You can do a lot to make that future good for you.

    P: Not with what I've done.

34. I: I think I've heard about everything—I've been around for a while. Let's talk about what got you kicked out of the house, the weird thing that you did while you were drinking, the stuff that you've held back throughout our session and that you look so shaken up about, so guilty, like the world's worst criminal.

    P: But I am.

35. I: [Sits up, walks over to the patient, pulls a chair close to him. The patient's body odor is strong.] I stick with you, Mr. S. What is it that tears you up?

    P: [Starts crying] I've committed the ultimate sin. [His shoulders shaking] It's unbelievable.

36. I: What is so unbelievable?

    P: I can't say it, I just can't.

37. I: How can I help you if you don't share?

    P: [Presses both hands against his chest] If it comes out from here I can't stop. It will wash me away.

38. I: Then tell me what do you gain by holding it back?

    P: You won't look at me like an animal.

39. I: What else?

    P: Maybe I can slowly forget.

40. I: Okay. [Pausing] And?

    P: And I don't have to put it in words.

41. I: You haven't convinced me yet that you're better off keeping your secret.

    P: Well, if you don't know what I've done, I don't have to fear that you'll despise me—that you just pretend to be on my side.

42. I: So you feel I'll just pretend and have phony pity?

    P: Something like that.

43. I: Why do you think that?
    P: Because everybody else turned their backs. My wife did. My daughter did.
44. I: I guess you have to take a chance. Now you're lonely.
    P: [His eyes filling with tears] I deserve it.
45. I: So you deserve loneliness and punishment? You suffer from guilt if you talk to me?
    P: I'll be shamed to death.
46. I: You have already shared your pain. You may as well share what you have done.
    P: How do you know that this will help me?
47. I: I don't know, but we'll face your problem together and then . . .
    P: [Interrupts] I was drunk. My wife has arthritis and Crohn's disease . . .
48. I: So, you were drinking—were you in a down mood?
    P: Oh, no, I was flying high. I got a bonus and a promotion at my job.
49. I: So what is your ultimate sin?
    P: [Stands up, turns around, hits the desk with his fist, and moans] I forced myself on my 11-year-old daughter like an animal. I can't stand it. [Starts crying, walks across the room, and sits down on a sofa away from the interviewer]
50. I: [Eventually, the interviewer encourages the patient to detail the incestuous act. Amid tears, Mr. S. reports that he had felt sexually attracted to young girls for a long time, but that he could push these thoughts out of his mind, because "such thoughts are not right." Now the memories of him abusing his daughter haunt him in flashbacks and dreams.]

Mr. S. volunteered symptoms of depression and bipolar disorder. However, because he was unable to disclose his secret, rapport was stymied and prevented the interviewer and Mr. S. from building an alliance against his problems. The interviewer's massive reassurance and support prompted Mr. S. to name his fear as one of being rejected because of an unforgivable crime that he had committed, one that was robbing him of his future (A. 30–35). The patient's statements explained what disadvantages he perceived would come from disclosure; the interviewer then invited the patient to name the advantages of concealing (A. 38–40). Mr. S. complied by stating that if he kept his secret concealed, he wouldn't be swept away by shame, might be able to slowly forget his crime, wouldn't receive phony pity, and wouldn't be looked at like an animal (A. 38–43). These statements allowed the interviewer to understand how the patient weighed the advantages of confession versus concealing. She then made him aware of the fact that he had already implemented his own punishment by being lonely and by enduring pain and guilt, feelings he had already shared with the interviewer (Q. 44–46). This empathic feedback tipped the scale in favor of disclosure (A. 47–49). This disclosure (A. 49) allowed rapport to evolve.

Countertransference

The patient's hygiene repelled the interviewer. She dealt with her negative feeling by bargaining for time. She modified the permissive and flagging steps and assessed the patient's symptoms of an affective disorder rather than focusing on the patient's concealed problem. After she garnered enough empathy for her patient, she could genuinely express her support for him (Q. 31). The interviewer's father had had a drinking problem. She remembered her own helplessness when he came home inebriated, or when her friends told her that they had seen him drunk in a ditch. Therefore, by dealing with this patient, she dealt with her own experiences, even though she had never been incestuously molested. The patient's shame and guilt helped her to overcome her countertransference.

Step 5: Approve

51. I: I'm glad you let it out. We both can't change the past, but we can try to work on the future.
    P: I have no future. I don't want to have a future. I want to be gone. I couldn't kill myself but I sure wish I was dead.
52. I: I can understand your feelings.
    P: I can't sleep. I see my daughter's face. I see my wife's face when she found out.
53. I: You mean in your dreams?
    P: In my dreams and during the day and when I wake up. Dr. B. gave me ECT [electroconvulsive therapy]. He did it twice a day. It made it worse. I didn't even remember that I was in the hospital but I still remembered what I had done.
54. I: Today, we saw that you can't bottle it up. You can't forget it. So, let's understand it.

In the process of approving, the interviewer reinforced the advantage of the patient's disclosure. Furthermore, she provided a road map for future therapy in the form of understanding (Q. 51–54).[1]

Differential Diagnosis

1. Alcohol abuse.
2. Major depressive disorder.

---

[1] It is beyond the scope of this book to discuss the reporting duties and legal issues of interviewing a patient with pedophiliac incest.

3. Rule out bipolar II disorder.
4. Pedophilia.

6. Concealing and the Plus-Minus Approach in Psychiatric Disorders

Concealing is pervasive. It occurs in many psychiatric disorders and for many reasons:

1. *Self-censorship.* Patients with major depression, obsessive-compulsive disorder, and obsessive-compulsive personality disorder experience internal censorship. They feel that some of their actions are objectionable and therefore decide to conceal them.
2. *Ambivalence.* Patients conceal because their thinking and feelings are polarized. Patients with bipolar disorder engage in a constant internal battle of revealing (manic episode) or guilt-ridden concealment (depressed episode). In obsessive-compulsive disorder, patients vacillate between giving and retaining, and in borderline personality disorder, between loving and hating.
3. *Anxiety.* A patient with high anticipatory and situational anxiety and self-doubt inflates her fear of repercussion and rejection even about minor infractions. She may have panic disorder, posttraumatic stress disorder, social phobia, agoraphobia, obsessive-compulsive disorder, generalized anxiety disorder, avoidant personality disorder, or obsessive-compulsive personality disorder.
4. *Guilt.* A patient who experiences intense guilt tends to conceal but not falsify if he considers his activity to be a sin, as may occur in patients with eating disorders, substance-related disorders, impulse-control disorders, and sexual and gender identity disorders.
5. *Distrust and suspicion.* A distrustful patient conceals information from you. Such a patient may have delusional disorder, schizophrenia, paranoid type, mood disorder with psychotic features, or paranoid personality disorder.

The clinical observation that concealment is a common characteristic of patients with an anxiety disorder, depressive disorder, or somatization disorder is supported by the finding that concealment as measured by the Self-Concealment Scale (Larson and Chastain 1990) correlated positively with self-report measures of anxiety, depressive, and bodily symptoms.

The plus-minus approach has broad application. Whenever a patient is about to decide about a behavior, he is rejecting one option in favor of another. The patient's decision making is a continuous process. In most cases, you are in a better position to provide unbiased help than any family member or friend because they may be directly affected by the patient's decision. You can help to bring to the patient's awareness short- and long-term risks and benefits to prevent unfavorable habits and short-sighted decisions. Therefore, review decisions by weighing their advantages and disadvantages. Typical decisions involve seeking out certain friends and dropping others, changing one's marital status, changing jobs, or giving up street drugs for abstinence. The plus-minus approach provides the format to reflect on the factors that determine the patient's decisions.

CHAPTER 13

FALSIFYING AND LYING

Summary

Falsifying expresses the patient's conscious intent to deceive the interviewer with lies, which effectively precludes rapport. The patient's double messages and inconsistencies in her history alert the interviewer to the presence of deceit. He introduces cross-examination, which dissects the patient's lies and exposes contradictions. The interviewer confronts the patient with them and persuades the patient to give them up and establish rapport.

◆ ◆ ◆ ◆ ◆

Lord, Lord, how this world is given to lying!

William Shakespeare
Henry IV, Part I

◆ ◆ ◆ ◆ ◆

1. What Is Falsification?

The ability to falsify is a human skill as old as language itself. Even apes and monkeys practice falsification, using what Byrne and Whiten (1988) described as "Machiavellian intelligence." Here is an example of tactical deception in primates: A juvenile baboon approaches an adult female who is digging for a root. He stops about 7 feet from her, looks at her, and then scans his environment. There are no other baboons in view. The youngster screams as if in distress. His mother, who usually defends him from attackers, comes running and chases away the adult female baboon over a ridge. When both adults are out of sight, the youngster helps himself to the food (Byrne and Whiten 1988).

In DSM-IV (American Psychiatric Association 1994), falsification is referred to explicitly in the diagnostic criteria for conduct disorder and antisocial personality disorder. In conduct disorder, criterion A11 under "deceitfulness and theft" states that the individual "often lies to obtain goods or favors or to avoid obligations (i.e., 'cons' others)" (p. 90). Under antisocial personality disorder, criterion C2 states that the individual practices "deceitfulness, as indicated by repeated lying, use of aliases, or conning others for personal profit or pleasure" (p. 650).

The falsifier replaces fact with fiction. He replaces chains of memories, feelings, thoughts, reflections, conclusions, and responses with a false chain of memories, feelings, thoughts, reflections, conclusions, and responses. The patient who is vague overlays the facts stored in his memory banks with a floating image of the event that he can amend, modify, revise, change, and fill. This fluid fabrication may have no resemblance to the facts. In contrast, the overdetailing patient tries to salvage as much reality as possible from his memory, then forges the critical links to form a new chain.

For these falsifications to work, they have to fulfill three criteria:

1. Consistency (i.e., they have to fit seamlessly, without contradictions)
2. Agreement with outside observations (i.e., they have to fit observations available to others and be congruent with the falsifier's personality)
3. Appearance of truthfulness (i.e., they have to ring true when reported by the falsifier)

If the falsifier violates any of the three criteria, his falsifications will be detected by a trained interviewer. In this chapter, we intend to sharpen your detection skills.

Falsification serves the following three purposes:

Falsification to cover up.   The person who uses a cover-up lie falsifies an action, event, or impulse. The cover-up lie exaggerates or downplays. Interviewers hear cover-up or protective lies all the time:

> I don't really drink as much as those five DWIs [drinking while intoxicated charges] may suggest.

> Mike is a better kid than the teachers report.

The intent behind such lies is obvious: to upgrade the culprit's standing. The falsifier may perceive criticism as unjustified because it exaggerates something that, in her opinion, is a minor or nonexistent fault. The patient may fear the truth will make the interviewer dislike her, reject her, and refuse to help her. Another falsifier may fear that any punishment will be disproportionate to her infraction. Therefore, she feels justified in covering up with a lie. If detected, she may still downplay the infraction but may express regret that she tried to mislead you. If she succeeds in deceiving you, she may express relief.

Falsification to divert responsibility.   The person who diverts responsibility admits the act but shifts the responsibility by changing labels—a mutually agreed-on sexual act becomes rape, or an accomplice turns into a victim and hostage. When a patient has committed an illegal act such as theft, assault, or physical or sexual abuse, he knows that if he admits his infraction he will be exposed to legal consequences and probably lose respect in his community or be ostracized altogether. Thus, he diverts responsibility. When caught, his amount of guilt determines whether he expresses shame about his infraction and deception or whether he still downplays the act and expresses anger that you suspected him. If he succeeds in his deception, he may feel relief or even enjoy the challenge of misleading you.

Falsification to slander.   The lying patient sometimes uses falsification to blame or hurt another person. Such slander can be either offensive or defensive. Some examples are

> To get revenge on her stepfather for grounding her, a female teenager accuses a male family member of rape

> To escape his mother's custody, a son falsely accuses her of beating him.

The falsifier in this case is clearly aware of the purpose of his falsification. He calculates the risks of his falsification and the consequences if it is detected.

A lying patient feels justified about his lying, about the act he is trying to falsify, and about the falsification itself. In his own mind, the falsifier feels that his falsification serves his higher purpose of justice. If such a falsifier is detected, his predominant emotion may be anger rather than anxiety or shame about either the falsified act or the falsification itself. On the other hand, if the falsifier manages to escape detection, he shows delight about his success and contempt for his victims, including the gullible interviewer. He may experience the excitement of the gambler who has hit the jackpot.

In practice, the act of falsification is rarely pure. Elements of concealment may become mixed in with the elements of hard-core falsification.

2. Falsification in the Mental Status

A patient's mental status is assessed by *observation, conversation, exploration,* and *testing* (Othmer and Othmer 1994) and notice the signs of falsification. These signs depend on how well the falsifier has prepared his falsifications and lines of speech. Thus, falsification will flood the mental status of the careless liar, or will only sporadically leak through the mask of the prepared and skillful falsifier. These leakages (Ekman 1992) show up in affect, psychomotor movements, and speech (Table 13–1). All these signs are valid only if compared with statements obtained regarding neutral and sensitive subjects for which you can exclude falsification. Thus, there is no absolute single sign of falsification. It is the difference in patterns of expression that occur during truth telling and falsification.

Double Message in Affect

The secret message is displayed in the components of affect—autonomic response, reactive movements, facial expressions, grooming, and voice (Table 13–1).

The emotional leakage of the truth in the form of the secret message usually precedes putting up the false front. The secret message is short lasting, flashes on and off, is incomplete, or may appear outside of your apparent visual field. It involves the autonomic and extrapyramidal nervous systems. It can only be controlled through imaginatory enacting, which takes planning, practice, and talent on the patient's part. The false front is deliberate, prolonged, and emphasized by the patient.

False emotions may be wooden, asymmetrical, exaggerated, and/or prolonged. They often follow the verbal expression, whereas the secret, true emotion precedes the verbal expression. Actors know that the emotion has to be developed in nonverbal cues before the line is delivered to bring the message across. They learn to develop a line by displaying the affect that goes with the line before saying it. Most deceitful patients are not trained or not talented enough to do this. Furthermore, true emotions show a natural crescendo and decrescendo, whereas artificial emotions are switched on and off without variation in intensity.

The concealing patient (Table 12–1) and the lying patient both have to deal with the leakage of the truth and with the anxiety about being detected, including the fear of the consequences and possibly guilt about the act. The difference between concealing and lying surfaces in the false fronts chosen by the concealer and the liar. The concealer merely wants to suppress the truth, whereas the liar actively tries to falsify the truth. For example, when the concealer is startled by a probing question, he tries to act relaxed. When the liar is startled by a probing question, he modifies the startle response into a response of intense interest. In the following sections, we describe the response of the falsifying and lying patient.

Table 13–1. Manifestations of falsification in affect

Expression	Leakage of truth	False front
Autonomic responses	Dilation of pupils, trembling, sweating, increased breathing rate, increased heart rate	Deflected responses displayed as excitement
Reactive movements	Startle	Acting intense and focused to deflect surprise
Facial expressions	Symmetrical	Asymmetrical, stronger on left side of face
	Micro affect Repressed affect	Opposite quality to micro affect Prolonged, distracted, incorporated in another affect
Grooming behavior	Fast, incomplete, broken off	Prolonged, deliberate, or repeated
Voice	Change in pitch, tremor, breaking	Firm, vigorous accentuation of consonants

Autonomic response.   Whereas the concealing patient suppresses autonomic responses, the falsifying patient tries to deflect and distort them. Patients who feel that you suspect them of deception attempt to suppress their arousal cues and display a positive demeanor. This clinical observation is supported by the results of Buller et al.'s (1991) study in which college students who were instructed to practice deceit responded to suspicious and probing questions with self-confident and positive behavior. The falsifying patient pretends to be excited about the subject you have introduced when in fact she is truly anxious about your question. For example, a patient who becomes angry because her falsification is being dismantled deflects her trembling and blushing into a high-pressured, detailed explanation of her position.

Reactive movements.   Reactive movements caused by surprise become falsified into a deliberate, goal-directed movement or into pretended interest in a topic. For example, a teenager is accused of forceful sodomy of a 10-year-old child, which he denies. When the interviewer enters his room, the teenager quickly looks away in avoidance, but then walks in the direction of his eye movement and says, "I'm looking for my score sheet for you to sign." Thus, he falsifies his reactive movement of escape into a goal-directed movement of following ward procedure.

Facial expressions.   The face shows a double message in affect by flashing on the true affect for a very brief time before switching to the intended affect. There are at least four reliable facial expressions of true affect that can only be voluntarily produced by 10%–15% of nonpsychiatric subjects (Ekman 1992). These are

- Corners of lips pulled downward without moving chin muscles, which expresses sadness, sorrow, or grief
- The omega sign, in which only the inner corner of the eyebrows are turned upward and the forehead is wrinkled, forming a fold between the eyebrows, which indicates sadness, grief, distress, and probably guilt
- Raising the eyebrows and pulling them together as an expression of fear and terror or, to a lesser degree, apprehension and anger
- Narrowing the lips, making the red nearly disappear, expressing anger

Thus, these facial expressions of grief, guilt, apprehension, and anger are giveaways for 85%–90% of patients who try to make you believe that they feel happy, easy, prepared, and content.

A falsifying patient may hide depressive and angry feelings behind a smile. However, the smile is often limited to the mouth area and does not involve the muscles around the eyes, or the smile may show an admixture of disgust, fear, contempt, or sadness (Ekman et al. 1988).

Grooming behavior. Spontaneous grooming movements increase if the patient becomes excited. A falsifying patient turns excited feelings into grooming mannerisms, such as taking off glasses and wiping them, or smoothing his hair. For example, a patient who was confronted with his heavy alcohol use scratched himself, massaged his neck, and shrugged one shoulder. Then he said in a calm voice that he was on the verge of heavy drinking but signed himself into the hospital to prevent progression into abuse. He then followed up his statement with overindulging in twirling his mustache to pretend comfort.

Voice. When stress and excitement heighten the pitch of the patient's voice, especially when you discuss a topic that he is lying about, he may conceal such stress by enthusiastic rapid talk. He may use pronounced articulation of consonants and a firm voice to falsify and hide his anxiety. But his articulation may sound pressed; he may talk through clenched teeth to stay in control.

Double Message in Psychomotor Movements and Speech

When caught by surprise, the suppressed secret message leaks out in gestures, symbolic signals, goal-directed movements, and speech (Table 13–1) before the patient can put up her false front. If she is well prepared, the suppressed motor response may merge with the pretended response. Confusing gestures, incomplete symbolic hand and facial signals, and slips of the tongue may emerge. Finally, the individual may give away a secret message by a goal-directed movement. For example, in 1992 during a televised presidential debate with candidate Bill Clinton, President George Bush looked at his watch, portraying his wish that the debate would end.

Gestures. Gestures may be more telling than words, especially in children and adolescents. Gestures that fit the patient's secret emotion and thought content may leak out and later be deflected and falsified. The deflecting gestures are often edgy, prolonged, and nonmodulated in intensity and speed and of deliberate quality.

Symbols (i.e., hand and facial signals). Abortive hand and facial signals can express the patient's helplessness, such as a one-sided shoulder shrug. A patient's wish to stay strong may be evident in his making a fist, which he keeps out of the interviewer's direct view. When he becomes aware of his fist, he may falsify his movements by cracking his knuckles pointedly, pretending that he is exercising his hand.

Goal-directed movements. Under questioning, the patient may look away from you, press her lips together, stare out the window or into open space, scoot around on the chair, or even get up. If she feels that her movements betray her intention to escape, she deflects attention from them—she may stretch and move deliberately, as if stiff from sitting so long.

Speech. The prepared deceiver delivers rehearsed phrases, smooth lines, and stories that contrast with the fluency and modulated voice of normal speech.

Verbal Strategies of Falsifying

Use of rehearsed statements. Because the patient is replacing a factual chain of events with a new one, he is afraid that the truth may slip out. So he rehearses his statements beforehand and may repeat them during the interview. In the 1969 political thriller Z, the investigation into a government conspiracy turned on the fact that two suspects, in separate interviews, used exactly the same unusual phrase to describe the man on whom they wished to pin the blame: "lithe and fierce like a tiger." In a custody dispute, a 9-year-old boy used the phrase "the joys of boyhood," a phrase apparently rehearsed by his caretaker relative (W. V. McKnelly, personal communication, 1994).

You can identify rehearsed statements by a change in the pace of the patient's speech. At first the patient may give you a truthful story with the hesitations, reformulations, and changes in tone of voice, speed, and emotional color that indicate natural speech. All of a sudden, the pace picks up. There are no more delays or pauses. The voice becomes monotonous. The patient's eyes stiffen. He looks at you straight without blinking, or stares at the wall while reeling off the rehearsed statement, as if the words were written there. He may even repeat the statement several times. The rehearsed part may be one line or a complex speech several minutes long.

Contradictions. A patient may have to create a new lie to support or augment an old one. In such cases, she may create details on the spur of the moment and will get lost in details, inconsistencies, and contradictions. There may seem to be a discrepancy between the judgment that the patient exercises while lying and her judgment when dealing with events other than those to which the lie applies.

Overly detailed information. An experienced liar knows that vagueness may raise a flag. Therefore, to gain credibility he provides an overdetailed story filled with irrelevant information.

> I know it was 3:00 A.M. because I heard the bell chime in the Episcopalian church tower over by the courthouse.

> I didn't see my husband hit my daughter because I happened to be looking down at my foot trying to get off my new shoe. I had just bought a pair of new black loafers that afternoon and the left one was pinching my big toe.

The patient gives important and unimportant details with the same emphasis, merging foreground and background.

Spin. Patients often provide a spin to a story. For example, a patient may say, "Rich people can get away with anything." The patient hopes that the interviewer will accept her spin and become favorably biased to her point of view and thus won't scrutinize her story too closely. In devoting her energies to creating that spin, she underestimates the task and falls short on details, thus creating contradictions between her spin and the facts.

Pretended cool. A patient may mask the signs of stress by slumping his shoulders, unclenching his fists and jaws, seeking eye contact, or cracking jokes—that is, pretending to feel cool and calm. However, this type of patient often overdoes it.

Defensive attitude. A defensive attitude may emerge in the form of one-sided, self-serving statements that cover up the role that the patient played in the situation. She diverts responsibility by pleading innocence or even by portraying herself as a victim. A defensive patient may not replace the chain of factual events with invented ones but may force a certain perspective on these events.

Opposition. When patients suspect you know they are lying, some will become uncooperative. They will talk with a sharp voice, show stern facial expression, give terse answers, criticize your questions, and launch into a tirade.

3. Technique: Cross-Examination

Judges need the truth so that they can render justice; therapists need it to make a diagnosis and to plan treatment appropriately. The technique of cross-examination, which dates back to the mid-seventeenth century, has been called "the greatest legal engine ever invented for the discovery of truth" (Degnan 1968, p. 908). This engine can also propel the psychiatric examination of the patient who falsifies.

Inevitably, the falsifying patient creates a story that conflicts with reality. Your challenge is to find out where. The more you ask the patient for a detailed account, the more likely it is that inconsistencies will show. Cross-examination slices up the patient's story into the smallest possible pieces, allowing the detection of inconsistent parts that do not fit into the larger picture. According to a German proverb, lies have short legs—it is easy to catch up with them. The basic technique of cross-examination is to limit the patient's answers to yes and no with closed-ended questions. Here are three advantages to this technique:

1. You can use your own concise questions rather than depend on the patient's vague, evasive words. Yes-or-no responses allow no room for freewheeling fantasies and evasions.
2. You can methodically direct the patient to the area where you suspect a lie.
3. You may, in true Socratic fashion, ask only those questions to which you can predict the answer.

Cross-examination in a psychiatric setting adopts the strategies of two adversaries—the direct examiner who permits the patient to tell the story in his own way (Steps 1 [listen] and 2 [tag]) and the cross-examiner who doubts the patient's story and exposes it to intense scrutiny (Steps 3 [confront] and 4 [solve]). Remember to take an adversarial stance against the lie, not against the patient. You are an empathic caregiver, not a hostile police interrogator. Make it clear that you are on the patient's side in battling the problem that causes him to lie. You are asking questions not to levy blame or impose punishment, but to discover the truth so that healing can begin.

Cross-examination is most useful with a patient who fabricates lies about a single event, such as with a malingerer who apparently fakes symptoms and signs to get compensation, or a patient who shifts guilt to avoid embarrassment or punishment.

Some readers of this book may feel uncomfortable with the idea of cross-examining patients. On the surface, it may appear that this approach places the interviewer in an adversarial position and risks being counterproductive. However, as we will show, skillful use of this technique may lead to a sharing of the problem and the development of rapport. Thus, we like to familiarize readers with this technique so that they can decide if and when to use it.

One advantage of psychiatric cross-examination is that it can serve as a dry run for the legal cross-examination that some patients with antisocial or borderline personality disorder may have to undergo. Not only does it prepare the patient for the grueling process ahead, it reveals any weaknesses in his history that need to be addressed.

Cross-examination appears justified to us if the lie in question is harmful to the patient or to others and threatens therapy. In such cases, recovery of the truth is helpful for the patient, his family, and perhaps a third party.

The decision to use cross-examination must be made on a case-by-case basis. Sometimes it is the last resort to let a patient realize the destructiveness of his behavior. Guiding the choice is the fundamental principle "Do no harm." The discomfort such an approach can cause is comparable with the discomfort of an injection, a surgical incision, or the side effects of medication: if the expected benefit is high enough, proceed with caution and confidence. Let the patient know at all times that you have empathy for his problem but have difficulties with the contradictions in his report.

Do not use cross-examination if the patient shows a chronic pattern of lying and you want to substantiate a general tendency toward lying. Other instances in which cross-examination is inappropriate include 1) if you suspect the patient is also lying to himself (i.e., is using self-deception); 2) if the patient has conversion or dissociative symptoms such as pseudoseizures, dissociative amnesia or fugue, or dissociative identity disorder (multiple personality disorder); or 3) if the patient's sense of reality is distorted by a psychotic process, such as in delusional (persecutory) thinking; hallucinatory perception; or psychotic muteness caused by depression, schizophrenia, or a cognitive disorder such as an amnestic syndrome or dementia.

Comparing the responses of the truthful with the lying patient during cross-examination shows that the truthful person answers promptly most of the time, except when he has to reconstruct a scene in memory precisely as it was. He remembers details coherently, and his attitude is usually friendly and cooperative. He may be proud of his ability to recall and show satisfaction about task completion and little defensiveness. His emotions and affect are congruent with the situation. For example, if the incident under scrutiny was embarrassing or painful, he will display normal and appropriate signs of embarrassment or pain.

In contrast, falsifying forces a patient to replace complex facts with inventions. The technique of cross-examination stretches the liar's imagination, logic, sense of reality, and intelligence. It is easier to tell the truth than to lie, because it is easier to reproduce facts than to spontaneously invent believable fiction to satisfy the interviewer's thirst for details. Successful lying requires intense concentration and an easy hand. Signs of struggle raise a flag. Ultimately, the patient will produce contradictory statements. To avoid doing so, he must bargain for time by delaying his response or requesting that the question be repeated to consider his response carefully. He may pretend not to understand, be vague, avoid details, or claim memory loss. For example, if the patient with antisocial personality disorder senses he is cornered, he may become hostile and try to escape.

Usually interviews with difficult patients follow through the five steps in a single session. For cross-examination, where the patient's resistance is strong, or where hostility or anxiousness may threaten the continuation of the interview, it is advisable to use the five-step process over several sessions. In your first interview, let the patient produce his falsification. Prepare your cross-examination. In the second session, try out some probing questions and proceed with the cross-examination.

4. Five Steps to Cross-Examine

Step 1: Listen.   How do you spot lying? Let the patient talk. Make her feel comfortable. Ask how you can help. Be empathic to both the patient and her story. Allow her to embellish to the fullest extent. Keep your questions open ended unless she diverts from the subject. Encourage her to elaborate. Do not give any indication yet that you doubt her truthfulness. If she asks you,

> Will you believe me? No one else does.

reassure her:

> I want you to tell me the truth. I think the more you trust me, the more you will be able to tell me what happened.

Keep a detailed record; if you don't trust your memory, give the patient a choice of your taping the interview or taking notes. Either method may interfere with rapport. Taping distracts initially; note taking disrupts eye contact during the interview.

When you prepare your cross-examination, you may need to examine the patient's background regarding her

- *General knowledge.* A mentally retarded patient who does not know what constitutes rape may falsely accuse someone of rape.
- *Intelligence.* A smart person may invent falsifications that a person with a low IQ is unable to do.
- *Memory function.* A patient with beginning dementia of the Alzheimer's type cannot give reliable testimony.
- *Special knowledge.* The patient should have the knowledge that only the culprit can have.
- *Interest in outcome.* The patient should benefit from falsifying.

In addition to signs of concealment (i.e., vagueness, distraction, and emotional discomfort), rehearsed phrases, contradictions, excess details, spin, and amnesia will emerge as indicators of falsification.

Step 2: Tag. Double-check for accuracy. Underscore the patient's key statements and ask her to repeat them with the aim of making her commit to a specific story.

Do I understand you right when you say? . . .

Is this what you want me to know? . . .

Then, fill in details.

Next, focus on and tag rehearsed phrases, contradictions, excessive detail, spin, and acting cool. Usually a defensive attitude and opposition do not emerge while you tag the suspect elements of the patient's story. However, if defensiveness and opposition do emerge, proceed to Step 3. Step 2 transforms rehearsed phrases, overdetailedness, spin, and amnesia into more details that do not fit into the larger picture.

Tag a rehearsed phrase. A rehearsed phrase "freezes" the patient's ability to respond. This is a weakness. Having spent her energy creating the rehearsed story, the falsifier may not be able to generate requested details spontaneously. She may reiterate the story or be forced to contradict herself. Let her elaborate and magnify her contradictions.

Tag the contradiction.   Make the patient aware that you are interested in something that does not quite add up or fit the whole picture. Show that you are puzzled, but be careful not to label her story a lie. Use nonjudgmental and nonthreatening language:

> I'm curious about something you said a moment ago.

> I'd like to take another look at the events of that evening. There's something about the sequence that I didn't quite follow.

Monitor the patient's emotional response to your tagging of the contradiction.

Tag excessively detailed descriptions.   Tell the patient that you are impressed with her good memory about an event that happened such a long time ago. Tell her that you would like to use that good memory to also reconstruct events that happened before and after her detailed account. Thus, use his overdetailedness to get a long, detailed account of the entire event. If she is falsifying the story, she is liable to contradict herself or the known facts.

Tag the spin.   When a patient offers a spin to a story, she hopes you will share her proposed prejudice, such as,

> Isn't that typical for a drug user?

Answer attempts to prejudice you with,

> Well, let's be fair. Let's examine the evidence and not jump to conclusions, just because a person abuses drugs.

Tag acting cool.   Tell the patient that it does not seem to bother her to talk about a certain subject. She may appear to be extremely confident and very relaxed. Sometimes it may be an effort for her to be that calm. Then you may ask the patient,

> Is that true for you?

Step 3: Confront. Zero in on the tagged areas of the patient's story and confront her with the inconsistencies—your evidence that she is falsifying. Say in a nonthreatening way,

I don't understand how A goes with B. Please explain that to me.

Now, you shift from direct examination to the preparation of cross-examination. Express your empathy for the patient's plight but not for her story. Scrutinize each single element and press for more details to flush out inconsistencies. Have her repeat it by asking probing questions:

Is this how things happened?

Is this the truth?

If you spot an inconsistency or contradiction, question the patient until she commits herself to one version.

Next, juxtapose the patient's contradictory statements and ask her what she thinks about the two stories. Does she notice that they don't match? Make her see that the event could not have happened the way she says. Then point out the undesirable consequences that will arise from falsifying. Remind the patient what is at stake for her. Heighten her awareness of her jeopardy to increase her guilt, apprehension at being detected, and fear of punishment if she is indeed falsifying. The mounting pressure to tell the truth usually forces the patient into one of six courses of action:

1. She admits the truth and gives a coherent history consistent with the facts. Then you have achieved the goal of the interview.
2. She pleads for your pity by crying or acting confused, helpless, or hurt in an effort to get you to quit your intensive confrontation.

What kind of therapist are you?

In response, separate your attack on her story from an attack on her person. Such a split keeps you empathic and supportive of the patient:

I'm not calling you a liar. I'm not interested in name calling. My difficulty isn't with you, it's with your story. I'm telling you my problem so that you clearly know where I stand. I'm being honest with you. I hope you will be honest with me too.

Or say,

> Your story does not work for me. There are too many unanswered
> questions. I would like you to give me all the details so I can understand
> what happened fully and clearly. That's the only way I'll be able to help
> you.

3. She claims amnesia for the events. At this point the patient may say,

   > You are pushing me too much. So far, I have tried to give you an accurate
   > account, but now I just can't remember.

4. She insists on her story. Even under intense questioning, the patient may
   maintain her original position without showing signs of doubt or
   weakness. Bear in mind that this may mean that you are wrong in
   assuming that she is lying or—perhaps more likely—that you have not
   convinced her that you have detected her falsification. She may even
   attack you, telling you she has had enough of you and that she hates
   you, and then clam up.
       At this point, you could again comment on the patient's position. For
   example, tell her you think that she does not seem to be impressed by
   what you are saying, and that she apparently does not feel the need to
   have you as an ally.
5. She may become tense, defensive, uncooperative, and argumentative.
   She may criticize you for your attitude or your approach. Bring out her
   hostile tendency and let her look into it. An obsessive or depressed
   patient with guilt and anger tends to become oppositional. The patient
   who opposes you is refusing to replace the event memory or semantic
   memory by falsifying. Address this change in attitude. State that you
   believe she is increasing her resistance against you. Tell the patient that
   she seems to be uncertain about lying but that you perceive that she has
   decided to stick with the lie. If her opposition continues to grow, she
   may end up in a tirade during which she gives away the truth in the form
   of unprepared, unrehearsed, and unplanned sentences. Slips of the
   tongue may aid her confession. In the movie *A Few Good Men* (1992),
   Jack Nicholson, who portrays a Marine commander, is provoked by Tom
   Cruise, playing a young interrogator, into such a tirade while being
   cross-examined. Nicholson's tirade exposes his network of lies.
6. She may overcompensate for her opposition. When the patient becomes
   aware that her resistance hurts her, she may try to hide her anger by
   pretending to be cooperative. Now eager to answer all questions, she

may assume a certain submissiveness. Regardless of the kind of evasive maneuvers, handle them:

> Your response is hurting you. People will think you are lying. They will either continue to push you for the truth or they will believe the other side.

Step 4: Solve. Cross-examination is the centerpiece of your efforts to confirm the patient's lie and reveal the truth.

First, you and your patient will need to agree on the ground rules for the cross-examination. Tell her:

> We both see that your story doesn't add up. We are missing some important details. We need to slow down and find a better way to make the story clear. I will try to use simple yes-or-no questions asking for one small piece of information at a time. If you can't answer with yes or no, just let me know and I'll rephrase the question. Do you understand? Can you do this with me?

With tightly focused, repeated closed-ended questions, zero in on the area where the patient presumably falsifies, and then inject verifying questions. Examples include

> Is this really the truth?
> Are you lying about this?
> Is there anything you are holding back?
> Is this all you can tell me?
> You are hiding something, aren't you?

This strategy helps your cause in several ways: For someone who falsifies, the yes-or-no format can become unbearable. To invent minute details over a long period of time is stressful. Even minor discrepancies erode credibility by forcing the patient to modify previous statements. Make sure she notices the discrepancy and is aware that you notice it as well. Now she may try to make you give up your cross-examination by creating an emotional uproar and making threats. Show empathy for her chagrin but stick to your method.

If you submit a patient who is not lying to a cross-examination, the examination will help the patient to clear herself. Her answers will have a normal latency of response. Pauses correlate with the difficulty of remembering certain details rather than with having to invent pieces that fit in an increasingly contradictory story. The patient's anger at having been wrongfully accused, which she may have expressed in an impatient, unfriendly, irritated, and annoyed way, gives way to signs of relief that she is being cleared of suspicion. You can help develop this feeling of relief by telling the patient how pleased you are that the pieces seem to fit and that your questions are being answered satisfactorily. Depending on the patient's personality, she may or may not express her understanding of why she was suspected of lying. She may be grateful that she had a chance to dissipate the suspicion, or she may remain angry at having been wrongfully accused. The latter response is more common in a grandiose, paranoid delusional, or narcissistic patient.

If you mistakenly vindicate a liar, your approval may provoke flashes of "deception delight" (Ekman 1992). A bluffing poker player may turn his cards in triumph to show his contempt for the others who he bluffed out of their better hands. The socially accepted form of deception delight and contempt for the victim is displayed in everyday kidding and putting somebody on.

Step 5: Approve. Your patient may feel ashamed and embarrassed after the cross-examination. Help her understand and accept her need to falsify. Convey that you understand her dilemma. Try to build an alliance that allows the patient to express relief that the truth has come out. Point out that, thanks to her, the stage is set for a solution of her problem.

5. Interview:
False Rape Charges by a Patient
With Traits of Borderline Personality
Disorder and Conduct Disorder

Rhea, a 16-year-old, single, white female, appears to have an acute posttraumatic reaction after purportedly being raped by Brian, a classmate, 5 weeks earlier. Her chief complaint at the interview is, "I was raped. I want to die." Her parents demand that she be hospitalized to be treated for the shock of the rape and her ensuing depression. The parents are pressing charges against Brian.

Rhea has a history of some drug and alcohol abuse. She has difficulties getting along with her younger sister, whom she beat several times when her sister used Rhea's tapes or her clothes or tattled on her. Her mother also reported other behavioral problems: truancy, violating curfew, stealing money, shoplifting, and frequent lying since age 9 years, even when lies offered no advantage. Rhea says she does not know why she lies. She admits that she sometimes lies to her father because she is afraid he'll hit her. Her father, a recovering alcoholic, often had punished her by beating her, but not since he began attending Alcoholics Anonymous meetings. Her mother expresses concerns about Rhea's truthfulness about the rape, because Rhea lied when she told her mother that she had not seen Brian again following the rape. Rhea's sister informed her mother that she had seen Rhea talking to Brian for a long time.

At the intake interview, Rhea is vague in her answers and given to angry outbursts. She clearly knows the difference between sexual intercourse and rape. The following question arises: Is Rhea a rape victim in need of therapy to prevent a posttraumatic stress reaction, or does she lie because she fears her parents and is in need of a better relationship with them? The patient agrees to have this interview audiotaped. (I = interviewer; P = patient)

Direct Examination

Step 1: Listen

1. I: Rhea, you came to the hospital last weekend, 5 weeks after you were raped. You must have gone through a lot.
   P: Oh, it was horrible. Dad has been yelling a lot. Mom and Dad treat me as if it was all my fault.
2. I: Your fault?
   P: Yes, the rape.
3. I: How did they find out about the rape?
   P: I came home late after school, and they asked me where I had been. I said I was at my girlfriend Janet's house doing homework. [Raises her right eyebrow] Later on that night they woke me up. My mom had found my panties.
4. I: Your panties?
   P: There was some blood on them and she knew I wasn't on the rag.
5. I: Hmmm.
   P: Dad called Janet's house and her mother said I hadn't been over there. He talked to Janet and asked if she knew anything. [Lips become thin] Janet told him I had left school with Brian.
6. I: And?
   P: So they yelled and screamed at me and they wanted to know what was going on.
7. I: Hmmm.
   P: So I told them what happened, that Brian had grabbed me by the throat, thrown me down, strangled me, pulled my panties down, and forced himself on me. [Lips become thin] But they acted as if they didn't believe me. [Pulls the corners of her mouth down and sniffles]
8. I: [Pausing] They didn't believe you.

P: [Lips becoming thin again] No. I swore to them that it was the truth. [Looking the interviewer in the eyes and pushing her chin forward]

9. I: Did they believe you then?

P: Yes, I guess. [Brief smirk, looks away] They told me that they were going to press charges against Brian and that he would be in a lot of trouble. They may throw him out of school and he may go to jail. [As the corners of her mouth sink down, the omega sign flashes onto her forehead; she starts to cry.] He hurt me. [Presses her lips together, cries more]

10. I: Rhea, it must have been really hard for you to go through all that. Do you like Brian?

P: [Blushing, head sinks down] No, not any more. [Bends her head further down so that her hair falls in her face, then bites her lower lip] I hate him! I hate him! [More crying]

11. I: I understand that if he hurt you and raped you, he should pay for it.

P: [Her sobbing is interrupted by a short grin, then she covers her face with her hands.]

12. I: Have you ever dreamed about it?

P: Dreamed about what? My father yelling? Sometimes. An angry man with a mean voice pops up in my dreams.

13. I: No, I mean dream about the rape.

P: Oh, no. That wouldn't be a dream, it'd be a nightmare.

14. I: Have thoughts about what happened to you ever popped into your mind suddenly when you are in school or when you are alone?

P: [Raising her eyebrows] No, of course not. I want to forget about it. I want to get it out of my mind. [Throws her head to the side as if throwing out some thoughts]

15. I: What do you remember of the rape?

P: [With impatience and higher pitch in voice] I remember Brian grabbed me by the throat, threw me down on the floor, strangled me, pulled my panties down, and forced himself on me.

From the start, Rhea's credibility was in doubt because she had a history of lying and shoplifting. She offered more details about how her parents detected the rape (A. 3–6) than about the rape itself (A. 7). When asked whether she was reexperiencing the rape in dreams (Q. 12–13), she misunderstood the question. Once she understood the question, she denied either dreaming about it or, in the next question (Q. 14), having intrusive flashbacks during the day (A. 13, 14). Her answers excluded two key symptoms of posttraumatic stress disorder.

This section of the interview contained several double messages: the patient's thin lips (A. 7) indicated either anger at being unfairly accused or, more likely, at being suspected (rightly) of falsifying her account. Her effort to look sad (end of A. 7) would support the latter interpretation. Rhea took a defiant stance against her being distrusted (A. 8). Her smirking (A. 9) might have indicated her satisfaction at being believed or her delight that her deception was successful. The latter interpretation is more likely because she tries to hide her smile by looking away. Her crying and involuntary sad facial expression (A. 9) may show guilt over Brian's possible punishment because she slandered him, or pain about her hurt, which she was expressing verbally. Because she changed her sadness into an expression of anger, it appeared that she intended to hide her sadness by falsification. Rhea's blushing (A. 10) covered by her veiling her face with her hair and biting her lip might indicate either shame of being caught or still liking Brian, which would make the rape charge more questionable. Her grin (A. 11), which she hid again, this time with her hands, strengthened the impression that she experienced deception delight. Her raised eyebrows—signaling surprise— reflected her true affect about flashbacks which she indeed might not have had, thus making questionable the diagnosis of acute posttraumatic stress disorder (A. 14). Rhea's statement about the rape in A. 15 appeared rehearsed (compare A. 7). On balance, Rhea's affective and verbal response pointed more to falsification than trauma.

Step 2: Tag

16. I: Would you mind telling me the whole incident, exactly how it all happened?
    P: [Thin lips] Do I really have to? I've had to tell it so often.
17. I: I really have to understand what happened so I can help you.
    P: [Angry] I've already told it to the police and to my parents and also to the social worker. Why don't you ask them? [Accelerated speech, increasing pitch] There isn't really that much to tell. Brian just grabbed me by the throat and threw me down on the floor. Then he strangled me, pulled my panties down, and forced himself on me.
18. I: Try to tell me everything from the beginning.
    P: Well, after school Brian forced me into his car. Then he took me to his house. When he got me inside he grabbed me by the throat, threw me down on the floor, strangled me, pulled my panties down, and forced himself on me. I already told you what happened after I got home.
19. I: Can you tell me how Brian forced you into his car?
    P: It was right after school. I was just passing by the parking lot and there was Brian in his car. His friend Paul was with him. So there were the two of them. And they got me into the car and then Brian drove over to his house.
20. I: What happened to Paul? Did he go to Brian's house, too?
    P: [Frowns] I don't really remember. He must have dropped him off. I didn't see him anymore.
21. I: How did Brian get you into the house?
    P: Well, he has this garage door opener and he just drove into the garage and closed it.

22. I: Did he rape you then, in the garage?
    P: Oh, no, he made me go upstairs and then he grabbed me by the throat, threw me down, strangled me, pulled my panties down, and forced himself on me.
23. I: So, there was nobody in the house when he grabbed you?
    P: [With increasing pitch in voice] I don't know. I'm really getting tired and I have a headache. All these questions. I want to stop. I'm so sick and tired of it. [Looks angry, then starts crying]
24. I: Did he hurt you?
    P: No, Dad didn't hit me this time. But he questioned and questioned me like he thought I was lying. And that hurt my feelings.
25. I: No, you misunderstand. What I really wanted to know was whether Brian hurt you when he raped you.
    P: Of course he did. [With high pitch] Look what I'm going through. I'm in the hospital, aren't I?
26. I: I understand, Rhea, but did Brian also hurt you physically?
    P: [Angry] I told you he grabbed me. That hurt.
27. I: Can you tell me where you were in the house when he grabbed you?
    P: In his room, he did it in his room. I'm really sick of this. [Looks away from the interviewer]
28. I: You still remember everything that happened at Brian's house, don't you?
    P: How could I? It's been more than a month.
29. I: But you usually have a good memory, don't you?
    P: Not really. I really went through a lot.
30. I: But you would remember things that Brian did to you against your will?
    P: You're just trying to make me say things.
31. I: I only want you to say what really happened.
    P: [Starts crying] Can't we stop this now?
32. I: Just one more thing, Rhea. How did you get home from Brian's house?
    P: Brian's mother offered to drive me but Brian said he'd do it.
33. I: So, Brian's mother was in the house?
    P: Yes, she was.
34. I: When did she come home?
    P: [With an angry voice] I don't know. How should I know? I was in Brian's room. I'm getting all mixed up. It seems like all I've been doing for 5 weeks is answering questions—"What did Brian do?" "How did he do it?" and on and on and on! Stop it!
35. I: I see, Rhea, that it's painful for you to tell me the story again now.
    P: You're damn right.
36. I: I'll let you sleep on it and if you feel like it we'll get back to it another time.
    P: Again?

Preparation of the Cross-Examination

The interviewer has the above interview transcribed. In the margins he marks four of the indicators of falsification: vagueness (A. 19–21, 23, 25, 28,

29, 34), flight into emotion through outbursts (A. 10, 11, 23, 25, 27, 30, 31, 34–36), rehearsed statements (A. 7, 15, 17, 18, 22), and opposition (A. 16, 17, 23, 27, 31, 34). He notes that his tagging of her poor memory with leading questions (Q. 28–31) reinforced her oppositional attitude.

An analysis question by question yielded the following observations. When asked for details leading to the rape, Rhea became irritated (A. 20, 23, 26, 27), frowned (A. 20), and increased the pitch of her voice (A. 23, 25). She misunderstood a question, which showed that she focused more on her punishment by her father than on the alleged rape (A. 24, 25).

Based on these clues, the interviewer decides to use cross-examination. Empathy, support, and understanding could not draw out the truth. By concentrating with closed-ended, tightly jointed questions on her vagueness, inconsistencies, and contradictions, he hopes to persuade Rhea to surrender the facts. However, during the cross-examination proper, rapport remains an important goal. Even though you are engaged in an intense and relentless pursuit of the facts, these facts can be useful in reaching genuine rapport in preparation of therapy.

Step 3: Confront

Two days after the direct examination, the interviewer meets with Rhea for another session.

37. I: I promised you that I would come back and talk to you in more detail about what's happened to you.
    P: [Sarcastically] Great! Thanks.
38. I: Rhea, I know you hate to talk about it and I understand that. As you know, your parents have also asked me to find out whether you are telling the truth. They need to know if they should go ahead and press charges against Brian. Then the court may ask me to testify. You understand, Rhea?
    P: [Dropping the corners of her mouth] I guess.
39. I: Rhea, there's something that's even more important. I have to know the truth if I'm going to help you, you see?
    P: [Frowning, looks down] Whatever. [Wriggles in her seat and looks to the door]
40. I: Well, let me explain. Let's say the real problem isn't that Brian raped you but that you are scared of your dad . . . so that you don't dare tell him what really happened. That would change my job as your doctor, you see? Then we should talk about your relationship with your dad, right?
    P: [Blushing, rapidly blinks eyes, looks away] But I've told you the truth. [Shrugs her shoulders, wriggles them, looks at the door, whips her crossed-over leg]

41. I: Okay. Let's talk about something else. Maybe what's really going on is that you're mad at Brian and want to get back at him and that's why you say he has raped you. Then we have a different problem. We'd have to talk about your anger. Right?

    P: [Blushing more, then eyes form a slit] Brian really raped me. He did it, he did it. [Slaps twice with her hand on her knee]

42. I: All right, then we should talk about how to overcome that painful experience so you can learn to trust other boys without thinking they all are rapists. You see, Rhea, if I'm going to do my job well, I have to find out all the things that happened so that I can do the right thing for you. Do you understand?

    P: [Grimacing] I guess.

When asked about her trauma, Rhea's response was adversarial and hostile (A. 37, 38). Her goal-directed movements indicated a wish to leave (A. 39). When the interviewer suggested that she might be slandering Brian out of fear of punishment by her father, she showed anxiety of being caught and displayed guilt. Her movements indicated a wish to escape (A. 40). Guilt followed by reluctance surfaced again (A. 41, 42). Her responses displayed a double message of guilt followed by a denial.

Step 4: Solve

43. I: There is a good way to find out what happened. I will make it real easy for you. All you have to do is answer my questions with a yes or a no. Okay? I don't want you to say anything other than yes or no.

    P: Okay.

44. I: If I ask you a question that you honestly can't answer with yes or no, then just tell me so. Say, "Dr. O., I can't answer that question with yes or no." Then I will come up with another question that you can answer with yes or no. Do you understand?

    P: Yes.

45. I: Will you try it?

    P: Okay.

46. I: From now on just say yes or no. Let's try it again. Can you go along with this rule?

    P: Yes, I guess.

47. I: Careful—yes or no only.

    P: [Indignant, with a stubborn expression on her face] Yes.

48. I: Now you've got it. Okay, here we go. Rhea, you said Brian raped you on November 27, isn't that true?

    P: Yes.

49. I: That was the first time he'd ever done anything like that to you, right?

    P: Yes.

50. I: It happened after school, right?

P: Yes.

51. I: Brian drove his car to school that day?

P: Yes.

52. I: You saw his car?

P: Yes.

53. I: When you saw him after school, he was already in that car?

P: Yes.

54. I: So you must have walked across the school's parking lot so that you could see him in his car.

P: Yes.

55. I: Is that the shortest way for you to go home, to walk across the parking lot?

P: [Blushing; no answer; looks down, massages her earlobe]

56. I: Rhea, please answer.

P: [Startling] No, not really. The lot's on the other side of the school.

57. I: Just answer yes or no.

P: [Huffy] Sorry. No.

58. I: Just yes or no, Rhea.

P: [Seething] No.

59. I: So, Brian must have told you to come to the parking lot.

P: Yes, he told me at lunch that he had his dad's Thunderbird and that he wanted to drive me home.

60. I: That's fine, Rhea. But I still just want you to answer yes or no.

P: [Flinching] I've forgotten the question.

61. I: I asked you whether Brian had told you to come to the parking lot after school.

P: [Loud, with increasing pitch] Yes.

62. I: And you did what he told you. You went to the parking lot.

P: Yes, I was curious. I wanted to know if he really got to drive the Thunderbird.

63. I: Yes or no, please. You did what Brian asked you to—you went to the parking lot after school?

P: Yes.

64. I: So Brian didn't force you to come to the parking lot.

P: No. [Yawns]

65. I: You came on your own?

P: Yes.

66. I: Now, you said when you saw Brian's car he was already in it. Isn't that right?

P: [Fast and short] Yes.

67. I: Was it a four-door car?

P: [Frowns] No.

68. I: Was it a two-door car?

P: Yes. [Shakes head and grins]

69. I: When he saw you, did he get out of the car?

P: No.

70. I: So you had to walk up to the car?

P: Yes.

71. I: Did he ask you to get into the car?

P: No.

72. I: But at some point you got into his car, correct?
    P: Yes.

73. I: So he must have told you to get into the car.
    P: No.

74. I: So you got into his car without being asked?
    P: I can't answer that with yes or no.

75. I: Fair enough. Did somebody else ask you to get into the car?
    P: [Mechanically] Yes.

76. I: Did Brian have a friend in his car?
    P: [Blandly] Yes.

77. I: Did this friend ask you to get into the car?
    P: Yes, yes, yes.

78. I: Was there anybody else besides that one friend in Brian's car?
    P: No. [Frowns and shakes head]

79. I: Did the friend get out of the car when he asked you to get in?
    P: No.

80. I: Did this person grab you and pull you into the car?
    P: No.

81. I: Did he just ask you to come into the car without grabbing you?
    P: Yes.

82. I: Did you know that friend of Brian's by name?
    P: Yes, it's Paul.

83. I: You're doing well, Rhea, but just answer yes or no.
    P: Okay, but what was the question again?

84. I: Did you know Brian's friend by name?
    P: [Fast] Yes.

85. I: So, neither Brian nor his friend got out of the car, isn't that right?
    P: [Fast] Yes.

86. I: And neither of them pulled you into the car, is that right?
    P: [Fast] Yes.

87. I: And Brian's friend was the only one who asked you to get into the car, isn't that right?
    P: [Fast] Yes.

88. I: So neither Brian nor his friend used force to pull or push you into the car, isn't that right?
    P: I can't answer that yes or no.

89. I: I'll try it again: Did Brian or his friend pull or push you into the car?
    P: No.

90. I: Did you get into the car on your own?
    P: Well, not really. Paul opened the door for me.

91. I: Remember, just yes or no. Did you get into the car on your own?
    P: I don't know how to answer that.

92. I: So Paul opened the door and asked you to get into the car, isn't that right?
    P: Yes.

93. I: And you did what he said, isn't that right?
    P: Yes.

94. I: So you were not really forced to get into the car as you told me 2 days ago?
   P: [Lips narrow] I don't know how to answer that. [Shrugs her shoulders then stiffens her body]

95. I: Let's try it this way: neither Brian nor Paul used force to get you into the car, isn't that right?
   P: I felt like I was forced. [Looks the interviewer straight in the eye; her left hand drops in her lap and she shows the finger (indicating an expletive)]

96. I: Rhea, yes or no? Did Brian or Paul use any kind of physical force to pull or push you into the car?
   P: [Sighing] I guess not, no.

97. I: Only yes or no.
   P: [Looking down at her lap, blushing] No.

98. I: So, Rhea, you lied to me when you said Brian forced you into the car. There was no force. You went to the car because Brian asked you to, and you entered the car because his friend asked you to. You did all that of your own free will. Isn't that right, Rhea, yes or no?
   P: [Falling into a tirade] Yes, yes, yes! I've had enough of this. You treat me like my father, you treat me like a liar. [Starts to cry] I can't answer everything yes or no. There is more to it than that. I felt I didn't have any choice because Paul told me I had to go with Brian if I wanted to stay friends with him.

99. I: Friends?
   P: [Sobs]

100. I: You see, Rhea, your parents want to press charges against Brian. And when they do, Brian's lawyer will put you on the stand and ask you questions just the way I am. But that lawyer will ask a lot more questions than me. And he's not on your side. His job is to show that you are lying. He may accuse you and shout at you. But I'm on your side. And I don't want that to happen to you.

   Okay, let's take a deep breath and try to find out now what really happened so that you don't get all shaken up when you are in court. You see now that you'll have to change at least one thing in your story. You can't keep saying that Brian forced you into the car. You felt like you had to get in or risk his friendship, but that's not the same thing as being forced. So when you are in court you need to tell the truth, because Brian has a witness who can testify under oath that he did not force you to get in. Do you understand?
   P: Yes.

101. I: Now let's go on.
   P: Do we have to?

102. I: Yes. But I'll give you a break from the yes-or-no answers—answer any way you like for a while. Was Paul still there when you went into Brian's house?
   P: [Looking down, with a bland voice] Yes.

103. I: Did Paul go with you into Brian's house?
   P: [Bland voice] No.

104. I: Did Paul leave?
   P: [Bland voice] Yes.

105. I: Did Paul or Brian grab you or push you to go into Brian's house?
     P: [Bland voice] No.
106. I: Did Brian just ask you to come with him into his house?
     P: [Bland voice] No.
107. I: But you went into Brian's house?
     P: [Bland voice] Yes.
108. I: Did Brian ask you?
     P: [Bland voice] No.
109. I: I don't understand. Somebody must have asked you to go into Brian's house.
     P: No, that's not how it was. See, I didn't understand the math homework and I asked Brian if I could come in so he could show me how to do it. But he said he wouldn't—the creep. He knew I was flunking math. And I got desperate and started crying.
110. I: So you were really desperate?
     P: [With falling pitch] Yes.
111. I: So what did Brian say?
     P: He said he wasn't supposed to have girls in his room. He said he would get into trouble.
112. I: What did you say?
     P: I told him not to be such a worrywart. Nobody would find out and he should help me.
113. I: So what did he do?
     P: He didn't do anything. He said his father was in his office downstairs and if he came up and found me, all hell would break loose. But I said, "Your father knows who I am. He wouldn't mind if you were just helping me with my homework."
114. I: So Brian really didn't want to help you.
     P: Brian just does what Brian wants to do.
115. I: So what happened then?
     P: Brian said he'd go in first, and if nobody was around he'd sneak me in. I didn't really like it—that he had to sneak me in.
116. I: And then what?
     P: He told me to hide in the car and then he went in the house to check whether his father was there.
117. I: And then?
     P: Then he yelled, "It's okay. Come in."
118. I: What happened next?
     P: I got out of the car and went into the house. He said his father wasn't home, that he must have gone out to see a client, and his mother wouldn't be back before 5:30 P.M. or 6:00 P.M. And I said, "So, then we're okay," and I started to unpack my homework. And then all of a sudden Brian just grabbed me and forced himself on me and started to rape me. That's it. [Stands up and walks to the door]
119. I: Whoa, whoa, slow down. We need to explore this more carefully. Let's go back to the yes-or-no method, all right?
     P: [Turning around] I hate yat [sic].

120. I: I know you do, Rhea. But it's the best way for me to understand your story. So let's start again.
    P: Do we have to?
121. I: Yes.
    P: [Walks back to the seat and sits down]
    I: So . . . you unpacked your homework?
    P: [Impatiently] Yes.
122. I: Did Brian also unpack his homework?
    P: Yes. Yes.
123. I: Did you sit down at a table?
    P: [Nodding] Yes.
124. I: Did Brian sit opposite of you?
    P: [Shaking head] Nope. [Grinning]
125. I: Did he sit diagonally?
    P: No.
126. I: Did he sit beside you?
    P: Hmmm. [Grinning again]
127. I: Did he touch you then?
    P: I don't know how to answer that.
128. I: Did you feel any part of him touching you?
    P: Yes.
129. I: Was it his hand?
    P: No.
130. I: His elbow?
    P: No.
131. I: His leg?
    P: Yes. [Sitting up straight] My knee accidentally leaned against his leg.
132. I: Did you move your leg away?
    P: [Upset; raising her voice] I don't know. [Standing up] Can't we just stop this stupid thing. We were just doing our homework! [Mumbling what sounded like "shit"]
133. I: Try to be calm. Did Brian also touch you with his hand?
    P: No. He touched me first on my arm and then he started to kiss me.
134. I: Did you kiss him back?
    P: Yes. [Looking down and grinning]
135. I: Had you ever kissed before?
    P: Yes.
136. I: So kissing was nothing new.
    P: No. We'd been going steady. [Running her fingers through her hair]
137. I: So Brian is really your boyfriend.
    P: [Grins, looks down, pulls down her shirt] Yes, until he raped me; I broke up with him after that. [Looks at interviewer from the corner of her eyes]
138. I: Let's go back for a moment. Did you stop doing your homework after you kissed?
    P: [Grin] No. [Crossing over her legs and pressing them together]
139. I: You kissed for a while and then worked and then started kissing again?
    P: Yes.

140. I: Did he touch you on your breast?
    P: No.
141. I: What happened?
    P: We were trying to read the same book and then he said we should lie down on his bed because it would be easier to look at the book.
142. I: When you were on the bed, did you kiss again?
    P: He kissed me.
143. I: Did you kiss back?
    P: [Blushing, left hand massaging left shoulder] I don't remember.
144. I: Did you do homework again after he kissed you that time?
    P: No, everything went so fast. He just grabbed and pulled down my panties. Then he raped me.
145. I: Did you try to stop him?
    P: [Swallows] Of . . . of course, yeah.
146. I: He did it anyway?
    P: [Nodding] Yes.
147. I: Did you push his hands away?
    P: He's so strong. [Shrugging]
148. I: Did you scream?
    P: No, I . . . I was afraid . . . afraid his parents may be back and walk . . . walk in on us. He and I, we would get into big trouble.
149. I: You let him rape you so that he wouldn't get into trouble?
    P: It wasn't, wasn't like that! I, I was biting his sh . . . shoulder because he was hurting me.
150. I: You bit him?
    P: But then it didn't hurt anymore. I was trying to press my legs together.
151. I: You pressed your legs together.
    P: [Looks away from the interviewer] I thought this would force him out of me, but he didn't stop. [Grins and then shrugs shoulders, then eyebrows]
152. I: So? . . .
    P: And then I . . . I had . . . I don't want to talk about it any more. I hated myself because he raped me. Okay?
153. I: He raped you.
    P: I'm sick and tired of talking about this. I hate you . . . that you make me talk about it.
154. I: Do you think Brian really raped you?
    P: [Screaming] What? Are you deaf? He started it. He wanted it. It's his fault.
155. I: Okay, let's go back because I still don't understand your story. Let's say we're in court and you can only answer yes and no, and I ask you, "Did you say no when Brian was pulling down your panties? Did you tell him no?"
    P: I don't know how to answer that.
156. I: Did you tell him, "I don't want you to pull my panties down."?
    P: [Shrugs shoulders] I was trying to get away.
157. I: But did you tell him not to?
    P: I don't remember. It all went so fast. Lisa had told me sex is fun, it feels good. [Grins] But he was hurting me. [Painful expression in face] So I pressed my legs together.

158. I: If you are the judge, Rhea, would you call that rape?
  P: [With a low voice, leaning forward] I don't want you to tell my parents.
159. I: Do you want your parents to take Brian to court?
  P: [Shrugs with her left shoulder] I can't stop them.
160. I: Do you want me to talk to them?
  P: I don't want them to be mad at me.
161. I: Your sister said that you went to see Brian after the rape. What did you talk about?
  P: Things in general.
162. I: Did you talk about the rape?
  P: I told him that I was sorry I'd said what I said. But I was afraid of my parents, I'm scared of what they'd do to me if they knew we'd made love together. He told me, "It's okay, don't worry."

Rhea's main claim was that Brian had raped her in his house. Part of this claim was that she was, first, incidentally walking by his car; second, forced into the car; and, third, forced into his house. With tightly stacked, closed-ended questions, the interviewer secured the details about the way Rhea had met Brian after school. These details contradicted her vague, previously implied assertion that she had accidentally met him after school. These details disproved that Rhea had just accidentally walked by Brian's car (Q. 51–65), was forced into his car (Q. 66–100), and then forced into his house (Q. 101–118). The interviewer also established that Rhea resisted Brian's advances only minimally or not at all (Q. 118–157).

These confrontations led to Rhea's anxiety about being caught (A. 55, 56); to suppressed hostility against the interviewer (A. 57, 58, 60, 61), which she deflected into an expression of boredom and hostility by a monotone, mechanical tone of voice (A. 75, 76); and to rapid answers (A. 84–87), indicating that she wanted to escape this line of questioning. When the details again revealed her falsification, her displaced hostility emerged in a symbolic (expletive) gesture (A. 95). Finally, she admitted to the lie about being forced into the car, underscoring her confession by sighing and blushing (A. 96, 97). When the interviewer confronted her by summarizing her lie (Q. 98), she fell into an angry tirade (A. 98) but deflected it into a nonverbal plea for pity and mercy (A. 99). The interviewer rewarded her by explaining why his cross-examination would help her in the future (Q. 100). Also, he released her temporarily from the yes-or-no format (Q. 102) in the hope that she might be forthcoming with the truth.

When the interviewer scrutinized Rhea's statement that she was forced into Brian's house (Q. 103–118), she responded first with suppressed (A. 102–108) and then with sad affect (A. 108–110) and finally admitted to her active role in entering the house (A. 111–118).

Then she fell back into falsifying by repeating her rehearsed statement about the rape (A. 118). When Rhea abandoned her detailed account of her meeting with Brian and tried to take a shortcut to her rehearsed rape statement, the interviewer redirected her to the yes-or-no format (Q. 118–119). This format would allow him to collect as many details as he needed. Rhea responded with anger and a slip of tongue (A. 119)—a fusion of "hate you" and "hate that."

However, she complied and appeared to be truthful from A. 121 to A. 131 and even enjoyed recalling the amorous situation (A. 124, 126). Then she suppressed her enjoyment (A. 131) and launched into a tirade (A. 132), during which she expressed her annoyance at being found out. She sent a double message that contradicted her statement and watched the interviewer to see whether he would buy into her story (A. 137).

When there were too many possibilities for how the sexual encounter had developed, the interviewer broke with the yes-or-no format in favor of an open-ended style, which indeed produced a telling detail (Q. and A. 141). But then Rhea resisted further detailing by claiming amnesia and returning to her rehearsed statement (A. 143, 144). Her nonverbal behavior (e.g., blushing, massaging her shoulder) appeared to contradict her claim. Because Rhea had shown enabling cooperation with Brian, the interviewer accepted her rape statement but focused on her resistance. Her claim of resisting Brian was weak and was contradicted by nonverbal messages (A. 145, 147, 151). When she realized that she had contradicted her rape claim, she directed her anger against the interviewer (A. 153, 154), but without claiming resistance against Brian's advances (A. 155–157). Furthermore, her resistance was more directed against the pain of first penetration than against the intercourse itself (A. 149, 157). These statements prepared the interviewer to ask Rhea whether she as judge would call her sexual involvement with Brian "rape." Rhea evaded the answer but expressed her anxiety of punishment by her father if the interviewer did not call it rape (A. 158–160).

Step 5: Approve

163. I: It seems to me you really like Brian.
     P: I loved him and I wanted to marry him, but my parents would never let me. Especially now.
164. I: Rhea, I'm glad that you told Brian that you were sorry that you accused him of having raped you.
     P: Yeah, I guess I was pretty angry that he got me into that mess. And he got away with it.

165. I: Hmmm.
     P: Hmmm what?
166. I: I'm confused.
     P: [Sarcastically] You are?
167. I: If we really take a good hard look at what happened, Rhea, how much would you say he was responsible for what happened—and how much of it was your doing?
     P: [Neck stiffens; looks at interviewer with hostility]
168. I: Rhea, don't answer! I don't want to accuse you. But it may help you to look into your heart and find out for yourself.
     P: [Relaxes]
169. I: I notice that Brian didn't seem to be angry that you accused him. He said he understood. He sounds like a real friend.
     P: [Biting her lower lip, silent]
170. I: Does Brian think he raped you?
     P: He loves me and I love him.
171. I: What are you really saying?
     P: I wanted him to make love to me.
172. I: Hmmm.
     P: I teased him.
173. I: What do you mean?
     P: When Brian told me that he loved me, I said, "How are you gonna prove it?" I took his hand and put it on my breast. He got all red and took his hand away. Then I said, "I knew it—all talk," and I pulled my shirt up.
174. I: You did?
     P: I told you I teased him.
175. I: [Nods]
     P: I was just angry the way it turned out. I'm scared of my father.
176. I: Do you think your father will understand if you tell him that things happened this way because you love Brian?
     P: I don't know. At first Dad was so pissed at Brian I thought he was going to kill him. But it was strange. Dad dragged me over to Brian's house to tell him we were pressing charges. And Brian did something I thought was kind of cool. Instead of denying everything, he admitted we'd had sex. Brian told Dad, "I love her. I didn't think I raped her. I would never do that to anybody. But if Rhea says it was rape, then I guess that's what it seemed like to her, and I'm really sorry." Dad was impressed by what Brian said. And I feel it made him think that I was lying.
177. I: Hmmm. Do you think you can tell your Dad how you feel about Brian? Will that help?
     P: [Shows painful expression in her face]
178. I: Maybe in your family session we can talk about it.
     P: Are you mad with me now?
179. I: Why would I be mad at you?
     P: Because I lied, and then I lied about lying.
180. I: You lied to me because you thought I'd be like your father.
     P: Yeah.

181. I: Well, Rhea, I'm glad that you helped me to get the story straight.
     P: Me too.
182. I: And I think we can work it out with your parents too.

In Step 5, the interviewer rewarded Rhea's truthfulness by focusing on her love for Brian. He then persuaded her to give a more accurate account of her participation in the sexual encounter. Her elaborations (A. 173) convinced him not just that she was pressured into tolerating the sexual act but that she had actively provoked Brian. This admission left the interviewer with the task of reducing Rhea's fear of her father, a fear that had led to her lying (A. 177–181).

If Rhea had stuck to her lie, she would probably have experienced guilt. She would also have lost a friend, one she cared about. The conflict with her parents would still have existed because Rhea would have missed the chance to defend her own needs against her parents' wishes. Her parents would have sued a boy who was innocent of rape but who, for whatever reasons, felt compelled to accept his guilt. And Rhea would have learned the wrong lesson: lies work. By helping Rhea to tell the truth, the interviewer averted these damaging outcomes.

Crucial to your success in interviewing a falsifying patient is your ability to show empathy for the patient's point of view. Demonstrating your understanding of the patient's need to lie is often all it takes to encourage the patient to admit the truth and free herself from the emotional burden of lying.

Remain sensitive to the immediate pain that a cross-examination may cause the patient. Also, become aware of your own punitive or even sadistic feelings that you may harbor against a patient whom you suspect of lying. Explore the reason for such negative countertransference. For the patient's sake, either resolve your feelings or consider referring the patient.

What if cross-examination fails? In the above example we viewed falsification as intentional and as possibly harmful for others involved. An alternative approach is to resolve the falsification by telling the patient that she is not being forthcoming and that for this very reason you cannot continue to work with her. This approach is effective in a patient who depends on a statement or some other type of support from you.

A second alternative is to wait it out. In the meantime work with other aspects of the patient's disorder until she is ready to level with you, but tell her that passage of time is working against her.

If the patient repeatedly falsifies as part of her personality disorder, consider analysis of her transference pattern toward you. Furthermore, you may choose a cognitive approach and ask her to reveal her self-talk as described in Chapter 15, "Self-Deceptive Behavior." This cognitive approach could lead toward the plus-minus approach featured in Chapter 12, "Concealing." Finally, consider polygraphic or voice-stress analysis as described in Chapter 14, "Factitious Behavior."

Diagnosis

The patient's symptoms do not fulfill criteria for posttraumatic stress disorder because she neither has the symptoms or signs of the disorder nor did she experience the alleged trauma. The patient has an acute adjustment reaction with mixed disturbance of emotions and conduct—not due to the alleged rape but rather due to her parents finding out about sexual activities they do not approve of and her fear of punishment by them. Thus, the patient's mood is depressed and anxious, and she lies.

A second diagnosis of conduct disorder is suspected from the history. However, to establish this diagnosis was not the focus of the interview.

6. Falsification and Cross-Examination in Psychiatric Disorders

Like concealing, falsification is ubiquitous—it can occur in all Axis I disorders. It is common in substance-related disorders when the patient downplays the amount of substance abused and its negative effects. It occurs in major depression when the patient lies about his suicidal plan to avoid psychiatric commitment, to avoid close observation on the inpatient ward, or to avoid restriction of a therapeutic pass, or lies to preclude interference with his suicide. The patient with grandiose delusions may lie about his suicidal tendencies because he wants to defeat the doctor or because he feels he will magically survive death. Patients with eating disorders lie about starving, vomiting, and self-torture. Patients with anxiety disorders lie about their embarrassing obsessions, compulsions, or phobias. Patients with impulse-control disorders lie about their physical violence, their gambling, or the physical abuse of a spouse, a child, or an elderly person. To remain an acceptable member of society, perpetrators may lie about sexual abuse of minor dependents or about incestuous or repulsive sexual practices.

Falsification is common in patients with a cluster B personality disorder. In antisocial personality disorder, a patient lies to cover up infractions (criterion A2). The possible antecedents of antisocial personality disorder in childhood and adolescence also include blaming (oppositional defiant disorder [criterion A5]) and lying (conduct disorder [criterion A11]) as criteria. In borderline personality disorder, a patient, fearing abandonment (criterion 1), uses lies to increase her acceptability. She lies to validate her idealization or devaluation of others (criterion 2). Her impulsivity lets her engage in self-damaging acts (criterion 4), which she covers up with lying. Also, she uses lies to get revenge for her intense anger (criterion 8). In histrionic personality disorder, the patient lies to become the center of attention (criterion 1) and she exaggerates her emotions (criterion 6) and her intimate involvement with others (criterion 8). In narcissistic personality disorder, a patient lies to enhance her self-importance (criterion 1) and exaggerates her success, power, and brilliance (criteria 2 and 3). She is uninhibited and lacks empathy (criterion 7) in exploiting others by using lies to reach her goals (criterion 6).

In the narrowest sense, the method of cross-examination targets lying. However, you can use this technique also outside of lying. Patients who are under the influence of a strong emotion are often unable to organize their thoughts. For example, patients who have just escaped a trauma, who experience severe anxiety, or who are vague, dramatic, or suspicious may be able to give you a clearer account if you help them with focused yes-or-no questions. In such cases, you do not search for inconsistencies but you assist the patient to organize his emotionally charged experiences. Rather than letting him struggle in an open-ended, unstructured interview, you provide the patient with a railing that guides him along a path toward clarity and resolution.

FACTITIOUS BEHAVIOR

Summary

A patient with factitious behavior or fabrication attempts to create (preferably) physical evidence that she herself or a family member has a severe disorder or has been a victim of a traumatic event. In a discussion about that evidence, the interviewer may use repeated voice-stress or polygraphic analysis to detect the physiological evidence of stress signals in the patient's answers as indicators of fabrication. The interviewer can then confront the patient with this evidence and convince her to give up fabrication in exchange for help in reducing pending legal and social consequences.

385

◆ ◆ ◆ ◆

A un dottor della mia sorte queste scuse, signorina!
Vi consiglio, mia carina, un po'meglio a imposturar,
meglio, meglio, meglio, meglio . . .
Ferma la, non mi toccate, ferma la no mi toccate!
No, figlia mia, non lo sperate ch'io mi lasci infinocchiar.
To a doc of my accumen do you offer lies and ruses?
I advise you in the future to tell better lies by far . . .
Do you hear? You can't deceive me . . .
Yes, my lady, you are clever, but I'm smarter than you are.

Dr. Bartolo's Aria, *The Barber of Seville* (1775)
Libretto by Cesare Sterbini

◆ ◆ ◆ ◆

1. What Is Factitious Behavior?

Factitious behavior represents a special form of deceit. In DSM-IV (American Psychiatric Association 1994, p. 474), the following diagnostic criteria are listed for factitious disorder:

1. Intentional production or feigning of physical or psychological signs or symptoms.
2. The motivation for the behavior is to assume the sick role.
3. External incentives for the behavior (such as economic gain, avoiding legal responsibility, or improving physical well-being, as in Malingering) are absent.

The patient actively produces physical evidence of an illness. A patient who fabricates signs and symptoms of a psychiatric or physical disorder in himself has factitious disorder, also called *Munchausen syndrome;* if he manufactures the symptomatology in another person, it is called "factitious disorder by proxy" (in DSM-IV specified as factitious disorder not otherwise specified). Between 10% and 25% of mothers who have factitious disorder by proxy also have actual factitious disorder themselves (Rosenberg 1987).

The syndrome gets its name from Baron Münchausen, originally Karl Friedrich Hieronymus, Freiherr von Münchausen of Germany (1720–1797). The baron traveled the world as a hunter, sportsman, and soldier fighting Russians and Turks. On his return, he became famous for telling fantastic stories about his adventures. In 1951, Asher attached Munchausen's name to factitious disorder; in 1977, Meadow coined the term *Munchausen syndrome by proxy* to describe those individuals who induced illness in another person (Forsyth 1991).

The fabrications of such patients differ from malingering in one essential aspect: fabricating patients receive no apparent reward for their stories, whereas malingering patients expect a specific benefit. The fabricating patient frequently challenges a professional. For example, she may present a bloody urine specimen to a physician, bloodied from a finger prick. She may call the police to her house, who will find her gagged and tied yet somehow able to call the police. The patient prefers to fabricate objective physical signs over reporting subjective psychological symptoms. The signs are her physical evidence. She only has to conceal their authorship.

The pathological fabricator of the Munchausen type knows the advantages of truthfulness, yet clinical experience shows that these patients continuously relapse into fabrications and lies. They do not show guilt, shame, or regret about their fabrication. To the contrary, they are angered when suspected. When caught, and even when convicted, they still try to salvage parts of their fabrication. Thus, in their double role they black out the fabricator in favor of the victim. This explains their flat affect as they seemingly ask the interviewer,

> Don't you see what I went through? How can you be so insensitive and focus on who did it when it is clear how much I'm suffering [even though through patient's own doing]?

If such a patient is not found out, she neither experiences guilt nor anxiety over her doings, but feels compelled to escalate her fabrications. Thus, if you do not recognize and diagnose the fabrication early, you become a victim too, as you become tangled up in the patient's web of lies and inadvertently enable the patient to victimize others. (The risk is real.

Later in this chapter we meet a patient whose pathology resulted in a health risk for her young child.)

Such patients do not level with the interviewer unless they are caught in the act. The patient-interviewer roles remain adversarial throughout all phases of the interview. These patients do ask for your help but only for their invented physical disorder, not for the fabricating factitious disorder that they truly have. Typically, for example, such a patient will fail to inform you that for years she has been in regularly scheduled psychotherapy with other caregivers. She may check herself (often on Friday evenings) into a hospital in a neighboring town complaining of factitious medical or psychological symptoms while under psychotherapy with you. She will suck you into her pathology, using you also to escape legal prosecution and punishment.

Why do patients fabricate illness in themselves or others? What kind of suffering is so powerful that it makes fabrication an attractive alternative? Some possibilities include

- Childhood neglect
- Desire for attention
- Hurting for love (Schreier and Libow 1993)
- Sociopathic plotting
- Obsession to fake symptoms and signs
- Self-punishment to overcome depression

The list of theories about the condition is long; the list of facts is short. It remains true that for a patient with a factitious disorder, deception is an irresistible urge that appears to be beyond "free will."

In factitious disorder, fabrication is defined as a symptom, not as a moral failing. Such a definition regards behaviors that are harmful to others and maladaptive to the patient as targets for treatment rather than punishment. Such a shift in perspective opens the door for healing.

2. Factitious Behavior in the Mental Status

A New York City lawyer calls the interviewer at a university center and asks for help. His client, Ms. W., has a history of factitious disorder by proxy. She is in danger of losing custody of her three children: Malcolm, age 5 years; David, age 3 years; and Cory, age 9 months. Ms. W. is currently in her fourth month of pregnancy.

Apparently, Ms. W. has given Malcolm laxatives and syrup of ipecac, which have induced vomiting and bloody diarrhea severe enough to require hospitalization. Criminal charges have been pressed and she has received media attention. The interviewer studies her records and makes an appointment.

Ms. W., is a 27-year-old, African-American, 5'7", sturdy-looking, soft-spoken woman who works in the computer industry. When seen for the interview, her outfit is clean, plain, understated, and bland. She wears horn-rimmed glasses and no makeup. She appears relaxed and maintains eye contact for most of the intake interview. Results on the Kent Test (Kent 1946) show she is of average intelligence. In her statements she appears matter-of-fact, without any dramatic exaggeration or embellishments. Her affect is flat. She delivers her story in an organized way, except when she practices deception. Then she becomes vague but does not show any change in her affect. She describes her mood as tending to be depressed. She denies hallucinations and delusions.

Ms. W. admits to staging events and expresses some puzzlement about why she does it, but does not think it's a problem. She admits that it is difficult for her to stop once she starts. She is an old hand at faking drama. Two years earlier, she told police she had received hate mail; had been the target of a satanic cult and received harassing phone calls; had found her own undergarments cut up outside her house; and had discovered a blood-smeared doll pierced by needles, voodoo style, hanging on her back door. To find the culprit, local police set up 24-hour stakeouts and telephone surveillance, at a cost to taxpayers of over $45,000.[1] Ultimately a hidden camera proved that Ms. W. had orchestrated it all herself.

At that time, the court ordered weekly psychotherapy. The therapist used an empathic approach in the belief that the patient's deception and lying was a protest against neglectful parents and spouse. This dynamic approach, however, was ineffective at preventing relapse. Now, Ms. W.'s son, Malcolm, is the victim. Ms. W. displays one of the typical features of Munchausen syndrome: resistance to therapy.

Ms. W. was interviewed after being caught once by the police and once by the physicians, and after having been convicted by the legal system.

Double Message in Affect

In cases of factitious disorder and factitious disorder by proxy, the physical evidence that the patient fabricates is real. You will, therefore, not observe a double message in affect when the patient describes the physical evidence. However, you can provoke a double message when you question the authorship of the evidence: "Is this the sign of a true illness?" or "This

---

[1] See also Powell and Boast 1993, who illustrated in a dramatic case history the costs to society incurred by a patient with confirmed factitious disorder.

sign does not make any medical sense. Did you create it?"

At this moment, anger of being caught may flash across the face, or, if the sense of jeopardy is high, the patient may show a mixture of anger and anxiety. The patient's affect is displayed in autonomic signs, reactive movements, facial expressions, grooming, and tone of voice.

Autonomic signs

Autonomic signs—such as flushing, blanching, sweating, and fast breathing—are absent when Ms. W. reports her history and recapitulates her fabrications. Her breathing is regular while talking or listening. It becomes slightly faster and less deep only when she is asked directly, "Did you create this?"

Only twice, when such a question addresses a suspected fabrication, which is later confirmed, does her face blanch. She does not blush at all. Retrospectively, it appears that the blanching indicates anger over being suspected or possibly caught.

Reactive movements

Ms. W.'s reactive movements are dampened when she appears for a follow-up visit and expects to be subjected to a voice-stress interview. When the interviewer calls her from the waiting area, she reacts to her name with increased latency of response and only with a slight turning of the head.

Facial expressions

Ms. W.'s facial expressions are also diminished. She presents a calm and cool exterior as long as she is not directly confronted with the critical question "Did you fabricate this?" Whenever she is asked such a question, she flashes on anger.

Grooming behavior

Grooming movements are absent in Ms. W., whether she talks about the signs and symptoms of the fabricated disorder, her marriage, or her social history or answers critical questions of authorship.

Voice

Ms. W.'s tone of voice is even in pitch, timbre, rhythm, and intensity. All qualities of her voice appear to be dampened and slowed down. Her voice becomes higher in pitch and slightly louder only when she attempts to save some elements of her fabrication as mentioned below under "Gestures."

Double Message in Psychomotor Movements and Speech

Ms. W. suppresses the fact that she is the fabricator of the disorder. She pretends that the signs indicate the presence of a natural psychiatric or medical disorder. Usually, she avoids the topic of origin. So she does not ask the question, "Doctor, what kind of illness do I have?" Instead, she focuses on delivering the signs or making sure the authority finds the physical evidence. She displays a double message only when she is suspected of authoring the signs.

Gestures

Usually Ms. W. uses only a few illustrative gestures. They seem to appear at a critical point in the interview—namely, when she is trying to convince the interviewer that certain signs of an illness are natural and not created by her. For example, she was convicted by the physicians of inducing diarrhea in one of her children while the child was hospitalized. When reviewing this incidence, Ms. W. insists that the first bout of her child's diarrhea was natural. The doctors had not caught her on that. She used slapping hand movements on the desk to emphasize this point. However, the stress in her voice was high, and she retracted her statement later when confronted with this high-stress response. Thus it appears that the patient may use illustrative movements when attacked and when she tries to save part of her fabrication.

Symbolic movements

Ms. W. does not make any symbolic hand, facial, or body movements in response to questions about her social history, college years, or marriage. No peripherally or incompletely displayed symbols are observed in her other than a one-sided shoulder shrug in lieu of saying "I don't know." Such a nonverbal response occurred within the context of a topic about which she was practicing deceit; by shrugging her shoulder instead of responding, she avoided revealing any stress in her voice-stress pattern.

Goal-directed movements

Ms. W.'s goal-directed movements are rare. Usually, she sits with both feet firm on the floor, and does not cross her legs or whip her foot. She does throw a quick glance at the door when she believes she is not being observed when questioned about her authorship of certain signs such as "Is this the truth?" or "Are you lying?" or "Did you fabricate this?"

Speech

Ms. W.'s speech is controlled and her words are well chosen: she searches for the correct word and corrects herself if she finds a better word. She commits herself to a version of an event and defends it even in the light of contradictory evidence. If accused of authorship, the latency of her responses increases. She may shrug her shoulders and say, "I don't know." However, her preferred response is to point toward evidence that she could not have authored. For example, Ms. W.'s high school peers had once reported mutilation of a black doll. Ms. W. pointed out that when this happened when she was out of town.

Verbal Strategies of Fabrication

Detailed knowledge

Ms. W. does not use rehearsed statements. She does not falsify a story or invent signs because the signs are truly there. She can describe them in detail without any contradictions. She shows unusual knowledge about the names of different medications and their milligram dosages, whereas details about other general subjects appear to be lacking (Schreier and Libow 1993).

Assumption of the victim role

Ms. W. plays a double role of persecutor and victim. She conceals the persecutor role but elaborates on the victim role. When she is confronted about her fabrication, she is vague, imprecise, and short on detail as her methods of fabrication are discussed. However, she elaborates and becomes emotionally more invested when her victim role is discussed. Even when she is forced to admit that she has fabricated a sign, she shows neither regret nor guilt, but still talks about the very sign as if it is a sign of a genuine illness not brought on by herself. She does not own up to her fabrication.

Cooperation with the experts

Ms. W. views her fabrications not as despicable lies that endanger her children and cost the police department and the taxpayer money but as artistic work and creations. Ms. W. assisted the police in helping to point out all the signs of harassment and has assisted the physicians in bringing all her child's symptoms and signs to their attention. Also, she appears to cooperate even in her voice-stress interviews in a calm way. However, she produces no insight into the reasons for her actions. She merely says, "I don't know." She gives the same answer when asked to interpret other factitious disorder by proxy or factitious disorder cases discussed in New York City newspaper clippings.

The only insight she gives is that once she starts, she escalates the production of signs and symptoms and cannot stop, thus giving the disorder the formal characteristics of an addiction to fabricate.

Defeat of the investigation

In the case of her previous fabrication about being stalked, Ms. W. had made sure that the authorities failed to detect the origin of the mail, phone calls, disarray of undergarments, and so on. Also, she was the one who had suggested that her house be surveyed from a parked car across the street. However, at that point the "break-in" occurred from the back, and a decapitated naked doll was found in the back of the house. In the current case, her son continues to have diarrhea even though antibiotics and Kaopectate have been administered.

Mimicking

The patient has a tendency to copy signs of an illness or a crime that come to her attention. For example, Ms. W. got the idea to cause diarrhea in her son after she had observed diarrhea in a neighbor's child and witnessed the worrying and medical attention that resulted.

3. Technique: Voice-Stress Analysis

The goal of your interview is to detect and prove fabrication. In interviewing patients like Ms. W., attention, empathy, and support do not work. In fact, patients exploit an understanding attitude and prey on the interviewer's gullibility. On the other hand, the rules of clinical interviewing require you to interview with empathy and not with disdain. What is needed is a firm grasp of the nature of the patient's pathology and her need to create turmoil by assuming the role of patient or victim. In the following, we describe how to interview such a patient using voice-stress analysis.

When under scrutiny, fabrication causes stress for the patient. Experienced falsifiers suppress leakages of fabrication in their behavior, but they have less control over their autonomic nervous system. Therefore, physiologists have developed methods to measure autonomic responses. For example, the polygraph records subtle changes in breathing, heart rate, body temperature, and sweating that may not be visually evident.

Another measure of stress that accompanies deception is change in voice pattern, which can be detected through voice-stress analysis. This technique detects subsonic frequencies in the muscles of the voice apparatus and prints them out as a chart. One device for measuring these vibrations is the psychological stress evaluator (PSE), which analyzes the human voice from a tape-recorded interview. Unlike the polygraph, the PSE uses no sensors attached to the patient's body. All that is required is a recording of the patient's voice on a good-quality cassette tape. The recording captures not just the words that the speaker generates voluntarily, but the involuntary vibrations of the vocal cords as well. These involuntary vibrations, inaudible to the human ear, indicate stress. A trained interpreter can discriminate between the degrees of stress and interpret their meaning.

Before you start the voice-stress analysis interview, receive the patient's informed consent. The elements of this consent include

- A description of the purpose and procedures of voice-stress analysis, specifying that the technique can detect the patient's deception or lying against his will.
- A statement spelling out the risks, hazards, and consequences of continued lying. For example, the patient with factitious disorder by proxy may be told that she will lose custody of her children if the interview confirms that she is lying about the way she has induced symptoms in her children.
- An explanation of alternatives to voice-stress analysis, such as continued interviewing, amobarbital interviews, polygraph interview, or cross-examination.

A standard clinical interview used to screen for all psychiatric pathology takes a broad, open-minded approach. In contrast, the voice-stress analysis interview uses cross-examination techniques (see Chapter 13, "Falsifying and Lying").

If the patient is truthful, the initial stress response fades away as a similar question is repeated several times. However, if the patient is practicing deception, the stress level will rise and the stress patterns will register.

Find a laboratory in your area that routinely does PSE analysis. Tape your interview using recorders that capture your and the patient's voice. Although no special microphones or leads are needed, the better the quality of the recorder and the tape, the more reliable the results. You then send the tape to the laboratory to be analyzed. An experienced analyst studies the printout and marks the areas that show characteristics of stress, tension, or discomfort.

When you receive the report about the arousal profile, it becomes your task to interpret the results. Rather than following blindly the analysis of the polygrapher or the PSE evaluator, analyze the results within the context of the patient's disorder, personality, and mental status at the time of the interview.

The polygraph method and the voice-stress method are most effective when the person being tested believes the following:

1. That the device is able to detect lies. If the patient does not believe the method is effective, then results will become questionable. Thus, for a polygraph or voice-stress test to succeed, the tester must convince the testee that the technique is valid.
2. That something important or very dear to the falsifier is at stake. If the consequences of detection are severe, the patient is usually much more aroused and shows clearer changes during his responses in the autonomic system and in his voice than if the consequences of being found out do not matter.

To increase the validity of the results, the analyst of polygraphic as well as voice-stress measurements uses control questions (see Chapter 12, "Concealing," or the discussion of the guilty knowledge technique [Lykken 1981] in the next section). Expected stress levels are indicated in Table 14–1.

Table 14–1. Stress levels in a voice-stress analysis interview

Questioned item	Sample question	Stress level
Fact	Have you ever watched a baseball game	+
Embarrassing fact	Have you ever lied to a friend who trusted you?	++
Challenge of embarrassing fact	You lied to a friend, really?	+
Requested lie	What is your name? (as instructed, patient lies about true name)	+++
Challenge of requested lie	This is not your name. Why do you lie to me?	++++
Lie	Have you been raped by your stepbrother?	+++++
Challenged lie	Are you lying now?	++++++

Note. + = no stress; ++ = mild stress; +++ = moderate stress; ++++ = marked stress; +++++ = severe stress; ++++++ = extreme stress.

Specific Methods for the Polygraphic or Voice-Stress Interview

Sequence of questions. During the interview, jump back and forth between factual and embarrassing questions, questions aimed at lies, and requested lies. With a patient who has factitious disorder, you have to direct the voice-stress or polygraphic interview toward questions like

> Did you create this symptom?
> Did you create this sign?

to catch her fabrication. Questions such as

> Did you receive this obscene letter?
> Was there blood in the urine?
> Did you have a high temperature?

fail because the patient made sure that these signs indeed occurred.

Insist on yes-or-no answers. Tell the patient that you will ask the control questions and all questions in such a way that he can answer either with a single fact, such as his birth date, or with a single word, such as yes or no. Whenever he gives you a simple answer, challenge it with such questions as

> Is that true?
> Are you lying?
> You are lying, aren't you?
> Do you know what will happen to you if you are found out to be lying?

Set the stage for lying. Instruct the patient to lie about her first name. (For example, ask Nancy to state that her name is Mona.) Tell the patient the purpose of this strategy is to produce responses to control questions that challenge her known lying.

Conduct an unrecorded trial interview. Proceed along the following lines: (I = interviewer; P = patient)

I: Are you ready for a trial interview?
P: Yes.
I: Have you watched a baseball game?
P: Not for the last 2 years.
I: Please try to answer with yes or no if you can. Do you understand?
P: Yes.

I: Have you watched a baseball game?
P: Yes.
I: Is this true?
P: Yes.
I: What is your name?
P: Mona.
I: Is this really true?
P: Yes.
I: I know you are lying.
P: Of course I'm lying—you told me to.
I: Please, I want you to continue to lie. Let's try again. I know you are lying about your first name. Am I not right?
P: No.
I: Have you ever lied before?
P: Yes.

Investigators have criticized control questions as being deceitful, especially when you use false accusation and false praise, because in both instances you know the truth when the patient does not. Lykken (1981) has proposed the guilty knowledge technique, a method to detect the culprit of an infraction in cases where only the interviewer and the culprit know the details of the act. For example, $20 has been stolen from a locker room. Only you, the interviewer, and of course the thief know the sum. You have three suspects. You ask each of the three whether he would be richer by $5, $10, $15, $20, $30, or $50 if he had taken the money. You expect that only the culprit and not the two innocent suspects will show signs of stress when you mention the $20. In cases where the offense is known but you have to identify the culprit from a number of suspects, you can choose Lykken's guilty knowledge test, also known as the Peak of Tension (POT) test.

Instruments for analyzing deceitfulness.   Clinicians may encounter difficulties in uncovering double messages. There is excellent research that can help clinicians to detect deceit (Ekman 1992). In addition, polygraph technicians and voice-stress analysts can measure and record autonomic and voice signals of secret messages (Hanson 1993; Lykken 1981; Rogers 1988).

In 1983, the U.S. Office of Technology Assessment (OTA) released a report (Ekman 1992), which was developed at the request of the United States Congress, on the scientific evidence of the polygraph as a lie detector. According to the report, the OTA screened over 3,200 articles and books on polygraphs. Only 10% (approximately 320) involved research, and of that 10%, only 30 publications met scientific minimum standards. Field studies that compared polygraphic test results to court verdicts showed that liars were correctly identified in 71%–99% of the cases (with an average close to 85%), whereas truthful persons were correctly identified in 13%–94% of the cases (giving an average hit rate of slightly less than 80%). Analogue studies that tested laboratory lies were reviewed according to whether control questions or the guilty knowledge test was used. The control question technique identified 35%–100% of the liars (with an average of approximately 65%) and 32%–91% of the truthful persons (with an average of less than 60%). Lykken's (1981) guilty knowledge test identified 61%–95% of the liars (averaging slightly less than 80%) and 80%–100% of the innocent persons (averaging better than 95%). Thus, Lykken's test appears to be particularly powerful in identifying the innocent.

Similarly extensive studies are not available about any of the several voice-stress analyzers, namely the PSE, the Mark II Voice Analyzer, the Voice Stress Analyzer, the Psychological Stress Analyzer, the Hagoth, and the Voice Stress Monitor (Ekman 1992). Lykken's analysis seemed to show that analogue studies cannot identify stress. The field studies that showed a better result seem to be flawed according to Lykken (1981). Therefore, if established validity is a requirement for clinical evaluation, you may use the more intrusive polygraph rather than the voice-stress method.

For interviewing in the mental health field we consider lie detection by instruments only for a limited range of applications, namely to provide the patient with feedback about his statements in the hope that the "scientific" nature of the method may persuade the patient to replace his stressful responses by less stressful and more plausible responses—that is, admit the lies, refrain from them, and replace them with the truth.

Use of detection instruments in therapy.   Voice-stress and polygraph analysis may be used for psychiatric disorders other than factitious disorder. Potential candidates are patients who use lies malignantly to blame, use, abuse, or hurt someone else, or those who claim repeated emotional, physical, and sexual abuse without objective evidence to support their claim. In our practice we used this technique in treating a 16-year-old, manic-depressive young man with some features of antisocial personality disorder. He eventually admitted that he had stolen money and objects from his father. Voice-stress interviews involved him more honestly in the therapy process.

In another case we established genuine rapport with a teenager after we scrutinized with voice-stress analysis his denial of having bullied two young girls.

If you choose to incorporate voice-stress analysis into your practice, be clear about its purpose. Voice-stress analysis is only one of the determinants in the diagnostic process. Your goal is not to convict a deceitful person but to identify, understand, and treat the deceit.

4. Five Steps to Unravel Fabrication

Step 1: Listen. Invite the patient to tell her story. Use the techniques discussed in Chapter 12, "Concealing," and Chapter 13, "Falsifying and Lying," under "Step 1: Listen."

Step 2: Tag. Focus on the symptoms or behavior you feel the patient is fabricating. As in cross-examination, have the patient commit herself to one version of the story.

Step 3: Confront. Focus on the suspected fabrication. Tell the patient that it is absolutely necessary that she be able to convince you and often an outside agency—a lawyer, a judge, or a division of family services— that her claims are accurate. Make it clear, however, that if she is lying, there may be grave consequences. For example, she may be charged with her false testimony or may lose custody of her children.

Step 4: Solve. Explain the voice-stress analysis or the polygraphic procedure to the patient. Tell her what the focus of the interview is, which statements will be scrutinized, and why. Make it clear you will not surprise her with unexpected questions. Quite the opposite, tell her to expect certain questions. Her answers to factual questions such as "When were you born?" will be compared with her answers to embarrassing questions such as "Have you ever lied before?" Then proceed with the control questions as outlined in Table IV–1.

After explaining the test purpose, ask the patient for informed consent, either verbal or in writing, to having the interview recorded and analyzed. Within the interview, this consent serves a very important purpose: it increases the patient's feeling of jeopardy.

The patient may agree to the interview to demonstrate her credibility. Do not assume, however, that she will want to cooperate. The fact that you are considering voice-stress analysis signals to her that you do not trust her. She now sees you as her opponent, not as an ally. If she is honest, she may welcome the fact that you are now preparing a test to prove it. Whether or not the patient is deceiving you, persuade her to cooperate. Emphasize that you are pursuing a common goal: you want to help her to establish credibility.

When you begin, turn on the tape recorder. Ask the patient if she understands the purpose and procedure of the voice-stress method. Then record the patient's oral consent to the interview (if possible, have her sign a consent form as well). Next, open the interview with general questions about factual information, always following the question with a confirming question:

When were you born?
Is this true?
Where were you born?
Are you telling the truth about that?

Next, ask the patient about her false first name and challenge her about the truthfulness of her answers. (I = interviewer; P = patient)

I: What is your first name?
P: Mona.
I: Is this true?
P: Yes.
I: Are you lying about that?
P: No.
I: I know you are lying about it because I told you to lie about it.
P: My name is still Mona.
I: And we both know you are lying. Why don't you admit that you lie?
P: No.
I: Do you always lie when somebody tells you to lie? Be truthful now.
P: I am.

Next, introduce the subject that is the main focus of the interview: the patient's lie. Ask a potentially embarrassing question such as

Have you ever lied before?

Step 5: Approve. At the end of the interview, express empathy for the patient's situation. Repeat that it was necessary to scrutinize her statements because of the importance of the issue and the implications for her and others close to her. Use the results of the test to design the most appropriate therapeutic response.

5. Interview: Factitious Disorder by Proxy

We now continue with the case of Ms. W. What to do with a patient like Ms. W.? Two years of supportive psychotherapy did not prevent relapse; no medication is known to control this condition. Because she induces actual physical symptoms, Ms. W. is dangerous to her children and her husband. Should she go to prison? Should she lose her children to a guardian to protect them from her potentially lethal influence?

The questions to be answered in the interview are

> Is the patient still fabricating?
> Have we detected the full extent of her fabrications?
> Can we develop a reliable method to detect her fabrication and her intentions to fabricate in the future?

The interviewer decides to offer voice-stress analysis because the test is easy to conduct, without the need for monitor wires used with the polygraph. With Ms. W.'s recorded informed consent, the interviewer undertakes the following interview. He then has the tape analyzed for stress reactions in the patient's voice. The relevant analyst's interpretations of stress are indicated as "S" at key points in the transcript.

Steps 1–3

In this interview, Steps 1–3 are omitted because the patient's fabrications are documented in police records. The interviewer reviewed with her the children's treatment records from the pediatrician's office, covering every sign and symptom the children had ever shown; the interviewer was uncertain as to whether the frequent visits her children had made to the pediatrician were based on legitimate or fabricated symptoms and signs in her children. The interviewer decided to review these details while the stress in the patient's voice was being monitored.

Step 4: Solve

1. I: Hi, Ms. W. Do you remember yesterday that I explained how the CIA [Central Intelligence Agency] has developed a method that police and psychiatrists use to detect the level of stress in the voice?
   P: You told me that.
2. I: You see, the muscles of the vocal cords produce tiny vibrations. You are completely unaware of these vibrations and you cannot control them. These vibrations increase and show a certain pattern when you feel stressed. Experts feel that when a person practices deception—that is, when he lies—the voice reflects that stress. Do you remember that?
   P: Yes, I thought about it all night.
3. I: You have signed a consent form that says we can tape record this interview

and perform a voice-stress analysis to see whether you show stress and practice deception during the interview. Right?

P: Yes.

4. I: I've also instructed you to answer my questions with yes and no first, and then you may add your explanation. And you agreed to do so.

P: Yes.

5. I: I also asked you to lie about your name.

P: Yes. You told me to deny that my name is Ms. W. whenever you ask me about it during the interview. You want to know how it shows up when I lie about my name on this test.

6. I: And you know what is at stake here.

P: Yes. The court wants to take away my children and give them to a guardian. The court thinks I'm a danger to them. I may make them sick and get them into the hospital or even kill them accidentally.

7. I: That's right. If you lie and practice deception here in the interview, you may indeed lose your children.

P: Yes, I understand.

8. I: The court wants to know two things. First, why do you induce illness in your kids?

P: But what if I really don't know. I mean, if I really don't understand why I do it, is that going to show up as a lie?

9. I: No, not if you are as truthful as you can be. If you answer that you don't understand it and if that's the truth, that's fine.

P: Okay, so I'm not expected? . . .

10. I: Just be as truthful as you can be.

P: Okay.

11. I: Don't try to get tricky about it.

P: I guess that I'm not supposed to be able to figure all of this out by myself. I mean that's what you're here for, right?

12. I: Right. I want to help you and protect you from practicing deception.

P: Okay.

13. I: The second thing the court wants to know is whether you can tell the truth after I point out to you that, for example, a certain answer in your last interview was not correct, that you did not tell the truth. Could you tell the truth the second time around if we go over the same topic again in a follow-up interview?

P: Yes.

14. I: But it would be even better, of course, if you tell the truth the first time around, in this interview now.

P: I'll try.

15. I: Before I start, do you have any questions?

P: No.

This dialogue set the stage. It made the patient aware of what was in jeopardy. This raised the chances of detecting abnormal stress in her voice. Four things increased Ms. W.'s sense of risk:

1. Highlighting the method's scientific authority by mentioning that it was valid and that the CIA, the police force, and some psychiatrists used the technique (Q. 1, 2).
2. Asking the patient to answer each question with yes or no before elaborating on the answer (Q. 4). This was important because stress is best detected during these initial answers. (In this interview the patient is allowed to follow her yes and no answers with explanations because these may contain leads for further questions. Some experts recommend refraining from this practice and insisting on only yes or no to heighten the stress. See discussion on cross-examination in Chapter 13, "Falsifying and Lying.")
3. Asking her to lie about a simple fact such as her name. This emphasizes that the test can differentiate between truth and deception (Q. 5).
4. Reminding the patient about what is at stake for her and her family. Such stress induction can be defended on ethical grounds if the stress is not merely an empty threat the interviewer uses to manipulate the patient but is a reminder of what is really at risk (Q. 6, 7).

The interviewer attempted to build an alliance with the patient (Q. 12) when he said he wanted to protect her from practicing deception. He invited her to split off her tendency to practice deception from her healthy personality. The stress and discomfort that would result from the interview were justified because they resulted from a therapeutic procedure, like the pain that results from the surgeon's knife.

16. I: Let me ask you in general, have you ever lied to get out of trouble?
    P: Yes. [S: Normal amount of nervous stress]
17. I: Can you give me an example?
    P: Yeah. [S: Normal amount of nervous stress] I remember doing it as a kid, saying I didn't do something or if I was late getting home, coming up with some reason other than the real one.
18. I: Do you have a driver's license?
    P: Yes.
19. I: Have you ever watched a baseball game?
    P: Yes.
20. I: Have you ever lied to someone who trusted you?
    P: Yeah. My parents trusted me, my husband trusted me, and I've lied to them. [S: Normal amount of nervous stress]
21. I: Have you done anything during that time which you are now ashamed of?
    P: I guess. Sometimes I feel guilty about lying to my parents, you know, but it was usually pretty trivial or minor things. [S: Normal amount of nervous stress]

In this part of the interview, two types of control questions were illustrated: those that normally do not cause stress (Q. 18, 19) and those that cause some mild stress because they require the patient to admit to potentially embarrassing faults (Q. 16, 17, 20, 21). These questions made it possible to discriminate between different levels of stress in this particular patient.

22. I: And [do you feel guilty] if you think of what you have done with Malcolm?
    P: Yes, I'm real embarrassed about that. I feel guilty, ashamed. [S: Slight amount of abnormal stress]
23. I: And about the letters from the satanic cult?
    P: Yeah. It's hard for me to talk about it because, you know, this thing with Malcolm is more recent. I didn't stuff it down as far as I did with the letters. [S: Slight amount of abnormal stress] Yet I think some of the things to do with the letters I've stuffed down for so long I don't even . . . I really don't remember everything. [S: Large amount of abnormal stress. Interpretation: the patient is practicing deception because she does remember about the letters.]
24 I: Hmmm. Are you a person who can push things completely down and forget about them altogether?
    P: I don't know whether I can totally forget about it, I guess it's just not at the top of my mind where I think about it all the time, but yeah, I think I've stuffed my feelings in since I was a little girl. I didn't talk about things. [S: Abnormal stress indicating deception]
25. I: Let me ask you, is your name Ms. W.?
    P: No. [S: Mild amount of abnormal stress]
26. I: Is this the truth?
    P: Yes. [S: Moderate amount of abnormal stress]
27. I: You are now clearly lying, aren't you?
    P: No. [S: Increased amounts of abnormal stress]

When the patient used the phrase "I don't remember," she showed high stress in her voice. Therefore, the phrase might have been a giveaway for her deception (A. 23). Because of the patient's history and her vagueness, the interviewer knew that she was most likely lying in A. 23, 24 and was certainly lying in A. 25–27. Thus, he enabled the laboratory analyst to determine the threshold level of the voice-stress measurement for Ms. W. Any stress level higher than that shown in the response to Q. 23–27 would raise a suspicion of deception. Next the interviewer is ready to tackle areas where he is uncertain whether the patient will lie or not.

28. I: Okay. Here are several things that I read in the court report. I read here that Cory had a severe ear infection. Did you induce any of that?
    P: No. A lot of times I would take her to the doctor because she had a

temperature and I did not know she had an ear infection. The doctor detected that, you know, her ear was actually red and he could see the fluid in it. No, I did not create that. [S: No signs of abnormal stress]

29. I: Have you ever done anything to make the ear infection worse even though it was there by itself?

P: No, I haven't.

30. I: Not even one time?

P: No. To make it worse? No.

31. I: Okay, and you told me one time—I think it was with Cory—you wanted to have the pregnancy shortened, right?

P: Yeah, but I didn't want to lose her. [S: No abnormal stress]

32. I: You wanted to have labor induced?

P: Right. [S: No abnormal stress]

33. I: And then the doctor did not want to induce labor.

P: I think partly because he felt the baby was due in 2 or 3 weeks anyway, and they wanted to make sure her lungs were developed. I just wanted to get the pregnancy over with. I was anxious for her to get here. Having a small child satisfies a lot of needs for me. [S: Abnormal stress present, especially at the phrase "having a small child"]

34. I: Did you do anything to persuade the doctor to induce labor?

P: Yes. [S: No abnormal stress]

35. I: What did you do?

P: I took laxatives to create . . . and I also probably wasn't eating properly as I should have been.

36. I: Did you tell him that you took laxatives?

P: Only recently. I didn't at the time, no. [S: Mild stress]

37. I: Okay. So at the time you lied about it.

P: Yes, but just recently my husband thought it was real important that if something started going wrong with this pregnancy that I should tell the doctor what had happened before so that I could be checked out to make sure something like that wasn't going on again. [S: Mild stress]

38. I: Hmmm. Have you done anything with this pregnancy?

P: No, I haven't tried to create anything. [S: No abnormal stress]

39. I: Do you think you will create anything with your present pregnancy?

P: No. [S: Slight amount of stress, unusual voice stress pattern]

40. I: Hmmm.

P: I have no intention of creating anything.

In Q. 28–40, the technique of challenging the patient's honesty was demonstrated. First, the interviewer identified some of the symptoms and signs reported in the patient's children and herself, and second, he immediately questioned the authorship of these symptoms (Q. 28, 32, 34, 38, 39). When the patient denied authorship, he challenged her answers (Q. 29, 30, 38, 40). Ms. W. had indeed tried to create labor with laxatives; she admitted her authorship of this action. She showed abnormal stress only once (A. 33).

The patient called induction of symptoms "creations" (A. 28, 38, 40). This word choice showed the many faces of deception. From her point of view, what she presented to the world was not lying or deceiving. It was deceiving only from the viewpoint of others. Instead she saw it as an expression of an urge to create the world that she needed, a world in which she took center stage as the sufferer, the victim. To her, her whole situation—being hauled into court, being prosecuted, hearing experts testifying right and left, and facing the possibility of losing her children—seemed not to be a trial; rather it was a show that featured her in the starring role of "supervictim." Public attention and court procedures were exactly what the patient was striving for. With the voice-stress analysis technique, the interviewer appeared to be playing right into her hands, continuing to gratify her need for this ongoing drama.

The interviewer adopted her term "creation" in Q. 39 and retained it for the remainder of the interview to address the key symptomatology from the patient's point of view.

41. I: Now, David had infected ears several times. Is that right, that he had ear infections?
    P: Hmmm.
42. I: Reddening of the ears?
    P: Yeah, they kind of got red.
43. I: Did you create any of that?
    P: No.
44. I: Did you create any of the ear infections with Cory?
    P: No.
45. I: Did you create any of the ear pains with David?
    P: No.
46. I: Now, one time, I think it was David who had diarrhea and vomiting, and then your husband had chest pains. Did you create any of that?
    P: No, I did not.
47. I: Your husband was then admitted to the hospital?
    P: Yes, for a couple of days. They catheterized him.
48. I: Did you create that?
    P: No, I didn't. [S: Slight amount of stress, but not severe enough to indicate that the patient was practicing deception, possibly indicating that she was nervous about her husband being in the hospital, or perhaps that she was glad that he was in the hospital]
49. I: And did the doctors find out why your husband had this problem?
    P: I think they just told him he had the flu. I really don't remember. I don't even know what he could have had, I mean, what chest problems, but they didn't attribute it to some kind of heart disorder or anything like that.
50. I: Have you ever created anything in your husband, any kind of symptom?
    P: No.

82. I: If you were to do it, how would you do it?
    P: I don't know, that's probably why I didn't do it. I didn't know how to go about doing it.
83. I: Have you ever thought of killing any of the children?
    P: No. [S: No signs of abnormal stress]
84. I: Or harming them?
    P: No. I mean, I know I did with Malcolm, so I suppose, but . . .
85. I: Yes?
    P: I mean, I didn't do it to intentionally hurt him.
86. I: Did you know when you did it that it could harm him?
    P: I knew it was making him vomit and giving him diarrhea. Even after he was out of the hospital and back home with us, my husband told me that it could have killed him. I didn't realize that at the time I was doing it to him.

The interviewer attempted to explore Ms. W.'s motive for "creating" symptoms, but he failed (Q. 71–86). Her answers appeared superficial. They did not explain the reason for her fabrication satisfactorily. She had stress at home and wanted some attention for her problems. She showed limited insight into the risk she caused for Malcolm in giving him laxatives and emetics. Ms. W. also endorsed symptoms of depression but denied being suicidal except for when her children were taken away from her. She denied being homicidal. In a self-defeating way she appeared to have created more problems for herself.

Diagnosis

The patient's symptoms fulfill criteria for factitious disorder by proxy. Criterion B of DSM-IV is difficult to assess because patients with factitious disorder rarely clearly admit that they seek, directly or indirectly, the sick role for themselves. Ms. W., for example, denies that she knows why she produces or feigns symptoms in herself and others. Thus, criterion B is fulfilled by exclusion of behavior that strives for an incentive—criterion B is not purely descriptive but is interpretative. As far as Ms. W. is concerned, it appears that her behavior is at least partly determined by her delight in deceiving others, because she calls her factitious behavior "creations and art work."

Follow-Up

As the clinical interview continued, Ms. W. admitted mainly to the acts that were a matter of record and concealed other problems. With the help of voice-stress analysis, however, she was later persuaded to be truthful.

Whenever the interviewer found evidence of lying, he pointed it out to her. He told her that he could not help her with her legal difficulties if she continued lying. He gave the patient a chance to revise her story. Gradually she gave up her lies until all elements of her story passed the voice-stress analysis.

Ms. W. started in therapy. The intensive weekly therapy, combined with voice-stress analysis, controlled her tendency to create but did not cure it. No further incidents of self-induced symptoms, persecution, or illness in family members occurred during this time. This innovative therapy kept the family together and the patient out of jail—but it did not cure her.

As with the symptoms of panic disorder, depressive disorder, or mania, a patient's urge to induce symptoms for herself or her family cannot be reduced merely to an unconscious psychological motive. Instead, this urge seems to be partly biological. It arises from that same physical source whence arise those other urges that make humans do things without knowing why, such as committing suicide, overeating, and abusing drugs or alcohol.

6. Fabrication and Voice-Stress Analysis in Psychiatric Disorders

In DSM-IV, factitious disorder is defined as a tendency to produce physical and psychological symptoms in order to assume the sick role but not to receive any secondary economic or social gain.

In the narrowest sense, fabrication occurs only in the group of factitious disorders that include

- Factitious disorder with predominantly psychological signs and symptoms
- Factitious disorder with predominantly physical signs and symptoms
- Factitious disorder with combined psychological and physical signs and symptoms
- Factitious disorder not otherwise specified

Only in these disorders does a patient intentionally produce, create, or feign physical and psychological signs and symptoms to assume the sick role or create the sick role in a dependent without obvious external incentives. It is the act of creation for the act itself. Thus, factitious disorder is distinct from malingering "in that the motivation for the symptom production in malingering is an external incentive" (DSM-IV, p. 474).

Ms. W.'s case illustrates that seeking the sick role is only one of several means to serve her purpose.

Rosenhan's (1973) famous experiment came close to the purpose of feigning disease. Rosenhan, a professor of psychology and law at Stanford University, and seven other nonpsychiatrically ill individuals presented to psychiatric emergency rooms in 12 different hospitals in five different states on the East and West coast, each reporting a single hallucination unspecific for any psychiatric disorder. The eight pseudopatients were admitted but not immediately released when they reported cessation of the hallucination to their providers. With deception delight Rosenhan reported the success in fooling the professionals and with deception contempt he exposed the foolishness of the experts who trusted him and the other pseudopatients. Rosenhan experimentally enacted factitious disorder but gave up this adopted disorder in exchange for being able to display to the world deception delight about their success in fooling the providers and contempt for the duped professionals. This human curiosity—whether or not one can succeed at deception at this level—and the delight about the success and the contempt for the victims appear to be a factor in Munchausen syndrome as if it was the Baron von Münchausen himself—we think.

Thus, the patient with factitious disorder initiates the deceptive behavior by asking herself curiously,

What would the professional [e.g., police] do if I get obscene phone calls?

She cannot rid herself of that curiosity. And finally she receives not just a phone call but also a letter, which provides physical evidence of an inflicted obscenity. Now she reports accurately without distortion how she received the letter. She helps to suggest how one should go about finding the culprit. Once started, she cannot stop until suspected or caught. Usually, patients with factitious disorder move away when their fabrication is suspected.

The patient with factitious disorder lays down a careful memory trace about all her symptoms and signs. She suppresses the memory trace of how she produced the signs. She looks very convincing and truthful when she reports them because she focuses solely on the characteristics of those signs. As long as she can maintain that tunnel vision, she can appear truthful because she is being truthful—the obscene letter indeed arrived in the mail. She can also assist the professional in how to go about detecting the culprit because her scotomatous memory allows her to play the game: "How would one find the culprit (as if the letter was sent by somebody real)?"

The nature of her disorder is the enacting of the "as if." Therefore, she reports all the feigned signs from a victim's perspective even after she has been identified as their creator. Her strong fixation on her victim memory appears to prevent her from enjoying fully—unlike Rosenhan—her deception delight and contempt.

Other disorders involve intentional creations by the patient. In antisocial personality disorder, a patient lies for the sake of lying without any apparent gain—this may come closest to the creations of the patient with factitious disorder. Other psychiatric patients create symptoms and signs with some gain in mind, which qualifies them as lies rather than as factitious acts:

- Malingerers expect to receive economic compensation, avoid legal consequences, or improve physical well-being.
- Patients with oppositional defiant disorder and conduct disorder expect to serve their aggressive purposes.
- Patients with alcoholism or who abuse drugs may invent elaborate schemes to express their particular disorder.
- Some patients are bewildered by their symptoms—they do not plan them consciously and voluntarily but have them more in a way of autosuggestion with limited awareness.
- Patients with conversion disorder create pseudoneurological symptoms that help them to avoid a task.
- Patients with dissociation have gaps in consciousness and identity that prevent them from facing unbearable problems.
- Patients with somatization disorder report symptoms that reduce the pressure to cope.
- Manic patients may invent elaborate histories out of a need for increased production and a breakdown of reality testing.

Patients' fabrications are not limited to the production of psychological and physical symptoms of disorders. Patients may portray themselves as victims of plagues of the times, such as being socially or sexually harassed by perverts. Because of that broader view, for our case example we chose a patient who did both: subject her children to the induction of physical symptoms and signs, and subject herself to be a victim of sexual harassment.

What if voice-stress analysis fails? The obvious alternative is a polygraphic analysis. Another option is a firm approach in which you point out the negative effects of the patient's persisting fabrications—for example, if you can prevent the patient from having custody of the children whom she harmed or from returning to a social situation in which she had practiced fabrication before. Obviously, the cross-examination technique is already a part of the voice-stress analysis interview. In cross-examination, you challenge the patient's claims by asking her to give a wealth of details, the accuracy of which is then assessed by closed-ended questions. If the patient's claim is false, you expect that the details will contradict each other and will not support the patient's claim. In voice-stress analysis, you also collect details. You want to identify those details that are fabricated. Fabricated details provoke—if repeatedly examined—increased stress in the voice or in the polygraphic recordings of the fabricator. Such patterns help you to spot fabrication. You scrutinize these suspicious details over and over again. In factitious disorders these details consist of symptoms and signs. Explore whether they were fabricated by the patient.

In selected cases you may consider the amobarbital interview (Marriage et al. 1988). However, because the patient's central pathology is fabrication for the sake of fabrication, such an approach may invite more fabrication rather than clarify existing ones.

Voice-stress analysis may be used in a broader sense than for lie detection. It may be useful for making those patients who have a tendency to suppress and deny their own stress experience aware of it. For example, patients who experience anxiety and panic may not be aware of their own stress experience. Voice-stress analysis may be a window into the patient's autonomic responses.

CHAPTER 15

SELF-DECEPTIVE BEHAVIOR

Summary

In self-deception, the patient deceives himself and others about his short-comings and failures. The interviewer invites the patient to identify his self-deception by discussing secret thoughts that he may have about his own behavior. Usually, such thoughts take the form of self-talk. This self-talk reveals the discrepancies between the idealized self-image and actual behavior. In exchange for his candid revelations, the interviewer praises the patient for his strength in facing his problems.

◆ ◆ ◆ ◆ ◆

Mein Freund, die Zeiten der Vergangenheit
Sind uns ein Buch mit sieben Siegeln.
Was ihr den Geist der Zeiten heisst,
Das ist im Grund der Herren eigner Geist,
In dem die Zeiten sich bespiegeln.
My friend, the times that antecede
Our own are books safely protected
By seven seals. What spirit of the time you call,
Is but the scholar's spirit, after all,
In which times past are now reflected.

Johann Wolfgang von Goethe
Faust (1808)

◆ ◆ ◆ ◆ ◆

1. What Is Self-Deception?

A patient practicing self-deception negates her failures and undesirable
personality traits because they clash with her self-image. This patient dilutes
her symptoms and deviant behaviors because she feels her image would be
destroyed if they were known. She does not trust anybody to understand
her suffering. She is convinced that if her secret is uncovered, others—even
family and friends—would reject her. Striving to be liked and loved, she
maintains relationships with others by hiding her suffering behind a wall of
deception. She suppresses her awareness of her shortcomings from herself
and from others rather than integrate them into her self-image. She fortifies
her suppressed awareness with a devaluation of her shortcomings as

insignificant, unimportant, and accidental. She sees them as glitches on an otherwise impressive track record. She cannot tolerate her self-deceptions and therefore denies them. Such a patient usually deceives herself with naïveté and pumped up conviction.

In DSM-IV (American Psychiatric Association 1994), deception and self-deception are not clearly distinguished. Deceptive or self-deceptive behavior is referred to most clearly in the text rather than in the diagnostic criteria. For example, in the discussion of substance-related disorders in DSM-IV, it is stated that individuals "incorrectly assure themselves that they will have no problem regulating substance use" (p. 189). As another example, within the discussion of bulimia nervosa in DSM-IV, it is stated that "individuals with bulimia nervosa are typically ashamed of their eating problems and attempt to conceal their symptoms" (p. 546).

Self-deception creates another problem—the patient becomes isolated from the people close to him. His deceit keeps him from forming open, honest relationships. Ironically, one of the most cherished needs of a dissimulator is to be close to others. Yet, such a patient also hides his symptoms from himself, deluding himself by claiming his problems are minor, transient, and without impact on his health or social life. However, his suppression of reality is incomplete because he still experiences discomfort from simmering conflicts on the fringes of his awareness. The self-deceiving patient is laden with apprehension and fear of having to face his own shortcomings. His discomfort increases when questions direct him toward his failures. Therefore, to push self-doubt aside, the patient overemphasizes his virtues.

Self-deception occurs for several reasons:

- To suppress memories of now embarrassing actions
- To keep in check unacceptable wishes, desires, and habits
- To protect oneself from one's personality defects

The mechanisms of self-deception operate in a fluid state on different levels of severity and awareness. Thus, we all practice some self-deception. It allows us to maintain hope in the presence of failure and adversity. Psychotherapists use reframing and supportive therapy to disperse hopelessness and reinstill energy in patients to work toward positive goals. Self-deception is harmful when it prevents us from facing up to more severe problems. For example, an individual who experiences chest pain that radiates into her left arm may tell herself that this is just her peptic ulcer acting up, thus depriving herself of a timely treatment for a possible cardiac condition. A patient who abuses alcohol may deceive herself about the impact of her abuse to avoid painful change.

Self-deception interferes with the interview because the patient filters his history. He presents you only with that segment of his problem that portrays him as a victim of environmental forces rather than as the originator of his defeat. Self-deception prevents you from receiving accurate information about the patient's history and his symptoms because he dissimulates them. He misleads you into drawing false diagnostic conclusions. Thus, the self-deceiver erects a wall of denial between the interviewer and himself. This wall serves two purposes: it seals off intrusive questions while creating a feeling of protection and safety for the patient. Basic interviewing techniques do not work here because they assume that the patient is truthful and cooperates in identifying his problems.

If you do not recognize self-deception, you may miss the presence and the severity of certain psychiatric disorders, personality disorders, psychiatric symptoms, problems, and conflicts.

2. Self-Deception in the Mental Status

The essence of self-deception is to concentrate on one's strength or to convert a weakness into a strength. Because the patient knows about her weakness, she overcompensates her strengths. Usually, the patient has worked out an internally consistent, noncontradictory self-image that she also wants to portray to others. She acts like a salesperson for her product.

How do you recognize self-deception? What alerts you? The mental status of the self-deceptive patient varies depending on how much she succeeds in convincing you and others.

Affect

The patient often portrays an elated affect. If challenged, he becomes even more emphatic about his successes, but flashes of anxiety or anger may precede or be intermingled with his positive affect and give you the double message of deceit. If you continue to challenge him, his affect turns into anger. When he finally faces up to his weakness, he may express guilt about his failures. He may accuse himself for having fooled himself for too long. Because this patient deceives not only you but also himself, he usually does not express guilt about deceiving you. Such quick and total changes in affect are the hallmark of the self-deceiving patient. They are reflected in autonomic responses, reactive movements, facial expressions, grooming, and tone of voice.

Autonomic responses reflect the affect that the patient positions himself to portray. He is prone to strong autonomic responses of blushing, increased breathing, and tears when he finally breaks down.

His *reactive movements* vary greatly. The patient suppresses reactive movements as if he wants to guard himself from outside interruptions while delivering his self-deceptive story. He may, however, exaggerate his reactive movements to invite a newcomer as audience for his inflated claims. Reactive movements may also increase if the patient is angered by your challenges. He may then respond briskly to an interrupting noise, seeking relief from your inquiries. However, he may ignore all interruptions after he has started a tirade against you and your challenges. Reactive movements may decrease if he finally faces up to his problems and gives room to depression and despair.

Facial expressions are both staged and genuine. If he can convince himself of the validity of his presentation, his facial expressions become intense and match the forceful tone of voice. However, he becomes irritated when interrupted and questioned but may hide these feelings behind a facade of confidence. He may experience anger if you steer him to recognize his self-deception. His affect displayed in facial movements mirrors the tension that he experiences when fighting for control.

The patient's *grooming behaviors* can be prolonged and continuous, such as massaging his neck or arms when he feels he is succeeding in getting his views accepted because he is pleased with himself. When he is challenged, rapid, short-lasting scratching, itching, or foot whipping may emerge just to be suppressed to hide discomfort.

The patient's *voice* may sound deep and overconfident. If the patient is challenged, his voice becomes louder and pressured and his words come faster, thereby heralding a pending outburst of anger. His pitch sinks with the collapse of self-deception.

Psychomotor Movements and Speech

The self-deceiving patient forces herself to believe in her strength, righteousness, and success. She supports that image in her self-talk. She suppresses gnawing thoughts that one could doubt her proclaimed accomplishments and behaviors. Therefore, her psychomotor movements and speech reflect the interviewer's attitude.

She uses various *gestures.* She underscores her assertions through emphatic head shaking or hand slapping on the desk. When challenged, she may freeze. If the challenge penetrates her self-deceptive armor, she may resort to angry fist pounding to scare you off. If the patient finally faces up to her failures, gestures may give away a motionless posture where she hangs down her head. A drama of self-condemnation may unfold in which she pounds her chest, clenches her fists, and looks up to the ceiling as if confessing to a higher power.

The patient also uses many *hand and facial signals.* When she presents her inflated view of herself, she may top her statement by making a V sign, symbolic of victory. Because a self-deceiving person emphasizes her strengths, you find symbols of such strengths at her disposal. The patient signals that she won't allow being trampled on. Behind that posturing, you frequently detect an insecure feeling reflecting self-doubt.

The patient wants to keep you as her attentive audience and therefore uses *goal-directed movements.* She may have a tendency to move toward you, especially when she feels that you start to doubt her and challenge her with disbelief. She may scoot her chair toward you. She may get up to come closer. However, if you succeed in making her face up to her self-deceptive behavior, she may retreat and collapse in her chair as if sinking into the ground.

The patient initially invests herself to present her view with fluent *speech.* If challenged, she becomes even more determined to make you see it her way by repeating her views and claims. She will try to silence you and say,

Absolutely not! This never crossed my mind! It never happened.

When you confront her with her self-deception, she may respond with tirades and spitting while talking, showing her uncontrolled excitement. She may remind you that

I have been most cooperative and friendly to you and what do I get for it? Accusations. Insult. Injustice. An unfair, distrusting interviewer. How dare you?

Now, signs of concealment and falsification surface on an emotionally charged background with ehs and uhs, convoluted speech, and slips of the tongue. Her speech turns into a cadence of falling pitch and deep sighs when she finally accepts her weaknesses. The pressure is off when she gets a glimpse of insight. Yet, her self-deceiving tendency may kick in again, and she may launch into a cascade of self-accusation, displaying the main tendency of the self-deceiver: overcompensation.

Verbal Strategies of Self-Deception

The verbal strategies of self-deception resemble defense mechanisms, except they may not operate in the unconscious (Table 15–1).

Most self-deceiving patients praise themselves and also flatter you. Self-glorification, a form of grandiosity, is the patient's effort to claim he is someone to be reckoned with. He may try to emphasize his honesty with statements such as

> To be perfectly honest with you. . . .
> To tell you the truth. . . .
> Let me level with you. . . .

Table 15–1. Signs of self-deception, psychiatric symptomatology, and defense mechanisms

Sign of self-deception	Definition of self-deception	Psychiatric symptomatology	Defense mechanisms
Self-praise	Inflation of strengths and accomplishments	Grandiosity, boasting	Reaction formation, idealization
Flattering	Praise of interviewer	Glorification, devotion	Idealization
Dissimulation	Diminishment of a weakness	Lack of insight, Pollyannism	Idealization, denial
Negation	Dispute of facts	Rejection of facts	Denial
Switching of topics	Overt and abrupt change of topic	Flight of ideas, tangentiality	Replacement
Blaming	Shift of responsibility to others	Accusing, finger pointing	Projection
Distrust	Expectation to be harmed	Ideas of reference and persecution	Projection
Refusal	Resistance to discussing topic	Anger, defiance	Suppression
Rejection	Criticism of others as inept	Accusations, tirades, sarcasm, threats	Externalization
Self-condemnation	Rejection of self	Self-hate, self-mutilation, suicidality	Introversion, introjection

I'll be candid with you. [A triviality follows]

The patient has limited insight into this self-deceptive behavior and wants to keep it this way. He may negate a problem, switch topics, and become distrustful of you. If you confront him with his self-deception, he may cut you off with emotionally laden statements sometimes followed by an intended final point such as

Is this clear?
I won't talk about it any more.

He may launch hostile tirades against you and refuse to discuss a sensitive topic.

All the signs of self-deception mark a sensitive area. A patient who starts to recognize his self-deception signals his discomfort by showing anxiety, guilt, or distress. He acts as if he is on the hot seat. He can run away from the interviewer but cannot escape from himself—and he is painfully aware of it. Trying to avoid discussing his problem, distracting the interviewer, becoming hostile, or using self-glorification does not do the job for him. He experiences too much guilt to slip out of the situation. He feels stuck. If he finally admits his weaknesses, he may show shame and guilt and indulge in self-condemnation.

The patient's social history often alerts you to his psychiatric problems. It may be peppered with unexplained relocations, frequent job changes, jobs that seem beneath his educational and intellectual level and that contrast with his self-portrayed competence, or unemployment. There may be frequent partner changes, separations, or divorces that betray his assertion of being a family man. His explanations for failures in job and marriage may be directed toward the company, his supervisors, or his spouse rather than toward his poor judgment or impulsivity.

His medical history may provide giveaways as well. Elevated liver enzymes, poor pulmonary functions, high cholesterol levels, and hypertension may indicate alcohol and nicotine abuse, poor dietary habits, and a lack of exercise despite the fact that he may emphasize his high level of health consciousness.

3. Technique: Cognitive Analysis of Self-Deception

Self-deception is the patient's way of dealing with her past failures and present weaknesses. It occurs through forgetting and verbal touch-ups of one's self-image. The patient thinks about herself in a more positive way than is justified by her actions. The goal of your interview is to detect her self-deception by tapping into the thoughts she has about herself.

Cognitive therapists refer to a person's reflections about her own behavior as *self-talk*. Self-talk precedes, accompanies, and follows feelings, reactions, and maladjusted behaviors (Dobson 1988). However, the patient is often deaf to this self-talk. To increase patients' awareness and control over their thinking and feelings, cognitive therapists teach patients to recognize and reconstruct their self-talk and to crystallize their feelings such as anxiety and embarrassment in words. This cognitive technique helps to expose patients' self-deception and to improve their communication with their therapist.

First, invite the patient to reconstruct her self-talk about the image that she wants to project to herself and others. For example, ask her what she tells herself about her control of drinking. Ask her how she ideally would like to appear to herself and to others. Let her paint a glowing picture of herself. Praise her for both her ideal and her achievements. Realistic reassurance and honest, genuine praise support the patient's self-esteem. With this cognitive approach you ally yourself with the patient's wishful thinking that forms the center of her pathology. Split her idealized self-image from the denied weaknesses that conflict with this self-image (Othmer and Othmer 1994). Rather than criticizing her self-deception, praise the goals reflected in the false claims. For example, encourage a patient who boasts that she has been dry since Christmas to stay completely sober.

Second, when the patient reveals her self-talk, she may begin to notice her inflated expectations, such as a sense of entitlement, a need for perfectionist performance, or self-pity. Point out that most people's self-talk sounds grandiose, irrational, embarrassing, or even silly. Cautiously ask her how close she comes to living up to her ideal.

> What do you tell yourself about how you want to be and what weaknesses you may still have?

With this question you implement the split between the idealized self-image based on self-deception and the actual behavior. By encouraging her self-talk, make her detect and describe her shortcomings that she hides not only from others but from herself. Keep her in a cooperative mode while she is describing her weaknesses, and assure her of your support in facing these problems.

Third, if the patient discloses her weaknesses and her self-deceptive behavior, she may compensate for this admission with promises to improve by contractual agreements. For example, in the case of a patient who abuses alcohol, help her understand that both her abuse and the deception and self-deception that she practices about this abuse will be a lifelong problem rather than a here-and-now conflict that can be put to rest with a one-time commitment or contract. Caution her not to set herself up for failure. Point out how humbling and anxiety- or anger-provoking it often is when realizing how far one is removed from one's desired image. Tell her that it may take a lifelong effort to deal with weakness by more effective coping methods than self-deception.

What if the cognitive method fails? In that case praise the patient for her accomplishments. Your acceptance softens her control and she may more openly volunteer her concerns. She may then look at her weaknesses. Patients with narcissistic personality disorder are particularly responsive to this accepting and praising approach. Alternatively, you may focus on the patient's defenses and on her transference patterns, if you are familiar with the psychodynamic principles of interviewing.

4. Five Steps to Unmask Self-Deception

A patient who deceives himself is sensitive to criticism and interventions. His self-confidence is fragile. Therefore, when you detect one or more signs of self-deception, you need to decide at what time to address them. You cannot conduct a successful diagnostic interview without understanding what the patient is denying. You may temporarily ignore it rather than jeopardize rapport because the patient may have sufficient openness about other aspects of his disorder. However, self-deception may frustrate you; you may lose empathy for the patient. Therefore, address this self-deceptive behavior sooner rather than later.

Step 1: Listen. Listening flushes out the patient's different strategies of self-deception, such as self-praise for accomplishments, dissimulation of symptoms, negation of problems, avoidance of admitting to a weakness, blaming others for failures, and feeling persecuted when criticized. Study the range of his self-deceptive behaviors. Allow the patient to express himself without interruption so he begins to feel comfortable.

Allow him to apparently succeed with his strategy, and state your clarifying questions in a casual manner. If he dodges a question, either repeat it or change the subject. Allow him to have the lead. If he, for example, dissimulates his substance abuse and then introduces a new topic, simply say,

> We got off our original topic. I would like to come back to our previous point.

Do not object if the patient changes the subject. Accept it as accidental, but remember it for future reference. Avoid hinting that you suspect a purpose behind the distraction. If the patient makes grandiose claims, such as inflated future income, invite him to explain and to give more details:

> It is helpful to me to learn from you in which areas you see your potentials.

Accept his self-deceptive behaviors even when he overplays them. Such a permissive posture keeps the patient's anxiety level low.

Step 2: Tag. Tell the patient that you recognize certain behaviors, but still do not indicate that you suspect a purpose in those behaviors or that you plan to address it. Thus, the patient can continue his self-deception, but is alerted that you notice his behavior. For example, say to a patient who continually changes topics on you,

> We always seem to get sidetracked. We don't seem to get an answer to that question. I wonder why we always get from A to C without having finished A or touching on B.

You may also express your puzzlement by repeating an answer,

> Hmm, so you say that has never occurred to you.

or

> I'm surprised about your answer.

Also use nonverbal expressions:

- Raise your eyebrows.
- Send the patient a questioning look.
- Shake your head slowly.
- Wait silently for the patient to continue.

Thus, you can steer the patient to follow up on a topic and take the lead instead of your having to do so. Make him realize the tag.

Step 3: Confront. It is tempting to address the patient's self-deception directly and communicate to him that you think it is in his best interest to overcome it. However, signs of self-deception are more easily recognized by you than by the patient. Usually the patient gets angry when directly confronted. Therefore, focus on the patient's signs of self-deception in an empathic, understanding, and accepting way. In a gentle yet firm way, make him aware of his behavior. Avoid the connotation of "I got you!" Instead, convey,

> I sense something that we may need to discuss. Let's explore that further.

At this point, summarize your understanding of what the patient feels is sensitive for him and where he sees his strengths. Explore and probe with the goal to learn how the patient views his problems. Thus, you prepare the stage to split off the problem from the patient's healthy self and build an alliance against his problem.

Step 4: Solve. Propose to the patient a change of perspective. Tell him that up to this point he was concerned about how he projected his problems to you. Now you would like to know how he views them, how he talks about them to himself (e.g., his drinking, his sobriety). When he starts to idealize himself again, you may remark,

> This sounds more like talking to me about it. How do you talk about it to yourself?

Tell the patient that the source of his embarrassment or guilt is, in your opinion, understandable. Suggest that the two of you discuss these feelings so that he can integrate them into his self-image, rather than trying to deny them and ban them from awareness. Ally yourself with the patient's critical self-talk. Offering an alliance strengthens the patient in his attempt to sort things out. Your body language and statements give the patient the feeling that he has a confidant. Make the patient feel that his alliance with you is worth giving up secretiveness. If the patient continues self-deception, ask,

> What do you tell yourself about why you hide your problem from others? What reason do you give yourself for not talking with me about it?

Get his attention by provoking his curiosity about your view of him. Doing so often makes him leave his defensive stance. During the interview you might sit in your chair, shake your head, and after a long pause say,

> I just wonder.

Of course, you have to mean what you say. If you come across as phony or rehearsed, you cannot expect the patient to tune in. Be genuine in your comment and the patient will wonder what you are wondering about. For example,

> What are you telling yourself about me that makes you insist on giving me a story that doesn't make sense to me or to anybody else—not even to you? Try to look at what's happening with an objective eye—like a referee. What are you telling yourself?

The patient will become surprised, curious, angry, hurt, or amazed. He may ask you suspiciously,

> Why do you act like that?
> Why do you say that?
> Don't you believe me?
> Do you think I'm lying to you?

You may reply with a variety of open-ended answers:

> I was surprised about your statements.
> I thought you would answer differently.
> Your answer gives me the message you don't want to talk about it right now.

The patient may stay in his self-deceptive pattern:

> You're pressuring me to tell you something I can't tell you because I'm telling you the truth. There's nothing more to say.

Then you might say,

> Well, we went over that before. The only thing that I can assume about why you insist on your story is that you must think I'll do something terrible to you if I discover the truth.

This approach works if you are open and friendly with the patient while continuing to disbelieve his story. If you see he is concerned that you may reject him if you learn the truth, give reassurance that this will not be the case. You have directed him to focus on his self-deception—an area of concern has been identified.

Apologize when you have provoked him to anger and respect his suspiciousness. If he is exceedingly hostile or suspicious, manage this behavior by addressing it directly. Thus, you may respond by saying,

> I notice that something made you angry . . . [Pause]
>
> I notice that something seems to prevent you from telling me . . . [Pause]

If the patient does not respond, you might say,

> Is there anything I said or asked you that annoyed you? I'm sorry if I did. Please help me understand what it was.

If the patient explains the reason, usually you get a clearer picture of the area of self-deception and of his technique. If the patient remains angry, hostile, or suspicious, back off:

> It seems we have touched a very sensitive spot. Let's talk about something else.

Backing off until a later time is essential if the patient is delusional about a topic.

With cognitive analysis of self-talk, the patient usually gains some insight and overcomes the obstacles to disclosure. Solving means the patient allows you to discuss his self-deceptive strategies so he realizes why he uses self-deception and what he is trying to hide. It does not mean that he will or can give it up. Such a change in behavior is the goal of therapy and difficult to achieve as outcome studies on the treatment of substance abuse, for example, demonstrate (Goodwin et al. 1984; Institute of Medicine 1990; Moos et al. 1990).

Step 5: Approve. In Step 5, you attempt to soothe the wounds caused by the patient's painful self-disclosure. He has temporarily relinquished a defensive strategy that has helped him to maintain his self-image—he is in pain. Tell him that you understand his dilemma and that you see how troublesome his problem is. Empathize with his reasons for using self-deception, and allow him to feel justified with them.

Next, tell the patient how the disclosure has helped you in making an accurate diagnosis and treatment plan. Help him to integrate his problem into his awareness about himself.

You have succeeded in Step 5 when the patient expresses relief or gratitude that his secret was discussed.

5. Interview A: Alcohol Abuse

Mr. W. is a 37-year-old, black, married, overweight engineer. (I = interviewer; P = patient)

Step 1: Listen

1. I: Hi, Mr. W. How can I help you?
   P: The shit hit the fan. I'm so fucking mad. Everybody turns against me.
2. I: Can you tell me who?
   P: Well, Mr. L., who was working for me, is jumping ship.
3. I: Hmmm.
   P: He's going to my worst competitor. Just for a few cents more. And he was like family to me. We were together from the start. But there's no thank you, I guess.
4. I: What kind of business did he help you with?
   P: We are construction consultants. My company is known all over the United States. We've done work in every state. But business is down in this shitty economy.
5. I: Well, can you survive?
   P: I'm not sure. We are doing a hell of a job. I just hope things will be picking up.
6. I: You said everybody is turning against you. What else is going on?
   P: My wife moved out. She and the kids are back at her mother's. She doesn't know what she wants to do. [With a sarcastic smile] Wants to find herself. Even talks about going back to school for a nursing degree.
7. I: What brought that about?
   P: Who knows? It's just one of those damn woman things. We have a nice house, two great kids—the most expensive house in a white neighborhood—moved in 5 years ago.
8. I: And she's leaving you.
   P: Yap [sic].
9. I: How were you getting along with her?
   P: Just great, I thought. Took my boy to the baseball game and my girl to her soccer games. They are 11 and 9.
10. I: Any reason why your wife leaves all that behind?
    P: I guess it's that woman's crap. Maybe, her mother is behind that. She never liked me. She likes the house and all that.

Step 2: Tag

11. I: You are telling me that you have a well-known consulting firm and you've gotten known all over the United States.
    P: That's right.
12. I: That you are a family man, and that you are pretty successful, being able to afford the best house in a good neighborhood. But that your key employee and your wife are leaving.

P: Yeah.
13. I: That's what makes you mad?
P: That sums it up.

The patient blamed his employee (A. 2), his wife (A. 6), women's issues (A. 7, 10), and his mother-in-law (A. 10) for his anger and the economy for his lack of business success (A. 4, 5). He glorified himself as a successful consultant (A. 4) and good family man (A. 9). This discrepancy showed the hallmark of self-deception. The interviewer verified the patient's views in tagging (Q. 11–13).

Step 3:   Confront

14. I: What's your wife telling you?
P: Some kind of bull. And I know that's not really it.
15. I: If I called her, what would she tell me on the phone?
P: I've given up guessing her mind.
16. I: Let's try it. I'm curious what she's coming up with. What's the number at her mom's house?
P: Oh, you don't have to listen to her. I can tell you what kind of crap she'll be putting out.
17. I: Okay. Let's hear it.
P: She'll give you some shit about me having a drink. Stupid. A drink! That's about the only thing that keeps me going. But I guess that woman doesn't understand what pressure I'm under.
18. I: So, what does alcohol do for you?
P: It makes me more of a man.
19. I: Can you give me an example?
P: Yeah, I do work for people all over the country. They owe me over $86,000. When I'm drunk, I call 'em up and ask 'em "When do I get my bills paid?" I can't do it otherwise.
20. I: Okay. That sounds fine to me. What else does alcohol do for you?
P: I'm under a lot of stress with my work. And when I drink it relaxes me. So, I feel good.
21. I: That's great. Indeed alcohol does a lot for you.
P: But I don't like the taste of it.
22. I: What do you like about alcohol then if you don't like the taste?
P: Well, the way it makes me feel. It makes me feel good.
23. I: It makes you feel good. Okay. After all, it makes you feel like a man.
P: [With surprise] Do you recommend that I should continue drinking?
24. I: It depends. I want to find out what's best for you.
P: But I hear drinking isn't good.
25. I: Says who?
P: My wife. She's disgusted with me and she's filing for divorce.

As an inroad to the patient's assumed self-deception, the interviewer used the criticism by the patient's wife. The patient negated and dissimulated the negative effects of alcohol (A. 17) and glorified its positive effects (A. 18–23). In Step 3, the focus of the interview shifted from self-pity and anger about the loss of the key employee to the more sensitive area of self-deception. Yet, the interviewer did not address the self-deception itself.

Step 4:　Solve

26. I:　So what do you tell yourself about your drinking?
　　P:　What I told you. That it relaxes me. That it makes me feel like a man and that I feel up to calling customers for my money.
27. I:　And what else would you like alcohol to do for you?
　　P:　Exactly that! In less than an hour I can feel good, even after a bad day at the office. It makes me forget things.
28. I:　Anything that you don't like about it?
　　P:　It can be too much at times if I don't watch it.
29. I:　I agree. You hit on all the good things with alcohol. It appears that alcohol can help you out a lot.
　　P:　So you're not all against it?
30. I:　You told me what a good role alcohol plays in your life. How far do you think alcohol really comes to fulfilling all these expectations?
　　P:　[Puzzled] I'm not sure.
31. I:　So, what do you tell yourself when you are alone and when you think about drinking?
　　P:　Depends when.
32. I:　Okay, you said at times you drink too much. When do you drink too much?
　　P:　When I feel bad and I need to feel good.
33. I:　How much do you need to feel good?
　　P:　About a quart.
34. I:　And what do you do after you've had a quart?
　　P:　I drink another quart the next day. And the next, and the next. And after 4 or 5 days, I'm just sitting at home and letting the effect wear off.
35. I:　And then?
　　P:　Then I stay sober for 2 weeks and try to catch up on my work, and I never want to drink again. And then the thought pops into my mind it would be nice to have a drink.
36. I:　So you give in?
　　P:　No, I fight the thought all the way to the liquor store. Even when I grab the door handle, I say to myself, "I don't have to do it anymore." I even say it when I buy the quart of vodka. I say this time I have just one drink. But it never works.
37. I:　And what do you tell yourself then?
　　P:　Then I tell myself, "Goddamnit! I did it again and I didn't want to. I have to learn to cut down," and I feel bad when I can't.
38. I:　But it makes you feel like a man.

P: Well . . . people can tell when I'm drunk. They don't want to talk to me when I'm drunk. I don't make sense.

39. I: But they pay you, don't they?

P: Not really. They tell me to sue 'em, and if I do I get only fifty cents on the dollar.

40. I: How's that?

P: Well, I make so many mistakes when I work while I'm drunk.

41. I: And that's why they don't want to pay you?

P: That's what they say.

42. I: Okay. As long as you can get by, what do you care?

P: Well, I'm losing my business over it. I had 12 employees. My name meant something all over the country. Last Friday, I had to let go of my last employee because I couldn't pay him.

43. I: Okay. So, you're losing your wife because she doesn't understand what alcohol does for you and you are losing your business. But that really doesn't matter because, after all, alcohol is worth it, it makes you feel good.

P: But I just told you how much trouble I got into with the drinking. I lost my job and now I am losing my wife.

44. I: Sure, it has a price, but it's worth the price, you say.

P: You can't mean that!

45. I: Why not? You meant it all the way or you wouldn't drink. You're losing your job—that's usually the first thing—and then you lose your wife.

P: That's right. But I don't want to lose her.

46. I: But it may well be worth it, you say.

P: I don't say this! How can you talk like that?

47. I: You say it through your actions. I just want to find out what's best for you, Mr. W. And so far, you were always willing to pay the price—your job, your wife. . . .

P: No, no! I like the money that I can get from my job. I always had a better car than my brothers and a bigger house—at least until now.

48. I: So what? These things didn't make you feel as good as alcohol does.

P: You don't understand. I would give my right foot if I could stop drinking.

49. I: [Laughing] I don't want your right foot—that's not good enough. Your right foot does not make you drink.

P: Then what do you want?

50. I: I want to work with that part of your brain that makes you enjoy the alcohol. What you have to give up is the fun that alcohol gives you. That's the only deal I would make.

P: I can't do that. When I drink, I have that temporary insanity that makes me keep drinking, as it says in the big book.

51. I: I'm not talking about when you are drinking. I'm talking about before you drink. You have control over only your first drink.

P: But that idea always pops into my mind and it can come back any time even if I'm sober for 7 years.

52. I: That's right. What I can give you is a 3-day grace period. When the idea of a drink pops into your mind, I can give you a 3-day grace period to make up your mind whether you want to drink again.

P: How's that?
53. I: I can give you Antabuse [disulfiram]. I can give you enough of it that it will make you sick when you drink. But you only have to stop Antabuse for 3 days and you can drink again.
P: I have to think about that.
54. I: You don't even have to tell me that you want to stop Antabuse so that you can drink again. You can lie to me, or tell me that you want to stop drinking without the Antabuse crutch. You can tell me that Antabuse makes you sick to your stomach, or that you can't sleep on it, or that it makes you impotent. I've heard it all. But we also can just dry you out, let you have some rest, and then you can keep drinking. You decide what is best for you, if you are willing to pay the price for drinking—job, wife, life.
P: I don't want to pay that price.
55. I: Well, Mr. W., you are not paying it all at once. You pay it little by little.
P: What can I do to change it?
56. I: By telling yourself every day that you will have to pay with everything you got if you go close to the liquor store to buy that quart.
P: I have a terrible vice—alcohol.
57. I: Maybe there's one that's worse.
P: What's that?
58. I: Bullshitting yourself about it.

The interviewer invited the patient to describe his self-talk about his drinking (A. 26, 27). His focus was to ask the patient to reveal what he told himself and not others. Furthermore, the interviewer enhanced the patient's honesty in his self-talk by accepting the patient's self-deceptive statements as true and believable. Thus, the interviewer induced a role reversal in which he became the defender of alcohol and the patient, the challenger. This role reversal usually opens up a patient's confession of the ill effects of alcohol. Yet, it does not make him quit the bottle's spirit. (Only a technique of interviewing still unknown to us could do that. If detected, it truly would deserve the Nobel prize.)

The role reversal prepared the patient to discuss more honestly the negative effects of alcohol (A. 28–44). It initiated the process of Mr. W. helping himself to detect and admit his self-deception and inability to control his drinking (A. 35–37, 48). Next the interviewer could point out a greater weakness than loss of control of drinking—the patient's deceiving himself about that loss of control (Q. 58).

Step 5: Approve

P: I do, don't I?
59. I: Well, remember what you told me at the beginning of the interview about your wife and your employee?

P: Thanks for reminding me. Doc, I feel ashamed. I feel like a fool.

60. I: It's often hard to look at our own weaknesses. Today you were able to face up to your problems. Such honesty with yourself will help you in your treatment.

P: I want to sign a contract with you that I'll never drink again.

61. I: I don't want you to do that.

P: Why not?

62. I: Because it's too easy. About 90% of alcoholics drink again within a year after quitting. I want you to tell yourself that alcohol is your problem, not your wife, not your employee. I want you to join AA [Alcoholics Anonymous], join a 12-step program and stop drinking as soon as you can after you start, if you do drink again. You know that to stop drinking is not a one-time contract matter. Every day you will feel the temptation and every day you have to win against it.

With empathy, the interviewer praised the patient for his ability to overcome his self-deception (A. 60). Yet, the patient remained self-deceptive about his ability to stop drinking (A. 60). The interviewer attempted to correct the patient's overconfidence with a more realistic view (Q. 62). Self-deception about drinking as well as drinking itself is a chronic behavior that interferes with the patient's progress. A patient cannot overcome self-deception in a one-time diagnostic interview, but the therapist can help him recognize his self-deception and keep it in focus for the remainder of his treatment. Mr. W.'s awareness of both his drinking problem and his self-deceptive attitude provided the insight necessary for successful interviewing and treatment.

Diagnosis

Axis I.   Alcohol abuse.

5. Interview B: Bulimia Nervosa

Ms. V. is a 17-year-old, white, slim girl who is a junior in high school. (I = interviewer; P = patient)

1. I: Hi. I'm Dr. O. What kind of problem brought you to see me?

P: [Looks up to the ceiling] No problems. [Shakes her head] I don't have any problems. I shouldn't even be here. [Scoots back and forth in her chair]

2. I: But you are here.

P: [Shrugs her shoulders] Yeah, I know. [Forces a grin] Isn't that stupid? [Bobbing her head back and forth] I kind of get into things.

Usually an interviewer initiates rapport by expressing empathy for the patient's suffering. Ms. V., however, denied suffering by withholding her chief complaint. Therefore, the interviewer could not express empathy. This put the interviewer on the alert. Disorders to consider at this point should fulfill two criteria: 1) the patient's lack of insight that she has a disorder and 2) the patient's self-deceit about her disorder. Among the diagnostic possibilities were embarrassing obsessions and compulsions, agoraphobia or other phobias, or sexually deviant behavior.

This brief exchange contained signs of deceit: contradiction (the patient arranged to see the psychiatrist but stated she was in the wrong place), opposition, emotional discomfort, distraction, and a defensive attitude (A. 1, 2; see Chapter 13, "Falsifying and Lying").

Therefore, the interviewer switched gears to the five-step approach.

Step 1: Listen

3. I: Well, what was on your mind when you called for an appointment?
   P: [Blows air out through her nose, shrugs her shoulders] Nothing in particular. I just did it. [Keeps her shoulders pulled up]
4. I: Maybe you can just tell me what you're worried about.
   P: [Shaking her head] You see, that's just it. I'm not the one who's worried about anything. [Contracts her eyes to a slit] I'm a straight-A student, I lead the football cheerleading squad. My mom even likes my boyfriend. He's the high school quarterback.
5. I: You mean, somebody else might be worried?
   P: [Frowning] Yeah, maybe.
6. I: Who?
   P: [Blowing air through her nose again] It's just my girlfriend. [Angles her head over her right shoulder] I guess I told her something and she just jumped to conclusions.
7. I: Conclusions? [Pausing] Like what?
   P: Like me having a problem.
8. I: Tell me about it. What is it that your friend thinks is a problem?
   P: I guess it has to do with the way I acted with her. It's really stupid. [Shaking her head] There isn't really any problem. She just misunderstood me. She blew things out of proportion. [Slapping her hands in her lap]
9. I: Do you care to tell me?
   P: [Flinching] Not really. See, it's all so stupid. It's really a long story, too long to get into it. I should just forget it. [Wiping her mouth with her hand]
10. I: You look stressed. It must be really difficult to talk about your problem.
    P: [Sarcastic] Maybe that's because I don't think I've got one.

Ms. V.'s mental status alerted the interviewer to the presence of denial and self-deception. She negated her problem and indulged in self-praise, an indication of self-deception (A. 4). However, she admitted a problem to her girlfriend—an indication of a double message (A. 6). The interviewer pressed for a chief complaint to gauge the degree of her resistance. His empathy (Q. 10) was met by a defensive patient. Her verbal and nonverbal negation of symptoms reinforced the impression that she was in denial (A. 4, 8, 10) because she used facial expressions and symbolic gestures (A. 3, 8) that were not spontaneous but under voluntary control and planted. Furthermore, a telling gesture slips out—she wipes her mouth with her hand as if to remind herself to be quiet (A. 9).

Step 2: Tag

11. I: I guess, then, we have to find out what exactly made you decide to call for an appointment. You did so for a reason, didn't you?
    P: Hmmm. I'm not sure. [Hovers down]
12. I: You mean you acted without a reason?
    P: [Raises her eyebrows] Not exactly. [Leaning forward] My friend and I had a conversation and she told my mother about it. They both pressured me to come here.
13. I: What was your conversation about?
    P: I really don't know if I want to get into all that. [Bites her left thumbnail]
14. I: You're reluctant to go into that?
    P: I guess. [Chewing her thumb]

The interviewer tagged the patient's resistance by insisting on a chief complaint. He put her in a double bind. She either functioned as a logical person—in which case she should have a chief complaint—or was illogical—in which case her behavior would raise concerns. In both instances, her visit with a mental health professional would be justified (A. 11, 12). The interviewer alerted her to the fact that she either appeared impulsive by arranging an appointment without good reason, or was being uncooperative at the interview. She blamed others for making the arrangement. Her desire to appear rational while at the same time showing irrational behavior produced pressure, anxiety, and discomfort, as expressed in her nonverbal responses (A. 13, 14). Ambivalence and indecisiveness are signs of major depression and obsessive-compulsive disorder.

Step 3: Confront

15. I: Let me summarize what we have learned so far.
    P: [Despondent] We haven't learned anything, have we?
16. I: Oh, I think we have learned a lot.
    P: [Startled and frightened] We have?

17. I: Yes, we have. Let me summarize for you. You live way out, across the state line. You made an appointment and came all this way to tell me that you are a straight-A student and a cheerleader and have the quarterback as a boyfriend.

    P: [Shrugs shoulders and throws her head back in defiance]

18. I: What do you tell yourself about being a straight-A student and a cheerleader?

    P: I don't talk to myself. I'm not psychotic.

This confrontation was limited to a short exchange. It brought into focus what had been indirectly implied in Step 2—namely, that there was another side to Ms. V.'s proclaimed success story.

Step 4: Solve

19. I: I don't mean talking aloud. I mean the silent talk that we all engage in when we think about something.

    P: [The angles of her mouth sink, she flashes on a depressive expression.] I think it's good. Many girls are envious of me. [Leans backward, chin in the air crossing her legs]

20. I: Okay, I can see that you are quite proud. You've done it. You are very successful. You did what other girls just dream about. What else do you tell yourself?

    P: [A depressed facial expression flashes on again, she sits up straight] What do you mean? What else should I tell myself?

21. I: What about your future?

    P: [Without enthusiasm] Well, it's still a year off. I'll go to college. Study English, or maybe premed or prelaw.

22. I: And I guess you'll have a 4.0 GPA [grade point average]. You are the quarterback's girlfriend, a cheerleader, slim and trim—the American success story. Everything seems to be possible for you.

    P: [Her face and shoulders drop, then she smiles and says with a hollow voice] I'm looking . . . looking forward to that.

23. I: [Raises eyebrows]

    P: Why do you make such a face?

24. I: [Frowning] Hmmm.

    P: Why do you go "hmmm"?

25. I: I just wonder how you feel about that future college success. You really don't look that happy when you talk about it. What do you tell yourself about it?

    P: [Frowning] It'll take a lot.

26. I: But you did it all through high school. You are on top of your class. You're in with the guys—you got the quarterback.

    P: [Looks out the window as if daydreaming, then looks at the interviewer] I'm sorry, what were we talking about?

27. I: About how successful you've been and will be.

    P: [Looks down in her lap]

28. I: What's missing?
   P: [Looks up, then shakes her head] I'm sorry, I was just thinking about what got me here.
29. I: Oh?
   P: Okay. [Pause] My friend and I went to have a pizza and I was pretty hungry. So after we had one, I ordered two more mediums. My friend said, "My God, you're eating them both? I don't understand how you can eat so much and stay so slim." And that's what really started it all.
30. I: So what did you tell her?
   P: I told her that I've always been able to eat a lot. It doesn't seem to affect me.
31. I: What do you mean, it doesn't affect you?
   P: Well, she asked me why don't I get fat if I eat so much.
32. I: So, that's what started it all. You eat a lot but you don't gain weight. And that made your friend think you should see a psychiatrist?
   P: Yeah—see what I mean? Isn't that ridiculous?
33. I: Yes, if that's all, then it is indeed ridiculous. But maybe there's something else that made your friend wonder?
   P: Like what? There's nothing.
34. I: There isn't?
   P: No, not really.
35. I: We better talk about that some more. What do you do to stay so slim after eating two and a half pizzas?
   P: I don't eat that much all the time.
36. I: Are you telling me you were bingeing?
   P: I never said that. You're putting words in my mouth.
37. I: You're right, I did do that. But I hope those words tell it like it is. So, let's get back to your bingeing.
   P: I just eat when I'm hungry. And when I'm not hungry, I don't eat that much.
38. I: How do you feel when you eat that much?
   P: I feel good. Relaxed.
39. I: At what point do you feel relaxed?
   P: Oh, right away.
40. I: And what do you think about then? What do you tell yourself when you have all that food in your stomach?
   P: No, no, no! Leave me alone! They are my thoughts. You have no right to get in my head and screw them up.
41. I: That's not what I want to do. I want to help you to understand and be aware of your thoughts.
   P: I don't think anything. I just eat.
42. I: But you stay so slim. If you binge, how do you stay slim? What do you do after bingeing?
   P: Nothing, I just won't eat for a while.
43. I: So you starve?
   P: Why do you call it starving? I just eat normally.
44. I: Will you help me understand? [Pause] You eat a lot at times—you binge eat. And then you eat normally. So what is your secret for staying so slim?
   P: I work out more.

45. I: When you exhaust yourself and starve yourself, what do you tell yourself?
    P: Not really anything.
46. I: You came here to talk about your problems, about how you eat and how you talk to yourself about it.
    P: [Hesitating] I don't know.
47. I: What's your self-talk?
    P: [Fumbles, shrugs her shoulders, and looks away]
48. I: Before you binge, what do you tell yourself?
    P: I feel anxious. Very anxious.
49. I: Hungry?
    P: [Shakes her head]
50. I: What are your thoughts? Tell me. Use all the words that come to your mind, whether they fit or not.
    P: Ravingly . . . hollow . . . empty . . . anxious . . . as if I'm not there.
51. I: So you eat and eat and eat. What do you tell yourself when you do that?
    P: I'm getting there.
52. I: When you eat, what do you think about?
    P: I think something will happen. Something big. I eat to find out what will happen. And then I'm full.
53. I: And you said you feel relieved?
    P: [Flinches again, wiggles]
54. I: You really don't look that relieved. What do you tell yourself?
    P: [Tense, presses her lips together] You're pushing me. [Takes a deep breath and keeps the air in]
55. I: Sorry I pushed you. You look ready to explode.
    P: [Retracts her head between her shoulders and squeezes the air out]
56. I: So what do you tell yourself when you are full of food?
    P: [Closes her eyes and shakes her body]
57. I: When you feel pushed and ready to explode?
    P: [Swallows rapidly]
58. I: What do you think?
    P: [Frowns]
59. I: What is so painful that you can't talk about?
    P: [Makes a noise as if ready to vomit]
60. I: What do you say to yourself?
    P: I really don't want to talk about it. It's gross.
61. I: I know. It's embarrassing for you . . . whether you should or shouldn't tell.
    P: I don't like it. You act as if you can read my mind.
62. I: I can't read your mind, Ms. V., but I can tell you what your behavior tells me. Your behavior tells me you're a binge eater and that you worry about it. So you do something about your bingeing but you are not ready to tell me what that is.
    P: Can't you understand that?
63. I: Yes, I understand that you are embarrassed about what you think. You have a problem in telling me.
    P: [Nods]
64. I: Your real problem is not what you tell or don't tell me, but what you told yourself after you binged with your friend.

P: No! No! Stop!

65. I: Ms. V., you make talking to me the problem. But you know it's not. What you tell yourself about the bingeing is the problem. So, what did you tell yourself after you binged with your friend?

P: [Suddenly talking rapidly] I thought, "Oh my God! She thinks I'm a pig. I'm a glutton. I'll be fat. She thinks I'm a big wastebasket. All this pizza will go in my waist and hips and legs. I'll be so bloated. I'll have to get rid of it. I have to spit it all out." So I went to the bathroom. But I don't want to tell you about that.

66. I: I can only help you if you tell me your thoughts.

P: I just vomit . . . I don't even have to put my finger in my throat . . . vomit until the blood comes up. Now, are you satisfied?

67. I: And you do this without asking for help?

P: Help? Who am I supposed to ask, my mother? Hah, a couple of months ago she read something about bulimia in a magazine. She just laughed and said, "How stupid can people be? Eat and then just puke it all out!?"

68. I: [Looking at the patient and then looking down in his lap]

P: Do you really think that she would understand that her own daughter does this stupid thing—eating and vomiting? Do you? [More urgently] Do you?

69. I: [After more silence] How long have you been doing this?

P: I don't know. Maybe 2 years.

70. I: How many times a week do you binge?

P: Two, three times . . . I don't know.

71. I: Have you done anything else to keep your weight down?

P: [Impatient] Yes, yes, yes. [Wrinkles her nose and exhales with a hiss] I take laxatives but they don't work anymore. Sometimes I'll go jogging until my knees collapse.

In response to the patient's self-serving and self-deceptive statements, the interviewer asked her repeatedly for her self-talk (Q. 20, 25, 40, 45, 47, 48, 50–52, 54, 56, 58, 60, 64–66). As more details emerge, solving of the patient's self-deception progresses in logical sequence. The interviewer started out by exploring what Ms. V. told herself about her success as a straight-A student and cheerleader. She responded with verbal self-praise, which contradicted her nonverbal facial expressions (A. 19–22). The interviewer picked up on her nonverbal message by using nonverbal expressions of disbelief and doubt himself (Q. 23–25). This response prompted Ms. V. to reduce her displayed self-confidence (A. 23–25). She admitted that she expected some difficulties. Thus, the interviewer had sliced off her most obvious layer of self-deceptive behavior.

After the patient admitted some difficulties, the interviewer propelled her self-revelation by using role reversal—namely, praising the patient himself. This allowed Ms. V. to experience some more self-doubt and she dissociated into a daydream (A. 26–28). When addressed, she started to admit some problems but dissimulated and minimized them. The interviewer responded with doubt (Q. 29–37). He translated her story into psychiatric symptom language (Q. 36, 43, 45).

Next the interviewer focused the patient on a critical situation, namely how she felt when she was filled with food. This activated the patient's anxiety and resistance to and critique of the interviewer (A. 40–45). The interviewer continued to focus the patient toward the feelings that she experienced before, during, and after bingeing. He also confronted her with the contradiction between the way she described her feelings and her body language. This prompted her to admit her suffering (A. 46–63) but not without critique directed toward the interviewer (A. 54, 60–62). The interviewer confronted her with this resistance (Q. 64–66). This confrontation persuaded Ms. V. to admit her pattern of bingeing and vomiting and reveal the severity of her bulimia (Q. and A. 64–71). She also showed a change in her mental status. She quit censoring her words and released her negative feelings. This change was paralleled by a switch in affect from a restricted (up to Q. 61) to a fuller range (after Q. 62). She began to show anxiety (A. 64), anger, shame (A. 66), and disgust (A. 71).

Step 5: Approve

72. I: Ms. V., I'm glad that you broke your silence. Maybe we should have a conference with you and your mother together. Would she come?

P: I don't know.

73. I: Well, she's concerned. She did send you here.

P: Not really. My friend told her that I have a problem, but she didn't say what it is.

74. I: Is that true?

P: Yes. Mom likes my friend. She trusts her. My friend told her I should first see a shrink just to find out whether there really is something wrong. Mom said she couldn't imagine what kind of problem her darling daughter could have, but she knows all teenagers have something wrong with them, so she said okay.

75. I: I feel you have made great progress in opening up about your bingeing. I'm glad that you came and that we could talk about it.

P: I guess. Most people wouldn't understand what I'm going through. They'd think I was a sicko if they knew.

76. I: So, you feel even your friends would dump you?

P: Yeah. I'll never tell.

77. I: Is this why you didn't want to tell me?

P: Of course! Mom and my friend will ask what I talked to you about. Now I'll have to tell them, unless I want to lie.

78. I: Is this what you tell yourself?

P: Isn't that right? Unless you want me to lie about what I told you.
79. I: Well, you could put the blame on me.
P: What do you mean?
80. I: You could tell your mother and your friend that I asked you not to discuss with them what we talked about.
P: Keep a secret from them?
81. I: You have been doing that for the last 2 years anyway. And that has isolated you, hasn't it? But now you and I will face your problem together. Maybe it'd better for you to talk with your mother and your friends about this after it's all over, not while we are still in the middle of trying to sort it all out.
P: That makes me feel better. Then I can talk to people without having to lie.

In Step 5 the interviewer gave positive feedback about the patient's disclosure. The patient assumed that she had to reveal her problem to everybody. The interviewer resolved her concern (Q. 80), thereby fortifying the bond with her. In this way, he erected a protective wall around the patient and himself, enhancing the patient's sense of trust and safety. This shared insight deepened the rapport and established a therapeutic alliance for the moment.

Diagnosis

This patient has bulimia nervosa, purging type. Her secret is binge eating, vomiting, laxative use, starvation, and strenuous exercise. Patients with bulimia nervosa may report depressive symptoms preceding or coexisting with their bulimia. A similar association exists with anxiety symptoms. The number of symptoms is often sufficient to make the diagnosis of one or more of the following disorders: dysthymic disorder, major depressive disorder, or any of the anxiety disorders, especially obsessive-compulsive disorder, which would explain our patient's stubbornness noticed early in the interview.

Two substances are preferentially abused by patients with bulimia nervosa—stimulants and alcohol. Patients explain their stimulant use as an attempt to control appetite and weight. Reasons for abuse of alcohol are less clear. Patients with bulimia nervosa often express how powerless they feel about the size of their appetites and their weight gain. Especially when their "compensatory behaviors" (DSM-IV, American Psychiatric Association 1994, p. 547) such as purging, starving, and laxative abuse fail, they experience feelings of anxious hopelessness. One may speculate that these patients drink alcohol in an attempt to overcome these feelings.

Impulsivity links bulimia nervosa with borderline personality disorder. According to DSM-IV, probably one-third to one-half of patients with bulimia nervosa have an associated personality disorder.

Sorting out this tangle for Ms. V., however, is a diagnostic task that must wait for the next session.

6. Self-Deception, Cognitive Analysis of Self-Talk, and the Defensive Functioning Scale in Psychiatric Disorders

Having a psychiatric disorder can be socially stigmatizing. Some afflicted patients may use self-deception to avoid thinking of themselves as "mentally ill." Thus, a patient who abuses drugs or alcohol may conceal his addiction from himself and others. Usually, his self-deception occurs at two different occasions: first, at the time when he drinks; second, at the time when his drinking is discussed.

One example is the alcoholic patient who has committed himself to sobriety because he knows that the first drink will release an avalanche of more drinking and ensuing social problems. When he reaches for the bottle again, he tells himself that he can stop after one drink. When he cannot, he tells himself that he drinks because this is the only way to cope with the stress at work, with his family, and with his financial problems. Then he continues drinking until he passes out. Thus, self-deception first takes place when he breaks his commitment and drinks again.

The second deception takes place when his counselor asks him if he has been drinking since the last session. He denies it, justifying his self-deception to himself in his self-talk such as,

> The counselor is a purist. He cannot understand what I'm going through. I really did well except for that one incidence. Therefore, it's more accurate not to report the drinking than to admit the relapse and look like a loser, when in fact I'm not.

Thus, a second layer of self-deception covers the primary one.

The patient stores two memories in his memory bank:

1. I drank and broke my commitment to sobriety.
2. I did not really drink. I maintained my ability to cope with my problems. If I did it by drinking, that was just coincidental.

When the patient recalls the drinking episode with his counselor, he addresses not his first but his second memory trace. He shows signs of self-deception, such as avoidance of and distraction from this topic. He glorifies his sobriety to suppress the memory trace of the relapse. Therefore, when you entice the patient to focus on the first memory trace rather than the preferred second one, you arouse his anger and his doubt in your allegiance to him.

Similar denial takes place in patients with other disorders:

- A patient who recovers from psychotic symptoms may deny them later.
- Patients with somatoform disorders deny that interpersonal conflicts contribute to their somatic symptoms.
- Patients with dissociative disorders show amnesia before they admit a social coping deficit that may have precipitated their dissociative state.
- Sexual deviations are prone to double denial, both to others and to patients themselves. Even though homosexuality is no longer viewed as a psychiatric disorder, homosexual individuals may hide their sexual orientation not only from others (by "staying in the closet") but also from themselves (self-deception). Some persons may admit to homosexual fantasies but then reject them as unacceptable (ego-alien).
- Patients with a paraphilia frequently hide this tendency from the public, admitting it only to consenting others, or suppress it from themselves.
- Double denial occurs in patients with an eating disorder who minimize the severity of their condition or their body image.
- Patients with an impulse-control disorder downplay the severity of their disorder, or deny its existence: "I don't remember. I must have been drunk when I beat my wife."
- A patient affected with a cluster B personality disorder may deny his failure in job, marriage, family, and community life. He does not want to discuss it. Yet, he wants relief from the stress. He feels tense, anxious, nervous, and anhedonic. He talks about his somatic complaints, but seals off their origin.

To make a patient aware of her self-talk is useful in all psychiatric disorders. Patients synchronize their pathological behaviors with automatic, unchallenged thoughts. The depressed patient, for example, tells herself her future is hopeless, and the agoraphobic patient, that the crowded supermarket is dangerous. Challenging these self-talks as illogical helps the patient to reflect on her feelings, impulses, and actions. Cognitive analysis of self-talk attempts to break the patient's automatic stimulus-reaction chain and gives her better adjusted choices. Initially, these choices may appear theoretical to her but constant reinforcement of rational and critical thoughts assists her in overcoming her irrational self-talk.

The Difficult Patient and the Defensive Functioning Scale

The Defensive Functioning Scale in Appendix B of DSM-IV (pp. 751–757) provides an approach to conceptualizing the patient with self-deceptive behavior in terms of his use of defense mechanisms. Other difficulties encountered with patients in this volume can also be viewed in terms of a psychological defense. This scale rates the patient's adaptive ability in terms of 31 defense mechanisms. They are organized into seven levels according to how they allow handling of the patient's stressors and conscious awareness of feelings, ideas, and their consequences.

The disorders that interfere most with the clinical interviewing are those in levels 2–7. Patients who use symptom language (Part I of this book) show the seven defense mechanisms of level 2. Patients with psychotic communication (Part II) show defense mechanisms of levels 5–7. Patients with cognitive impairment (Part III) may use defenses of level 4, especially when they deny or rationalize their cognitive deficit. Patients who conceal, deceive others, fabricate, or deceive themselves (Part IV) often show coping styles of levels 3 and 4.

Familiarity with these defense mechanisms may help you understand how a patient copes with his deficiencies and the stressors he is exposed to. It may also help you to improve your rapport with the patient and thus your interview.

EPILOGUE

◆ ◆ ◆ ◆ ◆

If knowledge is an artifact, will we go on inventing it, endlessly?

James Burke
The Day the Universe Changed (1985)

◆ ◆ ◆ ◆ ◆

The Interview as the Beginning of Therapy

Interviewing the difficult patient builds a bridge between diagnosis and therapy.

With the described approach and techniques, we have attempted to show how to create rapport. Rapport establishes trust in communicating between a patient in distress and an interviewer who strives to get in touch. In this book, we did not cover other difficulties that may inhibit rapport, such as differences in gender, age, or culture between patient and therapist. In addition, special difficulties arise from situational factors, such as interviewing in the emergency room or within the penal system. To master all of these difficulties we need rapport. Rapport is the basis of the diagnostic interview (as described in *The Clinical Interview Using DSM-IV, Volume 1: Fundamentals* [Othmer and Othmer 1994])—even more so in the interview with the difficult patient. However, it transcends both types of interviews. It determines the success of therapy. There is no success without rapport.

We aim to resolve conflicts, not exacerbate them. Some of the techniques we use are taken from the world of psychotherapy, such as the plus-minus approach, the cognitive method, free association, validation of unexplained somatic symptoms, and hypnosis. Some belong to the field of neuropsychiatry, such as focused neuropsychological assessment, some belong to the legal system, such as cross-examination and voice-stress analysis.

The interview techniques described require empathy toward patients who need attention the most—those with whom it is difficult to speak. Empathy helps us to communicate. It is the basis for the therapeutic relationship that lasts beyond the initial interview sessions described here. Thus, the interviewer's empathy is the foundation of care on which the healing process is built.

The Pyramid of Psychiatric Problems

Interviewing the difficult patient is the ultimate diagnostic task for a therapist who faces the pyramid of the patient's different layers of problems as represented in the five DSM-IV (American Psychiatric Association 1994) axes.

On the base of this pyramid lies the patient's *general medical condition,* represented in Axis III. Psychiatric care fails if somatic problems are not attended to. For example, unrecognized and untreated endocrine or neurological disorders will obscure psychiatric diagnoses and prevent successful treatment of psychiatric disorders. This book attends to this layer by teaching how to look out for subtle signs of dementia, delirium, and the amnestic disorders that often originate from general medical conditions. Furthermore, it deals with the patient who shows symptoms and signs that seemingly represent the medical layer, such as somatic and pseudo-neurological symptoms and altered states of consciousness.

The next layer in the pyramid represents psychiatric health or illness as summarized in the form of *clinical syndromes and personality disorders* on Axes I and II, respectively. Obviously, all chapters of this book address symptoms, signs, and behaviors of these disorders.

The third layer in the pyramid represents the impact that physical and psychiatric disorders have on the patient's life and how life stressors together with *psychosocial and environmental problems* afflict the patient's level of functioning. These stressors are addressed on Axis IV. On Axis V the patient's Global Assessment of Functioning (GAF) Scale score is shown. This book attends to these problems by showing you how to deal with patients who conceal and falsify their problems or deny them to themselves.

The tip of the pyramid represents the patient's *potential*—his or her unrealized ability. This potential is the promise for patients' futures. It is the highest level of functioning, the highest GAF Scale score that they can reach. We would like all patients to reach that goal. It is the therapist's ideal to strive to help patients overcome the impact of the medical and psychiatric disorders and assist them in dealing with psychosocial and environmental problems. Patients may then reach the level of internal peace and satisfaction that living up to their potential may give. This book was written in this spirit and with this hope in mind.

The Executive Interview (EXIT) and the Qualitative Evaluation of Dementia (QED)

The disturbance of executive control functions is an important diagnostic criterion of dementia as defined in DSM-IV (American Psychiatric Association 1994). Royall et al. (1992) developed an instrument, called the Executive Interview (EXIT), to measure these functions at the bedside. They also developed a rating scale, the Qualitative Evaluation of Dementia (QED; Royall et al. 1993), which separates dementia into two clinical types—the cortical type, which is characterized by disinhibition, and the subcortical type, which is characterized by apathy. Although it remains to be seen whether these represent homogeneous subtypes, they provide the clinician with an operational procedure to assess and describe qualitative differences in cognition and behavior.

The Executive Interview (EXIT)

Patient's name: _____

Date: _____

Age: _____

Sex: _____

Diagnosis: _____

Education level in years: _____

TOTAL TEST SCORE: _____

Global Testing Observations

During the interview, record signs and behaviors that indicate a disturbance of executive functions. Seven types of pathological behaviors can be observed:

1. Perseveration
2. Imitation behavior
3. Intrusion
4. Frontal release signs
5. Lack of spontaneity/prompting needed
6. Disinhibited behavior
7. Utilization behavior

Source. From Royall DR, Mahurin RK, Gray KF: "Bedside Assessment of Executive Cognitive Impairment: The Executive Interview." *Journal of the American Geriatrics Society* 40:1221–1226, 1992. Used with permission. Edited, adapted, supplemented, and reformatted for this book by Ekkehard and Sieglinde C. Othmer. We thank Drs. Royall et al. for granting us permission for use of this instrument here.

Notice that each of the 25 test items of the EXIT may reflect one or more pathological behaviors. We give short definitions of the seven types as they apply to the EXIT and examples for each below. (I = interviewer; P = patient)

1. Perseveration. Patient responds with a requested behavior but repeats it over and over, inappropriately.

Examples
Test Item 1:
    P: 1A, 1A, 1A.
    or, P: 1A, 1B, 1C.
    or, P: 1A, 2A, 3A.
Test Item 2:
    P: America, America, America.
Test Item 3:
    P copies one of the test examples or one of his/her own pictures over and over.

2. Imitation behavior. Patient repeats the interviewer's words (echolalia) or behaviors (echopraxia) rather than responding to them.

Examples
Test Item 1:
    I: 1A, 2B, 3—?
    P: 1A, 2B, 3—?
Test Item 2:
    P: People, pot, plan.
Test Item 3:
    Patient copies both test figures.
Test Items 16, 20, 25:
    Pathological response.

3. Intrusion. Inappropriately, patient includes items of a previous task in his/her response.

Examples
Test Item 2:
    Watch for intrusion from the local environment.
    P: America, axe, bird, chirping, nest . . .

Test Item 3:
  The patient starts one or two figures but then begins to draw related figures, such as cross, box, window, house, tree, car.
Test Items 6 and 7:
  Pathological responses.

4. Frontal release signs. These are reflexes that occur in patients with frontal lobe damage. Two of these frontal release signs, the grasp reflex and the snout reflex, are tested in test Items 10 and 13, respectively.

Examples
Test Item 10:
  Pathological response. Note when the patient's grasp is so firm that you can draw him/her out of the chair.
Test Item 13:
  Pathological response. Note if the patient, in addition to a snout reflex, shows puckering even before tapping (suck reflex).

5. Lack of spontaneity. The interviewer has to encourage the patient again and again to respond to the tasks. The patient responds with a long latency time. He/she gives only one response when a series of responses is requested.

Examples
Test Item 1:
  P: 1
  I: And what letter?
  P: A.
  I: What comes next?
  P: 2.
  Patient answers correctly but needs prompting to go on.
Test Item 5:
  Pathological response.
Test Item 22:
  P: December *[and looks at the interviewer]*
  I: Keep going!
  P: November *[then stops again]*

6. Disinhibited behavior. The patient responds as requested but ignores limiting test specifications.

Examples

Test Item 1:

The patient continues after the stop signal has been given, such as saying, "6F, 7G, 8H."

Test Item 2:

P: America, America *[starts singing "God shed his grace on thee, and bound thy good with brotherhood from sea to shining sea."]*

Test Item 4:

Pathological response.

Test Item 25:

P: *[Touches interviewer's wrist]* "Wrist."

7. Utilization behavior. The patient substitutes the logical or the requested response with a response that reflects a social habit or frequent usage.

Examples

Test Item 3:

P looks at the sheet and signs his/her name.

Test Item 11:

P: You are welcome.

Test Item 24:

Pathological response.

Materials Needed for the EXIT

- Stopwatch
- Three test cards with test Items 5 (cat chasing bird), 7 (brown), and 23 (four fish and shell)
- Two recording sheets for test Items 2 (word fluency) and 3 (design fluency)

Test instructions	0	1	2	Score
1. NUMBER-LETTER TASK I: I'd like you to say some numbers and letters for me like this: "1A, 2B, 3—What would come next?" P: C. I: Now you try it, starting with the number 1. Keep going until I say stop. P: 1A, 2B, 3C, 4D, 5E . . . . I: Stop.	No errors	Needs prompting	Does not complete task	
2. WORD FLUENCY I: I'm going to give you a letter. You have ONE MINUTE to name as many words as you can think of that begin with that letter. For example, with the letter *P* you could say "people," "pot," "plan," and so on. The letter is *A*. Go! *[Start stopwatch, record P's words on Recording Sheet 1 for word fluency (see p. 470) and stop after 1 minute.]*	10 or more words	5–9 words	Fewer than 5 words	
3. DESIGN FLUENCY *[Draw two pictures on Recording Sheet 2 (see p. 471).]* I: Look at these pictures. Each is made with only four lines. I'm going to give you ONE MINUTE to draw as many different designs as you can. They each must be different and be drawn with four lines. Now, go! *[Hand P Recording Sheet 2, on which you drew the two designs. Then start the stopwatch and stop after 1 minute. Correct figures can contain curves.]*	10 or more unique drawings, no copies of examples	5–9 unique drawings	Fewer than 5 unique drawings	

	No errors	One or more errors	Continues one or more sentences (e.g., "Mary had a little lamb whose fleece was white as snow.")
4. ANOMALOUS SENTENCE REPETITION I: Listen very carefully and repeat these sentences exactly: 1) I pledge allegiance to those flags. 2) Mary fed a little lamb. 3) A stitch in time saves lives. 4) Tinkle, tinkle little star. 5) A B C D U F G.	No errors	One or more errors	Continues one or more sentences (e.g., "Mary had a little lamb whose fleece was white as snow.")
5. THEMATIC PERCEPTION *[Show P the picture of the cat chasing the bird.]* I: Tell me what is happening in the picture.	Tells spontaneous story (story = setting, three characters, action)	Tells story with one prompt ("anything else?")	Fails to tell story despite prompt
6. MEMORY/DISTRACTION TASK I: Remember these three words: book, tree, house. *[Have P repeat words until they are registered.]* Remember them. I'll ask you to repeat them later. Now, spell *cat* for me. . . . Good. Now, spell it backward. OK. Tell me those three words we learned.	Names all three words correctly without *cat* *[I may prompt, "Anything else?"]*	Other responses (describe)	Names *cat* as one of the three words (intrusion)
7. INTERFERENCE TASK *[Show the card with the word* brown *and sweep index finger over all letters.]* I: What color are these letters?	Black	P: Brown *[Repeat question once]*; P: Black.	P: Brown *[Prompt]*; P: Brown (intrusion)
8. AUTOMATIC BEHAVIOR I I: Please, hold your hands forward, palms down. Relax while I check your reflexes. *[Rotate P's arms one at a time at the elbow as if to check for cogwheeling. Gauge P's active participation/ anticipation of the rotation.]*	Remains passive	Equivocal	Actively copies the circular motion

Note. I = interviewer; P = patient.

(continued)

Test instructions	0	1	2	Score
9. AUTOMATIC BEHAVIOR II I: Please, hold your hands out palms up. Just relax. *[Push down on P's hands—gently at first, becoming more forceful. Gauge P's active participation in the response.]*	No resistance, remains passive	Equivocal	Active resistance or compliance	
10. GRASP REFLEX I: Please hold your hands out with open palms down. Just relax. *[Lightly and simultaneously stroke both palms of P's hands from roots to fingertips with both of your hands palms up, fingers gently curved upward. Look for grasping/gripping actions in P's fingers.]*	Absent	Equivocal	Present	
11. SOCIAL HABIT *[Fixate on P's eyes. Silently count to 3 while maintaining P's gaze. Then say:]* I: Thank you.	Replies with a question (e.g., "Thank you for what?")	Other responses (describe)	P: You're welcome.	
12. MOTOR IMPERSISTENCE I: Stick out your tongue and say "aah" until I say stop . . . Go! *[Count to 3 silently. P must sustain a constant tone, not "ah . . . ah . . . ah . . ."]*	Completes task spontaneously	Completes task with I modeling task for patient	Fails task despite modeling by I	
13. SNOUT REFLEX I: Just relax. *[Slowly bring your index finger toward P's lips, pausing momentarily 2 inches away. Then place finger vertically across lips, touching lips, and tap the finger lightly with the other hand so that the crossed finger touches P's upper lip. Observe lips for puckering before and after the tapping.]*	Not present	Equivocal	Present	

14. FINGER-NOSE-FINGER TASK [Hold up your index finger.]

I: Touch my finger. [Leaving your finger in place, say:]

I: Now touch your nose.

Complies, using same hand	Other response (describe)	Complies, using other hand while continuing to touch examiner's finger

15. GO/NO-GO TASK

I: Now when I touch my nose, you raise your finger like this. [Raise your index finger (F).] When I raise my finger, you touch your nose like this. [Touch your nose (N) with index finger.]

I: Please, repeat my instructions. [Begin task. Leave finger in place while awaiting P's response. Circle P's responses. Left column shows P's correct responses.]

Interviewer	Patient	
F	N	F
N	F	N
F	N	F
F	N	F
N	F	N

Performs sequence correctly, e.g., N-F-N-N-F	Correct, requires prompting/repeat of instructions	Fails sequence despite prompting/repeat of instructions

16. ECHOPRAXIA I

I: Now listen carefully. I want you to do exactly what I say. Ready? Touch your ear! [Touch your nose and keep finger there.]

Touches his/her ear	Other response (describe). [Look for midposition stance]	Touches his/her nose

Note. I = interviewer; P = patient.

(continued)

Test instructions	0	1	2	Score
17. LURIA HAND SEQUENCE I I: Can you do this? *[In the air, make a single hammering-like movement with your arm, the hand forming a fist. Then repeat the arm motion with an open palm, making a cutting motion. Alternate between hammering and cutting hand motions. Stop movement. P may use either arm.]*	Four cycles without error after I stops	Four cycles with additional verbal prompt ("Keep going") or modeling	Unsuccessful despite prompting/modeling *[Watch for mid-position stances.]*	
18. LURIA HAND SEQUENCE II I: Can you do this? *[Model three hand movements on your knee or table surface: 1) slapping with palm, 2) hammering with fist, 3) cutting with edge of opened hand.]* I: Now follow me. *[Repeat the sequence of three movements.]* I: Keep doing this until I say stop. [Stop, let P repeat three cycles, then ask P to stop.]	Three cycles without error after I stops	Three cycles with additional verbal prompt ("Keep going") or modeling	Unsuccessful	
19. GRIP TASK *[With both hands, form a pistol (e.g., a fist with stretched index finger and erected thumb). Point both index fingers toward each other in front of yourself, leaving a 1-inch space between the index fingers.]* I: Squeeze my fingers.	Grips fingers	Other response (describe)	Pulls I's hands together	
20. ECHOPRAXIA II *[Suddenly and without warning, slap your hands together.]*	Does not imitate I	Hesitates, uncertain	Imitates slap	

Task			
21. COMPLEX COMMAND TASK I: Put your left hand on top of your head and close your eyes. . . . That was good. [*Remain aloof, quickly begin next task.*]	Stops when next task begins	Equivocal—holds posture during part of next task.	Maintains posture throughout completion of next task—has to be told to cease
22. SERIAL ORDER REVERSAL TASK I: Please recite the months of the year. [*Disregard P's errors.*] I: Now, start with January and recite them backward! [*Ask P to stop after September if correctly recited.*]	Recites January, December, November, October, September . . . . I: Stop!	Correct response but with prompting	Unsuccessful despite prompting
23. COUNTING TASK [*Show P the fish picture.*] *Tap each item in a clockwise direction.*] I: Please count the fish in this picture out loud.	Four	Fewer than four	More than four
24. UTILIZATION BEHAVIOR [*Hold a pen near its point and dramatically present it to the patient asking:*] I: What is this called?	P: Pen	Reaches, hesitates	Takes the pen from I
25. IMITATION BEHAVIOR (ECHOPRAXIA III) [*Hold your wrist up, flex it up and down, and point to it.*] I: What is this called?	P: Wrist	Other response (describe)	Flexes wrist up and down

SCORE

TOTAL SCORE

Note. I = interviewer; P = patient.

EXIT Recording Sheet 1 for Test Item 2:
Word Fluency

Write down all words that P gives you within 1 minute.

1. _____

2. _____

3. _____

4. _____

5. _____

6. _____

7. _____

8. _____

9. _____

10. _____

EXIT Recording Sheet 2 for Test Item 3:
Design Fluency

Draw two pictures using only four lines for each.

Exit Scores and Activity of Daily Living (ADL)

Exit scores ADL

0–10   Independent, normal, unsupervised living of control subjects (normal 11-year-old and older)

11–12   Equivocal

13–17   Living with minimal supervision in apartments, using parking space and kitchen appropriately (normal 8- to 10-year-old)

18–23   Group home, residential care, no driving, not institutionalized, common dining, no independent shopping or cooking (normal grade schooler)

24–32   Skilled nursing facility, institutionalized, nurses, charts, fed on the unit, rehabilitation activity (normal preschooler)

33–50   Dementia of the Alzheimer's type, special care units

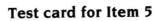

Test card for Item 5

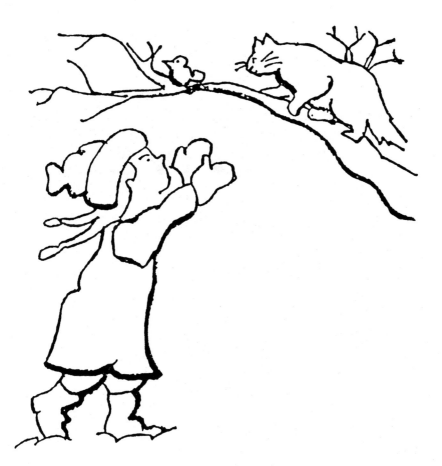

Test card for Item 7

brown

Test card for Item 23

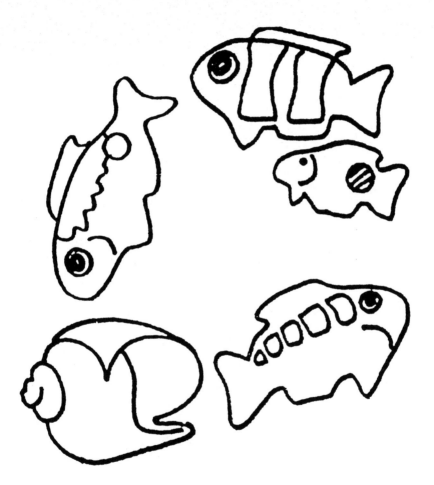

Qualitative Evaluation of Dementia (QED)

The Qualitative Evaluation of Dementia (QED) is an instrument designed to operationalize, standardize, and quantify the clinical concepts of cortical and subcortical dementia. The classical example of a predominantly cortical dementia is dementia of the Alzheimer's type; examples of predominantly subcortical dementias include vascular dementia and dementia due to major depressive disorder. This subtyping of dementia overlaps and parallels the subtyping of irreversible and reversible dementia, active and passive dementia, and disinhibited and apathetic dementia.

The QED discriminated patients with probable dementia of the Alzheimer's type ($n = 17$) from 1) those with no dementia as defined by criteria of the National Institute of Neurological and Communicative Disorders and Stroke (NINCDS) and the Alzheimer Disease and Related Disorders Association ($n = 22$), and 2) dementia patients without evidence of aphasia, agnosia, constructional apraxia, or memory deficits who did not improve with prompting ($n = 46$) (Royall et al. 1993). In another study, the QED distinguished 29 subjects with dementia due to major depressive disorder from 35 subjects with either dementia due to probable Alzheimer's disease ($n = 22$) or frontal lobe–type dementia ($n = 13$). The latter two cortical dementias could not be discriminated (Royall et al. 1994).

Source. Reprinted from Royall DR, Mahurin RK, Cornell J, et al.: "Bedside Assessment of Dementia Type Using the Qualitative Evaluation of Dementia." *Neuropsychiatry, Neuropsychology, and Behavioral Neurology* 6:235–244, 1993. Used with permission. We thank Drs. Royall et al. for granting us permission to reproduce this instrument here.

Directions

For each domain, first determine if an abnormality exists. If not, rate **NORMAL = 1.** If deficit is present, you **MUST** choose between the available alternatives. If insufficient information is available, rate as 1.

Domain	Clinical features			Score
	0	1	2	
Interview	Not spontaneous Short replies Little elaboration	Normal	Spontaneous and/or tangential. May be pressured	
Interview	Led to interview Little participation Prompting needed	Normal	Disinhibited Socially adroit but inappropriate	
Memory	Recalls 1–2 of 3 words spontaneously aided by prompting	Normal	Unable to recall 3 words after distraction. Not aided by prompts	
Orientation	Disoriented to time only	Normal	Disoriented to location or person	
Language	Word finding or mild comprehension deficits only	Normal	Paraphasias Poor comprehension Fluent or nonfluent aphasia, vague or empty speech	
Speech	Dysarthric Hypophonic	Normal	Perseverative, flat, effortful, or mumbling	
Frontal release	Gegenhalten or motor soft signs but no snout/ grasp	Normal	Snout or grasp present	
Judgment	Worried, complains, ruminates Says "I don't know" or "I can't"	Normal concern	Little insight Denies deficits Confabulates	

TOTAL PAGE 1 [ ]

Domain	Clinical features			Score
	0	1	2	
Constructions (See Mini-Mental State Exam [Folstein et al. 1975])	Recognizable but distorted by flattening or omissions	Normal	Unrecognizable Disorganized	
Praxis	Rarely initiates self-care/household chores, but does well if prompted	Normal	Tries to participate in self-care/household chores, but uses tools/appliances inappropriately	
Motor/gait	Shuffling Dyskinetic "Apractic" Prominent tremor	Normal	Spastic Hemiparetic or ataxic	
Mood	Depressed Apathetic Cries without provocation	Normal	Can be outgoing, even euphoric at times Sings, claps, can be prone to catastrophic reactions	
Behavior	Sits around Needs prompting or encouragement	Normal	Into trouble Habit driven Environmentally dependent Resists change Wanders	
Personal care	Cares for himself/herself, but disheveled, inattentive to details or appearance	Normal	Requires personal assistance in dressing, bathing, or toileting	
Community affairs	Rarely asks to leave house, room, unit	Normal	Goes out but needs constant supervision at home or in public Easily lost, anxious, or confused	

TOTAL PAGE 2

QED TOTAL

A QED score of 0 indicates pure subcortical dementia characterized by apathy, and a score of 30 indicates pure cortical dementia characterized by disinhibition. A score of 15 indicates normal function.

BIBLIOGRAPHY

Abrams R, Taylor MA: Catatonia: a prospective clinical study. Arch Gen Psychiatry 33:579–581, 1976

Abrams R, Taylor MA: Catatonia: prediction of response to somatic treatments. Am J Psychiatry 134:78–80, 1977

Abrams R, Taylor MA, Stolurow KC: Catatonia and mania: patterns of cerebral dysfunction. Biol Psychiatry 14:111–117, 1979

Akhtar S, Buckman J: The differential diagnosis of mutism: a review and a report of three unusual cases. Diseases of the Nervous System 38:558–563, 1977

Allport GW: Personality and Social Encounter: Selected Essays. Boston, MA, Beacon Press, 1960

Altshuler LL, Cummings JL, Mills MJ: Mutism: review, differential diagnosis, and report of 22 cases. Am J Psychiatry 143:1409–1414, 1986

American Medical Association: Polygraph: Report of the Council on Scientific Affairs. JAMA 256:1172–1175, 1986

American Psychiatric Association: Diagnostic and Statistical Manual: Mental Disorders. Washington DC, American Psychiatric Association, 1952

American Psychiatric Association: Diagnostic and Statistical Manual of Mental Disorders, 3rd Edition. Washington DC, American Psychiatric Association, 1980

American Psychiatric Association: Diagnostic and Statistical Manual of Mental Disorders, 3rd Edition, Revised. Washington DC, American Psychiatric Association, 1987

American Psychiatric Association: Diagnostic and Statistical Manual of Mental Disorders, 4th Edition. Washington DC, American Psychiatric Association, 1994

Anderson E, Trethowan W: Psychiatry, 3rd Edition. London, Ballière, Tindall, 1973

Arkonac O, Guze SB: A family study of hysteria. N Engl J Med 268:239–242, 1963

Asher R: Munchausen syndrome. Lancet 1:339–341, 1951

Baldwin B, Förstl H: Pick's disease—101 years on: still there, but in need of reform. Br J Psychiatry 163:100–104, 1993

Bandler R, Grinder J: The Structure of Magic: A Book About Language and Therapy, Vols I and II. Palo Alto, CA, Science & Behavior Books, 1975

Barkley RA, Grodzinsky G, DuPaul GJ: Frontal lobe functions in attention deficit disorder with and without hyperactivity: a review and research report. J Abnorm Child Psychol 20:163–188, 1992

Baron DA, Nagy R: The amobarbital interview in a general hospital setting—friend or foe: a case report. Gen Hosp Psychiatry 10:220–222, 1988

Barsky AJ: Somatoform disorders, in Comprehensive Textbook of Psychiatry/V, 5th Edition, Vol 1. Edited by Kaplan HI, Sadock BJ. Baltimore, MD, William & Wilkins, 1989, pp 1009–1027

Bell AD: The PSE: a decade of controversy. Security Management 25(3):63–73, 1981

Bell IR: Somatization disorder: health care costs in the decade of the brain (editorial). Biol Psychiatry 35:81–83, 1994

Bellak L, Black RB: Attention-deficit hyperactivity disorder in adults. Clin Ther 14:138–147, 1992

Bernstein EM, Putnam FW: Development, reliability and validity of a dissociation scale. J Nerv Ment Dis 174:727–735, 1986

Blank AS: The unconscious flashback to the war in Viet Nam veterans: clinical mystery, legal defense, and community problem, in The Trauma of War: Stress and Recovery in Viet Nam Veterans. Edited by Sonnenberg SM, Blank AS, Talbott JA. Washington, DC, American Psychiatric Press, 1985, pp 293–308

Bleuler E: Textbook of Psychiatry (1916). Translated by Brill A. New York, Macmillan, 1924

Bleuler E: Lehrbuch der Psychiatrie: Zwölfte Auflage neubearbeitet von M. Bleuler, 12th Edition. Berlin, Springer-Verlag, 1972

Boccellari AA, Dilley JW: Management and residential placement problems of patients with HIV-related cognitive impairment. Hosp Community Psychiatry 43:32–37, 1992

Bohurt AC: Toward a cognitive theory of catharsis. Psychotherapy: Theory, Research and Practice 17:192–201, 1980

Boon S, Draijer N: Multiple personality disorder in the Netherlands: a clinical investigation of 71 patients. Am J Psychiatry 150:489–494, 1993

Boor M: The multiple personality epidemic: additional cases and inferences regarding diagnosis, etiology, dynamics, and treatment. J Nerv Ment Dis 170:302–304, 1982

Bouchard TJ Jr, Lykken DT, McGue M, et al: Sources of human physiological differences: the Minnesota study of twins reared apart. Science 250:223–228, 1990

Bowers KS: Dissociation in hypnosis and multiple personality disorder. Int J Clin Exp Hypn 39(3):155–176, 1991

Braid J: Neurypnology, or the Rationale of Nervous Sleep, Considered in Relation With Animal Magnetism: Illustrated by Numerous Cases of Its Successful Application in the Relief and Cure of Disease. London, J Churchill; Edinburgh, A & C Black, 1843

Braun BG: Iatrophilia and iatrophobia in the diagnosis and treatment of MPD. Dissociation: Progress in the Dissociative Disorders 2:66–69, 1989

Braun BG: Multiple personality disorder: an overview. Am J Occup Ther 44:971–976, 1990

Brende JO: Electrodermal responses in post-traumatic stress disorders. J Nerv Ment Dis 170:325–356, 1982

Brende JO: A psychodynamic view of character pathology in Vietnam combat veterans. Bull Menninger Clin 47:193–210, 1983

Brende JO: The use of hypnosis in post-traumatic conditions, in Posttraumatic Stress Disorder and the War Veteran Patient. Edited by Kelly WE. New York, Brunner/Mazel, 1985, pp 193–210

Breuer J, Freud S: Studies on Hysteria (1895). Translated by Strachey J, Freud A. New York, Basic Books, 1957

Briquet PL: Traité de L'Hysterie. Paris, JB Baillière & Fils, 1859

Buchanan A, Reed A, Wessely S: Acting on delusions, II: the phenomenological correlates of acting on delusions. Br J Psychiatry 163:77–81, 1993

Buhrich N, Cooper DA, Freed E: HIV infection associated with symptoms indistinguishable from functional psychosis. Br J Psychiatry 152:649–653, 1988

Buller DB, Strzyzewski KD, Comstock J: Interpersonal deception, I: deceivers' reaction to receivers' suspicions and probing. Communication Monographs 58:1–24, 1991

Bumke O: Lehrbuch der Geisteskrankheiten: Siebente Auflage. München, JF Bergmann, Berlin, Springer-Verlag, 1948

Byrne RW, Whiten A: Tactical deception of familiar individuals in baboons, in Machiavellian Intelligence: Social Expertise and the Evolution of Intellect in Monkeys, Apes and Humans. Edited by Byrne R, Whiten A. Oxford, England, Clarendon Press, 1988, pp 205–210

Cadoret RJ: Psychopathology in adopted-away offspring of biologic parents with antisocial behavior. Arch Gen Psychiatry 35:176–184, 1978

Cadoret RJ, Cunningham L, Loftus R, et al: Studies of adoptees from psychiatrically disturbed biological parents, III: medical symptoms and illness in childhood and adolescence. Am J Psychiatry 133:1316–1318, 1976

Caro M: Mike Caro's Book of Tells: The Body Language of Poker. Secaucus, NJ, Lyle Stuart, 1984

Carroll BT: Catatonia on the consultation-liaison service. Psychosomatics 33:310–315, 1992

Cloninger CR: Somatoform and dissociative disorders, in The Medical Basis of Psychiatry. Edited by Winokur G, Clayton PJ. Philadelphia, PA, WB Saunders, 1986, pp 123–151

Cloninger CR: Diagnosis of somatoform disorders: a critique of DSM-III, in Diagnosis and Classification in Psychiatry. Edited by Tischler GL. New York, Cambridge University Press, 1987, pp 243–259

Cloninger CR, Guze SB: Psychiatric illness and female criminality: the role of sociopathy and hysteria in the antisocial woman. Am J Psychiatry 127:303–311, 1970

Cohen ME, Robins E, Purtell JJ, et al: Excessive surgery in hysteria. JAMA 141:977–986, 1953

Cohen RA, Sparling-Cohen YA, O'Donnell BF: The Neuropsychology of Attention. New York, Plenum, 1993

Coons PM: Iatrogenesis and malingering of multiple personality disorder in the forensic evaluation of homicide defendants. Psychiatr Clin North Am 14:757–768, 1991

Coons PM, Bowman ES, Milstein V: Multiple personality disorder: a clinical investigation of 50 cases. J Nerv Ment Dis 176:519–527, 1988

Cooper S: The Clinical Use and Interpretation of the Wechsler Intelligence Scale for Children—Revised. Springfield, IL, Charles C Thomas, 1982

Corsini RJ: Current Psychotherapies. With the assistance of Wedding D. Itasca, IL, FE Peacock, 1984

Cummings JL: Frontal subcortical circuits and human behavior. Arch Neurol (in press)

Curtin SL: Recognizing multiple personality disorder. J Psychosoc Nurs Ment Health Serv 31:29–33, 1993

Davidson JRT, Foa EB (eds): Posttraumatic Stress Disorder: DSM-IV and Beyond. Washington, DC, American Psychiatric Press, 1993

DeFazio VJ: Dynamic perspectives on the nature and effects of combat stress, in Stress Disorders Among Vietnam Veterans: Theory, Research and Treatment. Edited by Figley CR. New York, Brunner/Mazel, 1978, pp 23–42

Degnan RE: Evidence, in Encyclopaedia Britannica, Vol 8. Chicago, IL, William Benton, 1968, p 905–916

DeJong RN, Haerer AF: Case taking and the neurologic examination, in Clinical Neurology, Vol 1, Revised. Edited by Joynt RJ. Philadelphia, PA, JB Lippincott, 1992, pp 1–89

de la Pena A: Post-traumatic stress disorder in the Vietnam veteran: a brain-modulated, compensatory, information-augmenting response to information underload in the central nervous system, in Post-Traumatic Stress Disorder: Psychological and Biological Sequelae. Edited by van der Kolk BA. Washington, DC, American Psychiatric Press, 1984, pp 107–122

Denckla MB: Attention deficit hyperactivity disorder—residual type. J Child Neurol 6 (suppl):S44–S50, 1991

deVito RA: The use of Amytal interviews in the treatment of an exceptionally complex case of multiple personality disorder, in Clinical Perspectives on Multiple Personality Disorder. Edited by Kluft RP, Fine CG. Washington, DC, American Psychiatric Press, 1993, pp 227–240

Dew MA, Bromet EJ, Brent D, et al: A quantitative literature review of the effectiveness of suicide prevention centers: fifth biennial workshop for the psychiatric epidemiological/statistics training programs. J Consult Clin Psychol 55:239–244, 1987

Dilley JW, Ochitill HN, Perl M, et al: Findings in psychiatric consultations with patients with acquired immune deficiency syndrome. Am J Psychiatry 142:82–86, 1985

Dobson KS (ed): Handbook of Cognitive-Behavioral Therapies. New York, Guilford, 1988

Donlon PT, Hopkin J, Tupin JP: Overview: efficacy and safety of the rapid neuroleptization method with injectable haloperidol. Am J Psychiatry 136:273–278, 1979

Dubin WR: Rapid tranquilization: antipsychotics or benzodiazepines? J Clin Psychiatry 49 (suppl):5–11, 1988

Dubin WR, Feld JA: Rapid tranquilization of the violent patient. Am J Emerg Med 7:313–320, 1989

Dubin WR, Waxman HM, Weiss KJ, et al: Rapid tranquilization: the efficacy of oral concentrate. J Clin Psychiatry 46:475–478, 1985

Dubin WR, Weiss KJ, Dorn JM: Pharmacotherapy of psychiatric emergencies. J Clin Psychopharmacol 6:210–222, 1986

Dynes JB: Objective method for distinguishing sleep from the hypnotic trance. Archives of Neurology and Psychiatry 57:84–93, 1947

Edgerton JE, Campbell RJ III (eds): American Psychiatric Glossary. Washington, DC, American Psychiatric Press, 1994

Edwards RH, Simon RP: Coma, in Clinical Neurology, Vol 1, Revised. Edited by Joynt RJ. Philadelphia, PA, JB Lippincott, 1992, pp 1–44

Efron D: Gesture, Race and Culture. The Hague, Netherlands, Mouton Press, 1972

Egan V: Neuropsychological aspects of HIV infection. AIDS Care 4:3–10, 1992

Ekman P: Telling Lies: Clues to Deceit in the Marketplace, Politics, and Marriage. New York, WW Norton, 1992

Ekman P, Friesen WV, O'Sullivan M: Smiles when lying. J Pers Soc Psychol 54:414–420, 1988

Epstein S: The self-concept: the traumatic neurosis and the structure of personality, in Perspectives in Personality, Vol 3, Part A. Edited by Stewart AJ. London, Jessica Kingsley, 1991, pp 63–98

Erikson E: Youth, Identity, and Crisis. New York, Norton, 1968

Escobar JI, Burnam A, Karno M, et al: Somatization in the community. Arch Gen Psychiatry 44:713–718, 1987

Escobar JI, Swartz M, Rubio-Stipec M, et al: Medically unexplained symptoms: distribution, risk factors and comorbidity, in Current Concepts of Somatization: Research and Clinical Perspectives. Edited by Kirmayer LJ, Robbins JM. Washington, DC, American Psychiatric Press, 1991, pp 63–78

"Examination," in The New Encyclopaedia Britannica, 15th edition, Micropaedia, Vol III. Chicago, Benton & Benton, 1977, p 1021

Farley J, Woodruff RA Jr, Guze SB: The prevalence of hysteria and conversion symptoms. Br J Psychiatry 114:1121–1125, 1968

Feighner JP, Robins E, Guze SB, et al: Diagnostic criteria for use in psychiatric research. Arch Gen Psychiatry 26:57–63, 1972

Fein S, McGrath MG: Problems in diagnosing bipolar disorder in catatonic patients. J Clin Psychiatry 51:203–205, 1990

Fish F: Clinical Psychopathology. Bristol, England, John Wright, 1967

Fisher R, Brown S: Getting Together: Building Relationships as We Negotiate. New York, Penguin Books, 1988

Fisher R, Ury W: Getting to Yes: Negotiating Agreement Without Giving In, 2nd Edition. Edited by Patton B. New York, Penguin Books, 1991

Folks DG, Ford CV, Regan W: Conversion symptoms in a general hospital. Psychosomatics 25:285–295, 1984

Folstein MF, Folstein SE, McHugh PR: Mini-Mental State: a practical method for grading the cognitive state of patients for the clinician. J Psychiatr Res 12:189–198, 1975

Ford CV, Folks DG: Conversion disorders: an overview. Psychosomatics 26:371–383, 1985

Ford CV, Parker PE: Somatization in consultation-liaison psychiatry, in Current Concepts of Somatization: Research and Clinical Perspectives. Edited by Kirmayer LJ, Robbins JM. Washington, DC, American Psychiatric Press, 1991, pp 143–157

Ford CV, King BH, Hollender MH: Lies and liars: psychiatric aspects of prevarication. Am J Psychiatry 145:554–562, 1988

Forstein M: The neuropsychiatric aspects of HIV infection. Prim Care 19:97–117, 1992

Forsyth BWC: Munchhausen syndrome by proxy, in Child and Adolescent Psychiatry: A Comprehensive Textbook. Edited by Lewis M. Baltimore, MD, Williams & Wilkins, 1991, pp 1030–1037

Freimer N, Lu F, Chen J: Posttraumatic stress and conversion disorders in a Laotian refugee veteran: use of amobarbital interviews. J Nerv Ment Dis 177:432–433, 1989

Freud S: Gesammelte Werke chronologisch geordnet, Bd 1–17. London, Imago Publishing, 1952–1955

Freud S: Further remarks on the neuro-psychoses of defence (1896), in The Standard Edition of the Complete Psychological Works of Sigmund Freud, Vol 3. Translated and edited by Strachey J. London, Hogarth Press, 1962, pp 157–185

Freud S: Introduction to psycho-analysis and the war neuroses (1919), in The Standard Edition of the Complete Psychological Works of Sigmund Freud, Vol 17. Translated and edited by Strachey J. London, Hogarth Press, 1955, pp 205–215

Freud S: The defence neuro-psychoses (1924), in Collected Papers, Vol 1. London, Hogarth Press/Institute of Psycho-Analysis, 1950

Fricchione GL, Cassem NH, Hooberman D, et al: Intravenous lorazepam in neuroleptic-induced catatonia. J Clin Psychopharmacol 3:338–342, 1983

Frischholz EJ, Braun BG, Sachs RG, et al: The Dissociative Experiences Scale: further replication and validation. Dissociation: Progress in the Dissociative Disorders 3:151–153, 1990

Frost LH: Methylphenidate in Amytal-resistant mutism. Acta Psychiatr Scand 79:408–410, 1989

Fuller BF: Reliability and validity of an interval measure of vocal stress. Psychol Med 14:159–166, 1984

Gabel RH, Barnard N, Notko M, et al: AIDS presenting as mania. Compr Psychiatry 27:251–254, 1986

Gatfield PD, Guze SB: Prognosis and differential diagnosis of conversion reactions: a follow-up study. Diseases of the Nervous System 23:623–631, 1962

Gauld A: A History of Hypnotism. Cambridge, England, Cambridge University Press, 1992

Gelenberg AJ: The catatonic syndrome. Lancet 1:1339–1341, 1976

Gillem TR: Deming's 14 points and hospital quality: responding to the consumer's demand for the best value health care. Journal of Nursing Quality Assurance 2(3):70–78, 1988

Giller EL Jr (ed): Biological Assessment and Treatment of Posttraumatic Stress Disorder. Washington, DC, American Psychiatric Press, 1990

Goldberg DP, Bridges K: Somatic presentation of psychiatric illness in primary care setting. J Psychosom Res 32:137–144, 1988

Golden CJ: Screening Test for the Luria-Nebraska Neuropsychological Battery: Adult and Children's Forms. Los Angeles, CA, Western Psychological Services, 1987

Golden CJ, Purish AD, Hammeke TA: Luria-Nebraska Neuropsychological Battery (LNNB). Los Angeles, CA, Western Psychological Services, 1991

Goodwin DW, Van Dusen KT, Mednick SA (eds): Longitudinal Research in Alcoholism. Boston, MA, Kluwer/Nijhoff, 1984

Goodwin J: The etiology of combat-related post-traumatic stress disorder, in Posttraumatic Stress Disorders of the Vietnam Veteran. Edited by Williams T. Cincinnati, OH, Disabled American Veterans, 1980, pp 1–23

Graham JR: The Minnesota Multiphasic Personality Inventory: A Practical Guide, 2nd Edition. New York, Oxford University Press, 1987

Green BL, Wilson JP, Lindy JD: Conceptualizing post-traumatic stress disorder: a psychosocial framework, in Trauma and Its Wake: The Study and Treatment of Post-Traumatic Stress Disorder. Edited by Figley CR. New York, Brunner/Mazel, 1985, pp 53–69

Greenfield D, Conrad C, Kincare P, et al: Treatment of catatonia with low-dose lorazepam. Am J Psychiatry 144:1224–1225, 1987

Grinker RR, Spiegel JP: Men Under Stress. New York, McGraw-Hill, 1945a

Grinker RR, Spiegel JP: War Neuroses. Philadelphia, PA, Blakiston, 1945b

Guillain G: J.-M. Charcot 1825–1893: His Life—His Work. Edited and translated by Bailey P. New York, Paul B Hoebner, 1959

Guinagh B: Catharsis and Cognition in Psychotherapy. New York, Springer-Verlag, 1987

Gunderson EK, Rahe RH (eds): Life Stress and Illness. Springfield, IL, Charles C Thomas, 1974

Gunn J, Gudjonsson G: Using the psychological stress evaluator in conditions of extreme stress: brief communication. Psychol Med 18:235–238, 1988

Gutheil TG, Appelbaum PS: Clinical Handbook of Psychiatry and the Law. Baltimore, MD, Williams & Wilkins, 1991

Guze SB: The diagnosis of hysteria: what are we trying to do? Am J Psychiatry 124:491–498, 1967

Guze SB, Wolfgram ED, KcKinney JK, et al: Psychiatric illness in the families of convicted criminals: a study of 519 first-degree relatives. Diseases of the Nervous System 28:651–659, 1967

Guze SB, Woodruff RA, Clayton PJ: A study of conversion symptoms in psychiatric outpatients. Am J Psychiatry 128:643–646, 1971

Guze SB, Cloninger CR, Martin RL, et al: A follow-up and family study of Briquet's syndrome. Br J Psychiatry 149:17–23, 1986

Hafeiz HB: Hysterical conversion: a prognostic study. Br J Psychiatry 136:548–551, 1980

Haley J: Uncommon Therapy. The Psychiatric Techniques of Milton H. Erickson, M.D. New York, WW Norton, 1986

Halleck SL: Dissociative phenomena and the question of responsibility. Int J Clin Exp Hypn 38:298–314, 1990

Halstead S, Riccio M, Harlow P, et al: Psychosis associated with HIV infection. Br J Psychiatry 153:618–623, 1988

Hanson FA: Testing. Testing. Social Consequences of the Examined Life. Los Angeles, University of California Press, 1993

Harris D, Menza MA: Benzodiazepines and catatonia: a case report. Can J Psychiatry 34:725–727, 1989

Hathaway SR, McKinley JC: Minnesota Multiphasic Personality Inventory—2. Minneapolis, University of Minnesota Press, 1989

Health Care Financing Administration: HCFA Standard 482.61, form HCFA 1537 A, Law 42 CFR, in The Federal Register: Standards and Certification. Washington, DC, U.S. Government Printing Office, 1986

Hechtman L: Resilience and vulnerability in long term outcome of attention deficit hyperactive disorder. Can J Psychiatry 36:415–421, 1991

Hendin H, Pollinger A, Singer P, et al: Meanings of combat and the development of posttraumatic stress disorder. Am J Psychiatry 138:1490–1493, 1981

Hendin H, Pollinger Hass A, Singer P, et al: The reliving experience in Vietnam veterans with posttraumatic stress disorder. Compr Psychiatry 25:165–173, 1984

Hirsch SR, Walsh C, Draper R: Parasuicide: a review of treatment interventions. J Affect Disord 4:299–311, 1982

Hoch PH: The present status of narcodiagnosis and therapy. J Nerv Ment Dis 103:248–259, 1946

Hollien H, Geison L, Hicks JW Jr: Voice stress evaluators and lie detection. J Forensic Sci 32:405–418, 1987

Hollister LE, Csernansky JG: Clinical Pharmacology and Psychotherapeutic Drugs, 3rd Edition. New York, Churchill Livingstone, 1990

Holmes TH, Rahe RH: The social readjustment rating scale. J Psychosom Res 11:213–18, 1967

Hopkinson K, Cox A, Rutter M: Psychiatric interviewing techniques, III: naturalistic study: eliciting feelings. Br J Psychiatry 138:406–415, 1981

Horowitz MJ: Phase-oriented treatment of stress response syndromes. Am J Psychother 27:506–515, 1973

Horowitz MJ: Stress response syndromes: character style and dynamic psychotherapy. Arch Gen Psychiatry 31:768–781, 1974

Horowitz MJ: Psychological response to serious life events, in Human Stress and Cognition: An Information Processing Approach. Edited by Hamilton V, Warburton DM. New York, Wiley, 1979, pp 235–263

Horowitz MJ: Stress Response Syndromes, 2nd Edition. New York, Jason Aronson, 1986

Horowitz MJ, Wilner N, Kaltreider N, et al: Signs and symptoms of posttraumatic stress disorder. Arch Gen Psychiatry 37:85–92, 1980

Horvath TB, Siever LJ, Mohs RC, et al: Organic mental syndromes and disorders, in Comprehensive Textbook of Psychiatry/5, 5th Edition, Vol 1. Edited by Kaplan HI, Sadock BJ. Baltimore, MD, Williams & Wilkins, 1989, pp 599–641

Hurwitz TA: Narcosuggestion in chronic conversion symptoms using combined intravenous amobarbital and methylphenidate. Can J Psychiatry 33:147–152, 1988

Hutzell RR, Jerkins ME: The use of a logotherapy technique in the treatment of multiple personality disorder. Dissociation: Progress in the Dissociative Disorders 3:88–93, 1990

Iannuzzi JN: Cross-Examination: The Mosaic Art. Englewood Cliffs, NJ, Prentice-Hall, 1982

Institute of Medicine (U.S.), Committee for the Study of Treatment and Rehabilitation Services for Alcoholism and Alcohol Abuse: Broadening the Base of Treatment for Alcohol Problems: Report of a Study by a Committee of the Institute of Medicine, Division of Mental Health and Behavioral Medicine. Washington, DC, National Academy Press, 1990

Jackins H: The Human Side of Human Beings: The Theory of Re-evaluation Counseling. Seattle, WA, Rational Island, 1978

Jaffe R: Dissociative phenomena in former concentration camp inmates. Int J Psychoanal 49:310–312, 1968

Janet P: L'État mental des Hystériques (1911). Marseille, France, Laffitte Reprints, 1983

Janet P: The major symptoms of hysteria, in Fifteen Lectures Given in the Medical School of Harvard University. New York, Macmillan, 1907

Janoff-Bulman R: The aftermath of victimization: rebuilding shattered assumptions, in Trauma and Its Wake: The Study and Treatment of Post-Traumatic Stress Disorder. Edited by Figley CR. New York, Brunner/Mazel, 1985, pp 15–35

Janov A: The Primal Scream. New York, Dell, 1970

Jaspers K: General Psychopathology. Translated by Hoenig J, Hamilton M. London, Manchester University Press, 1963

Johnson HG, Ekman P, Friesen WV: Communicative body movements: American emblems. Semiotica 15:335–353, 1975

Jorm AF: The Epidemiology of Alzheimer's Disease and Related Disorders. London, Chapman & Hall, 1990

Kaplan HI, Sadock BJ (eds): Comprehensive Textbook of Psychiatry/V, 5th Edition, Vols 1 and 2. Baltimore, MD, Williams & Wilkins, 1989

Kardiner A: The Traumatic Neuroses of War. New York, Hoeber, 1941

Karp H: Dementia in adults (Chapter 32), in Clinical Neurology, Vol 3, Revised. Edited by Joynt RJ. Philadelphia, PA, JB Lippincott, 1992, pp 1–31

Kaufman AS: Intelligent Testing With the WISC-R. New York, Wiley, 1979

Keane TM, Zimering RT, Caddell RT: A behavioral formulation of PTSD in Vietnam veterans. Behavior Therapist 8:9–12, 1985a

Keane TM, Fairbank JA, Caddell RT, et al: A behavioral approach to assessing and treating post-traumatic stress disorder in Vietnam veterans, in Trauma and Its Wake: The Study and Treatment of Post-Traumatic Stress Disorder. Edited by Figley CR. New York, Brunner/Mazel, 1985b, pp 257–294

Kent GH: E-G-Y Scales. New York, Williams & Wilkins, 1946

Kernberg OF: Borderline Conditions and Pathological Narcissism. New York, Jason Aronson, 1975

Kerns LL: Falsification in the psychiatric history: a differential diagnosis. Psychiatry 49:13–17, 1986

Kestenbaum CJ, Williams DT (eds): Handbook of Clinical Assessment of Children and Adolescents, Vols 1 and 2. New York, New York University Press, 1988

Kinzie JD: Severe posttraumatic stress syndrome among Cambodian refugees: symptoms, clinical course, and treatment approaches, in Disaster Stress Studies: New Methods and Findings. Edited by Shore JH. Washington, DC, American Psychiatric Press, 1986, pp 123–140

Kirmayer LJ, Robbins JM (eds): Current Concepts of Somatization: Research and Clinical Perspectives. Washington, DC, American Psychiatric Press, 1991

Kluft RP: An update on multiple personality disorder. Hosp Community Psychiatry 38:363–373, 1987

Kluft RP: Playing for time: temporizing techniques in the treatment of multiple personality disorder. Am J Clin Hypn 32:90–98, 1989a

Kluft RP: Iatrogenic creation of new alter personalities. Dissociation: Progress in the Dissociative Disorders 2:83–91, 1989b

Kluft RP: Clinical presentations of multiple personality disorder. Psychiatr Clin North Am 14:605–629, 1991

Kluft RP: A specialist's perspective on multiple personality disorder. Psychoanalytic Inquiry 12:139–171, 1992

Kluft RP, Fine CG (eds): Clinical Perspectives on Multiple Personality Disorder. Washington, DC, American Psychiatric Press, 1993

Kohut H: The Analysis of the Self. New York, International Universities Press, 1971

Kolb LC: The place of narcosynthesis in the treatment of chronic and delayed stress reactions of war, in The Trauma of War: Stress and Recovery in Viet Nam Veterans. Edited by Sonnenberg SM, Blank AS Jr, Talbott JA. Washington, DC, American Psychiatric Press, 1985, pp 211–226

Kolb LC: Recovery of memory and repressed fantasy in combat-induced post-traumatic stress disorder of Vietnam veterans, in Hypnosis and Memory. Edited by Pettinati HM. New York, Guilford, 1988, pp 265–274

Kovner R, Lazar M, Perecman E, et al: Use of the Dementia Rating Scale as a test for neuropsychological dysfunction in HIV-positive IV drug abusers. J Subst Abuse Treat 9:133–137, 1992

Kraepelin E: Lectures on Clinical Psychiatry, Revised. Edited by Johnstone T. New York, Hafner, 1968

Krull F, Schifferdecker M: Inpatient treatment of conversion disorder: a clinical investigation of outcome. Psychother Psychosom 53:161–165, 1990

Krupnick J: Brief psychotherapy with victims of violent crime. Victimology: An International Journal 2:347–354, 1980

Krystal H (ed): Massive Psychic Trauma. New York, International Universities Press, 1968

Krystal H, Niederland WG: Clinical observations on the survivor syndrome, in Massive Psychic Trauma. Edited by Krystal H. New York, International Universities Press, 1968, pp 327–348

Kwentus JA: Interviewing with intravenous drugs. J Clin Psychiatry 42:432–436, 1981

Larson DG, Chastain RL: Self-concealment: conceptualization, measurement, and health implications. Journal of Social and Clinical Psychology 9:439–455, 1990

Lehmkuhl G, Blanz B, Lehmkuhl U, et al: Conversion disorder (DSM-III 300.11): symptomatology and course in childhood and adolescence. Eur Arch Psychiatry Clin Neurosci 238:155–160, 1989

Leonhard K: The Classification of Endogenous Psychoses, 5th Edition. Edited by Robins E. Translated by Berman R. New York, Irvington Press, 1979

Lifton RJ: Death in Life: Survivors of Hiroshima. New York, Basic Books, 1967

Lifton RJ: The Life of the Self. New York, Simon & Schuster, 1976

Lifton RJ: The Broken Connection. New York, Simon & Schuster, 1979

Lindeman E: Psychological changes in normal and abnormal individuals under the influence of Sodium Amytal. Am J Psychiatry 11:1083–1091, 1932

Lipowski ZJ: Delirium: Acute Confusional States. New York, Oxford University Press, 1990

Liskow B, Othmer E, Penick EC, et al: Is Briquet's syndrome a heterogeneous disorder? Am J Psychiatry 143:626–629, 1986

Little KY: Amphetamine, but not methylphenidate, predicts antidepressant efficacy. J Clin Psychopharmacol 8:177–183, 1988

Loewenstein RJ: An office mental status examination for complex chronic dissociative symptoms and multiple personality disorder. Psychiatr Clin North Am 14:567–604, 1991

Ludwig AM, Othmer E: The medical model of psychiatry. Am J Psychiatry 134:1087–1092, 1977

Ludwig AM, Surawicz FG: Restitutive therapies, in American Handbook of Psychiatry, 2nd Edition, Vol 5. Edited by Freedman DX, Dyrud JE. New York, Basic Books, 1975

Luria AR: Higher Cortical Function in Man. New York, Basic Books, 1966

Lykken DT: A Tremor in the Blood: Uses and Abuses of the Lie Detector. New York, McGraw-Hill, 1981

Magrinat G, Danziger JA, Lorenzo IC, et al: A reassessment of catatonia. Compr Psychiatry 24:218–228, 1983

Maier SF, Seligman MEP: Learned helplessness: theory and evidence. J Exp Psychol Gen 105:3–46, 1976

Maj M: Organic mental disorders in HIV-1 infection. AIDS 4:831–840, 1990

Marcos LR: Cautions regarding Amytal interviews (letter). Am J Psychiatry 140:510–511, 1983

Marcum JM, Wright K, Bissell WG: Chance discovery of multiple personality disorder in a depressed patient by amobarbital interview. J Nerv Ment Dis 174:489–492, 1986

Marriage K, Govorchin M, George P, et al: Use of an Amytal interview in the management of factitious deaf mutism. Aust N Z J Psychiatry 22:454–456, 1988

Martin RL: Diagnostic issues for conversion disorder. Hosp Community Psychiatry 43:771—773, 1992

Martin RL: DSM-IV diagnostic options for conversion disorder: proposed autonomic arousal disorder and pseudocyesis, in DSM-IV Sourcebook, Volume 2. Edited by Widiger TA, Frances AJ, Pincus HA, et al. Washington, DC, American Psychiatric Association (in press)

Martin RL, Yutzy SH: Somatoform disorders, in American Psychiatric Press Textbook of Psychiatry, 2nd Edition. Edited by Hales RE, Yudofsky SC, Talbott JA. Washington, DC, American Psychiatric Press, 1994, pp 591–622

Mason AS, Granacher RP: Clinical Handbook of Antipsychotic Drug Therapy. New York, Brunner/Mazel, 1980

Masterson JF: Psychotherapy for the Borderline Adult: A Developmental Approach. New York, Brunner/Mazel, 1976

Maultsby M Jr: Rational Behavior Therapy. Englewood Cliffs, NJ, Prentice-Hall, 1984

McCall WV, Shelp FE, McDonald WM: Controlled investigation of the amobarbital interview for catatonic mutism. Am J Psychiatry 149:202–206, 1992

McEvoy JP, Lohr JB: Diazepam for catatonia. Am J Psychiatry 141:284–285, 1984

McFarlane AC, Weber DL, Clark CR: Abnormal stimulus processing in posttraumatic stress disorder. Biol Psychiatry 34:311–320, 1993

Meadow R: Munchausen syndrome by proxy: the hinterland of child abuse. Lancet 2:343–345, 1977

Medoff MH: An evaluation of the effectiveness of suicide prevention centers. Journal of Behavioral Economics 15:43–55, 1986

Meichenbaum D, Cameron R: Stress inoculation training: toward a general paradigm for training in coping skills, in Stress Reduction and Prevention. Edited by Meichenbaum D, Jaremko M. New York, Plenum, 1983, pp 115–154

Merskey H: Psychiatric Illness, 3rd Edition. London, Ballière, Tindall, 1980

Merskey H: The manufacture of personalities: the production of multiple personality disorder. Br J Psychiatry 160:327–340, 1992

Mesulam M-M: Dissociative states with abnormal temporal lobe EEG. Arch Neurol 38:176–181, 1981

Mesulam M-M: Principles of Behavioral Neurology. Philadelphia, PA, FA Davis, 1985

Miller C, Swift K: The Handbook of Nonsexist Writing, 2nd Edition. New York, Harper & Row, 1988

Millon T: Millon Clinical Multiaxial Inventory—II. Minneapolis, MN, NCS Professional Assessment Services, 1976

Moos RH, Finney JW, Cronkite RC: Alcoholism Treatment: Context, Process and Outcome. New York, Oxford University Press, 1990

Morrison JR: Catatonia: prediction of outcome. Compr Psychiatry 15:317–324, 1974

Morrison J: The First Interview: A Guide for Clinicians. New York, Guilford, 1993

Murphy GE: Suicide in Alcoholism. New York, Oxford University Press, 1992

Navia BA, Jordan BD, Price RW: The AIDS dementia complex, I: clinical features. Ann Neurol 19:517–524, 1986

Neborsky R, Janowsky D, Munson E, et al: Rapid treatment of acute psychotic symptoms with high- and low-dose haloperidol. Arch Gen Psychiatry 38:195–199, 1981

Nemiah JC: Dissociation, conversion, and somatization, in American Psychiatric Press Review of Psychiatry, Vol 10. Edited by Tasman A, Goldfinger SM. Washington, DC, American Psychiatric Press, 1991, pp 248–260

Niederland WG: Clinical observations on the survivor syndrome. Int J Psychoanal 49:313–315, 1968

Orne MT, Dinges DF: Hypnosis, in Comprehensive Textbook of Psychiatry/V, 5th Edition, Vol 2. Edited by Kaplan HI, Sadock BJ. Baltimore, MD, Williams & Wilkins, 1989, pp 1501–1516

Ostrovsky V, Hoy C: By Way of Deception. Toronto, Canada, Stoddart Publishing, 1990

Othmer E, Desouza C: A screening test for somatization disorder (hysteria). Am J Psychiatry 142:1146–1149, 1985

Othmer E, Othmer SC: Life on a Roller Coaster: Coping With the Ups and Downs of Mood Disorder. New York, Berkley Press, 1991

Othmer E, Othmer SC: The Clinical Interview Using DSM-IV, Vol 1: Fundamentals. Washington, DC, American Psychiatric Press, 1994

Othmer E, Penick EC, Powell BJ, et al: The Psychiatric Diagnostic Interview. Revised by Penick EC. Los Angeles, CA, Western Psychological Services, 1988

Othmer SC: Berlin und die Verbreitung des Naturrechts in Europa: Kultur- und sozialgeschichtliche Studien zu Jean Barbeyracs Pufendorf-Übersetzungen und eine Analyse seiner Leserschaft [Berlin and the Expansion of the Philosophy of Natural Law in Europe: Cultural and Sociological Studies Concerning Jean Barbeyrac's Translations of Pufendorf's Works and a Historical Analysis of His Readers]. Berlin, Walter de Gruyter, 1970

Pajeau AK, Roman GC: HIV encephalopathy and dementia. Psychiatr Clin North Am 15:455–466, 1992

Parks RW, Zec RF, Wilson RS (eds): Neuropsychology of Alzheimer's Disease and Other Dementias. New York, Oxford University Press, 1993

Perley M, Guze S: Hysteria: the stability and usefulness of clinical criteria. N Engl J Med 266:421–426, 1962

Perls FS: In and Out of the Garbage Pail. New York, Bantam Books, 1969

Perry JC, Jacobs D: Overview: clinical applications of the Amytal interview in psychiatric emergency settings. Am J Psychiatry 139:552–559, 1982

Perry SW, Tross S: Psychiatric problems of AIDS inpatients at the New York Hospital: preliminary report. Public Health Rep 99:200–205, 1984

Peterson KC, Prout MF, Schwarz RA: Post-Traumatic Stress Disorder: A Clinician's Guide. New York, Plenum, 1991

Pettinati HM (ed): Hypnosis and Memory. New York, Guilford, 1988

Pincus JH, Tucker GJ: Behavioral Neurology, 3rd Edition. New York, Oxford University Press, 1985

Pincus JH, Cohan SL, Glaser GH: Neurological complications of internal disease, in Clinical Neurology, Vol 4, Revised. Edited by Joynt RJ. Philadelphia, PA, JB Lippincott, 1992, pp 16–18

Piper WE, Azim HFA, Joyce AS, et al: Transference interpretations, therapeutic alliance, and outcome in short-term individual psychotherapy. Arch Gen Psychiatry 48:946–953, 1991

Powell R, Boast N: The million dollar man: resource implications for chronic Munchausen syndrome. Br J Psychiatry 162:253–256, 1993

Price RW, Brew BJ: The AIDS dementia complex. J Infect Dis 158:1079–1083, 1988

Putnam FW: The switch process in multiple personality disorder and other state-change disorders. Dissociation: Progress in the Dissociative Disorders 1:24–32, 1988

Putnam FW: Recent research on multiple personality disorder. Psychiatr Clin North Am 14:489–502, 1991

Putnam FW, Guroff JJ, Silberman EK, et al: The clinical phenomenology of multiple personality disorder: review of 100 recent cases. J Clin Psychiatry 47:285–293, 1986

Putnam FW, Zahn TP, Post RM: Differential autonomic nervous system activity in multiple personality disorder. Psychiatry Res 31:251–260, 1990

Rapoport JL, Ismond DR: DSM-III-R Training Guide for Diagnosis of Childhood Disorders. New York, Brunner/Mazel, 1990

Raskin M, Talbott JA, Meyerson AT: Diagnosis of conversion reaction: predictive value of psychiatric criteria. JAMA 197:102–106, 1966

Reitan RM, Wolfson D: The Halstead-Reitan Neuropsychological Test Battery: Theory and Clinical Interpretation. Tucson, AZ, Neuropsychology Press, 1985

Riley KC: Unraveling hysteria: a neuropsychological investigation of Briquet syndrome. Unpublished doctoral dissertation, University of Texas at Austin, 1984

Rinsley DB: Borderline and Other Self Disorders: A Developmental and Objects-Relations Perspective. New York, Jason Aronson, 1982

Robins LN, Regier DA: Psychiatric Disorders in America: The Epidemiologic Catchment Area Study. New York, Free Press, 1991

Rogers R (ed): Clinical Assessment of Malingering and Deception. New York, Guilford, 1988

Rolin J: Police Drugs. Translated with a foreword by Bendit LJ, appendix on narcoanalysis by Saher EV. New York, Philosophical Library, 1956

Roman GC: Lacunar dementia, in Senile Dementia of the Alzheimer Type. Neurology and Neurobiology, Vol 18. Edited by Hutton JT, Kenny AD. New York, Alan R Liss, 1985, pp 131–151

Rosebush PI, Hildebrand AM, Furlong BG, et al: Catatonic syndrome in a general psychiatric inpatient population: frequency, clinical presentation, and response to lorazepam. J Clin Psychiatry 51:357–362, 1990

Rosenberg D: Web of deceit: a literature review of Munchausen syndrome by proxy. Child Abuse Negl 11:547–563, 1987

Rosenhan DL: On being sane in insane places. Science 179:250–258, 1973

Ross CA: Comments on Garcia's "The concept of dissociation and conversion in the new ICD-10." Dissociation: Progress in the Dissociative Disorders 3:211–213, 1990

Ross CA: Epidemiology of multiple personality disorder and dissociation. Psychiatr Clin North Am 14:503–517, 1991

Ross CA, Gahan P: Techniques in the treatment of multiple personality disorder. Am J Psychother 42:40–52, 1988

Ross CA, Norton GR: Suicide and parasuicide in multiple personality disorder. Psychiatry 52:365–371, 1989

Ross CA, Norton GR, Anderson G: The Dissociative Experiences Scale: a replication study. Dissociation: Progress in the Dissociative Disorders 1:21–22, 1988

Ross CA, Heber S, Norton GR, et al: Somatic symptoms in multiple personality disorder. Psychosomatics 30:154–160, 1989

Ross CA, Anderson G, Fleischer WP, et al: The frequency of multiple personality disorder among psychiatric inpatients. Am J Psychiatry 148:1717–1720, 1991a

Ross CA, Miller SD, Bjornson L, et al: Abuse histories in 102 cases of multiple personality disorder. Can J Psychiatry 36:97–101, 1991b

Rosvold HE, Mirsky AE, Sarandon I, et al: A continuous performance test of brain damage. Journal of Consulting Psychology 20:343–350, 1956

Rothman T, Sward K: Studies and pharmacological psychotherapy. Archives of Neurology and Psychiatry 75:95–105, 1956

Royall DR, Mahurin RK, Gray KF: Bedside assessment of executive cognitive impairment: the executive interview. J Am Geriatr Soc 40:1221–1226, 1992

Royall DR, Mahurin RK, Cornell J, et al: Bedside assessment of dementia type using the qualitative evaluation of dementia. Neuropsychiatry, Neuropsychology, and Behavioral Neurology 6:235–244, 1993

Royall DR, Mahurin RK, Cornell J: Bedside assessment of frontal degeneration: distinguishing Alzheimer's disease from non-Alzheimer's cortical dementia. Experimental Aging Research 20:95–103, 1994

Rubin TI: Shrink! The Diary of a Psychiatrist. New York, Popular Library, 1974

Rutter M, Bolton P, Harrington R, et al: Genetic factors in child psychiatric disorders, I: a review of research strategies. J Child Psychol Psychiatry 31:3–37, 1990a

Rutter M, Macdonald H, Le Couteur A, et al: Genetic factors in child psychiatric disorders, II: empirical findings. J Child Psychol Psychiatry 31:39–83, 1990b

Salam SA, Kilzieh N: Lorazepam treatment of psychogenic catatonia: an update. J Clin Psychiatry 49 (suppl):16–21, 1988

Salam SA, Pillai AK, Beresford TP: Lorazepam for psychogenic catatonia. Am J Psychiatry 144:1082–1083, 1987

Salano OA, Sadow T, Ananth J: Rapid tranquilization: a reevaluation. Neuropsychobiology 22:90–96, 1989

Sangiovanni F, Taylor M, Abrams R, et al: Rapid control of psychotic excitement states with intramuscular haloperidol. Am J Psychiatry 130:1155–1156, 1973

Sattler JM: Assessment of Children's Intelligence and Special Abilities, 2nd Edition. Boston, MA, Allyn & Bacon, 1982

Sbriglio R: The Amytal interview in emergency and psychiatric settings. Hospital Physician, October 1984, pp 91–99

Schatzberg AF, Cole JO: Manual of Clinical Psychopharmacology, 2nd Edition. Washington, DC, American Psychiatric Press, 1991

Scheff TJ: Catharsis in Healing, Ritual, and Drama. Berkley, University of California Press, 1979

Schilder FE: Treatment by systematic desensitization of a recurring nightmare of a real life trauma. J Behav Ther Exp Psychiatry 11:53–54, 1980

Schmidt U, Miller D: Two cases of hypomania in AIDS. Br J Psychiatry 152:839–842, 1988

Schreier HA, Libow JA: Hurting for Love. New York, Guilford, 1993

Schultz JH: Autogenic Therapy, Vols 1–6. Edited by Luthe W. New York, Grune & Stratton, 1969

Schultz SJ: Family Systems Therapy: An Integration. New York, Jason Aronson, 1984

Schweitzer I: The psychiatric assessment of the patient requesting facial surgery. Aust N Z J Psychiatry 2:249–254, 1989

Shatan CF: The grief of soldiers: Vietnam combat veterans' self-help movement. Am J Orthopsychiatry 43:640–653, 1973

Shatan CF: Stress disorders among Vietnam veterans: the emotional content of combat continues, in Stress Disorders Among Vietnam Veterans: Theory, Research and Treatment. Edited by Figley CR. New York, Brunner/Mazel, 1978, pp 43–55

Sheehan PW: Confidence, memory, and hypnosis, in Hypnosis and Memory. Edited by Pettinati HM. New York, Guilford, 1988, pp 95–127

Shekim WO, Asarnow RF, Hess E, et al: A clinical and demographic profile of a sample of adults with attention deficit hyperactivity disorder, residual state. Compr Psychiatry 31:416–425, 1990

Siegel M, Barthel RP: Conversion disorders on a child consultation service. Psychosomatics 27:201–204, 1986

Simon GE: Somatization and psychiatric disorders, in Current Concepts of Somatization: Research and Clinical Perspectives. Edited by Kirmayer LJ, Robbins JM. Washington, DC, American Psychiatric Press, 1991, pp 37–62

Slaby AE: Aftershock: Surviving the Delayed Effects of Trauma, Crisis and Loss. New York, Villard Books, 1989

Slater E, Roth M: Clinical Psychiatry, 3rd Edition. London, Ballière, Tindall & Cassell, 1969

Spiegel H: Hypnosis: an adjunct to psychotherapy, in Comprehensive Textbook of Psychiatry/II, 2nd Edition, Vol 2. Edited by Freedman AM, Kaplan HI, Sadock BJ. Baltimore, MD, Williams & Wilkins, 1975, pp 1843–1849

Spierings C, Poels PJ, Sijben N, et al: Conversion disorder in childhood: a retrospective follow-up study of 84 inpatients. Dev Med Child Neurol 32:865–871, 1990

Stefánsson JG, Messina JA, Meyerrowitz S: Hysterical neurosis, conversion type: clinical and epidemiological considerations. Acta Psychiatr Scand 53:119–138, 1976

Stekel W: The Interpretation of Dreams: New Developments and Techniques (2 Vols). Translated by Paul E, Paul C. New York, Liveright, 1943

Strub RL, Black FW: The Mental Status Examination in Neurology. Philadelphia, PA, FA Davis, 1977

Strub RL, Black FW: Neurobehavioral Disorders: A Clinical Approach. Philadelphia, PA, FA Davis, 1988

Strub RL, Black FW: The Mental Status Examination in Neurology, 3rd Edition. Philadelphia, PA, FA Davis, 1993

Sykes DH, Douglas VI, Morgenstern G: Sustained attention in hyperactive children. J Child Psychol Psychiatry 14:213–220, 1973

Takahashi Y: Is multiple personality disorder really rare in Japan? Dissociation: Progress in the Dissociative Disorders 3:57–59, 1990

Taylor MA: The Neuropsychiatric Guide to Modern Everyday Psychiatry. New York, Free Press, 1993

Taylor MA, Abrams R: The phenomenology of mania: a new look at some old patients. Arch Gen Psychiatry 29:520–522, 1973

Thigpen CH, Cleckley HM: The Three Faces of Eve. Kingsport, TN, Kingsport Press, 1957

Torgersen S: Genetic factors in anxiety disorders. Arch Gen Psychiatry 40:1085–1089, 1983

Trimble MR: Post-Traumatic Neurosis. New York, Wiley, 1981

Trommer BL, Hoeppner JB, Lorber R, et al: The go/no-go paradigm in attention deficit disorder. Ann Neurol 24:610–614, 1988

Tupin JP: Focal neuroleptization: an approach to optimal dosing for initial and continuing therapy. J Clin Psychopharm 5 (suppl):15S–21S, 1985

Van der Hart O: Is multiple personality disorder really rare in Japan (commentary)? Dissociation: Progress in the Dissociative Disorders 3:66–67, 1990

Van der Hart O, Boon S: Contemporary interest in multiple personality disorder and child abuse in the Netherlands. Dissociation: Progress in the Dissociative Disorders 3:34–37, 1990

van der Kolk BA (ed): Posttraumatic Stress Disorder: Psychological and Biological Sequelae. Washington, DC, American Psychiatric Press, 1984

van der Kolk BA, Boyd H, Krystal J, et al: Post-traumatic stress disorder as a biologically based disorder: implications of the animal model of inescapable shock, in Post-Traumatic Stress Disorder: Psychological and Biological Sequelae. Edited by van der Kolk BA. Washington, DC, American Psychiatric Press, 1984, pp 123–134

van der Kolk BA, Greenberg MS, Boyd H, et al: Inescapable shock, neurotransmitters and addiction to trauma: towards a psychobiology of post-traumatic stress. Biol Psychiatry 20:314–325, 1985

Van Gorp WG, Hinkin C, Satz P, et al: Neuropsychological findings in HIV infection, encephalopathy, and dementia, in Neuropsychology of Alzheimer's Disease and Other Dementias. Edited by Parks RW, Zec RF, Wilson RS. New York, Oxford University Press, 1993, pp 153–185

Victor M: Neurologic disorders due to alcoholism and malnutrition, in Clinical Neurology, Vol 4, Revised. Edited by Joynt RJ. Philadelphia, PA, JB Lippincott, 1992, pp 1–94

Wakefield H, Underwager R: Recovered memories of alleged sexual abuse: lawsuits against parents. Behavioral Sciences and the Law 10:483–507, 1992

Watzlawick P, Beavin JH, Jackson DD: Pragmatics of Human Communication. New York, WW Norton, 1967

Watzlawick P: The Language of Change: Elements of Therapeutic Communication. New York, Basic Books, 1978

Wechsler D: Wechsler Intelligence Scale for Children—Revised (WISC-R). New York, Psychological Corporation, 1974

Wechsler D: Wechsler Adult Intelligence Scale—Revised. San Antonio, TX, Psychological Corporation, 1981

Weitzenhoffer AM, Hilgard ER: Stanford Hypnotic Susceptibility Scale—Forms A and B: For Use in Research Investigations in the Field of Hypnotic Phenomena. Palo Alto, CA, Consulting Psychologists Press, 1962a

Weitzenhoffer AM, Hilgard ER: Stanford Hypnotic Susceptibility Scale—Form C: For Use in Research Investigations in the Field of Hypnotic Phenomena. Palo Alto, CA, Consulting Psychologists Press, 1962b

Wessely S, Buchanan A, Reed A, et al: Acting on delusions, I: prevalence. Br J Psychiatry 163:69–76, 1993

Whiten A, Byrne RW: Tactical deception in primates. Behavioral and Brain Sciences 11:233–273, 1988

Whitman BY, Munkel W: Multiple personality disorder: a risk indicator, diagnostic marker and psychiatric outcome for severe child abuse. Clin Pediatr (Phila) 30:422–428, 1991

Wilbur CB: Multiple personality disorder and transference. Dissociation: Progress in the Dissociative Disorders 1:73–76, 1988

Wilcox JA: Predictive variables in catatonia (abstract). Biol Psychiatry 29 (suppl):66A, 1991

Wilkinson CB: Aftermath of a disaster: the collapse of the Hyatt Regency Hotel skywalks. Am J Psychiatry 140:1134–1139, 1983

Willerman L, Cohen DB: Psychopathology. New York, McGraw-Hill, 1990

Wilmer HA: Post-traumatic stress disorder. Psychiatric Annals 12:995–1003, 1982

Wilson IC: Rapid Approximate Intelligence Test. Am J Psychiatry 123:1289–1290, 1967

Wilson JP: Identity, Ideology, and Crisis: The Vietnam Veteran in Transition, Vol 2. Washington, DC, Disabled Veterans, 1978

Wilson JP: Conflict, stress, and growth: the effects of war on psychosocial development among Vietnam veterans, in Strangers at Home: Vietnam Veterans Since the War. Edited by Figley CR, Leventman S. New York, Brunner/Mazel, 1980, pp 123–165

Wilson JP: New Theoretical Dimensions of PTSD (cassette recording). Dayton, OH, Serco Marketing & Human Resources Initiative, 1983

Wilson JP, Krauss GE: Predicting post-traumatic stress disorders among Vietnam veterans, in Post-Traumatic Stress Disorder and the War Veteran Patient. Edited by Kelly WE. New York, Brunner/Mazel, 1985, pp 102–147

Wise MG, Brandt GT: Delirium, in The American Psychiatric Press Textbook of Neuropsychiatry, 2nd Edition. Edited by Yudofsky SC, Hales RE. Washington, DC, American Psychiatric Press, 1992, pp 291–310

Woerner PI, Guze SB: A family and marital study of hysteria. Br J Psychiatry 114:161–168, 1968

Wolcott DL, Fawzy IF, Pasnau RD: Acquired immune deficiency syndrome (AIDS) and consultation-liaison psychiatry. Gen Hosp Psychiatry 7:280–292, 1985

Woods D: The diagnosis and treatment of attention deficit disorder, residual type. Psychiatric Annals 16:23–28, 1986

World Health Organization: International Classification of Diseases, 10th Revision. Geneva, Switzerland, World Health Organization, 1992

Worthington ER: Demographic and preservice variables as predictors of post-military service adjustment, in Stress Disorders Among Vietnam Veterans: Theory, Research and Treatment. Edited by Figley CR. New York, Brunner/Mazel, 1978, pp 173–187

Wright ME, Wright BA: Clinical Practice of Hypnotherapy. New York, Guilford, 1987

Young CB, McGlone J: Cerebral localization (Chapter 8), in Clinical Neurology, Vol 1, Revised. Edited by Joynt RJ. Philadelphia, PA, JB Lippincott, 1992, 1–97

Zachary RA: Shipley Institute of Living Scale, Revised. Los Angeles, CA, Western Psychological Services, 1986

Ziegler FJ, Imboden JB, Meyer E: Contemporary conversion reactions: clinical study. Am J Psychiatry 116:901–910, 1960

INDEX

*Page numbers printed in **boldface** type refer to tables or figures.*

materials needed for, 455
recording sheets for, 462–463
test cards for, 465–467
test instructions for, 456–461
Eye fixation hypnotic technique, 15
Eye test, of hypnotizability, 13

F

Facial expressions
  in concealing behavior, **322,** 323
  in factitious behavior, 390
  in falsifying, lying behavior, **353,**
    354–355, 368–369
  in self-deceptive behavior, 419
Facilitating, in psychotic acting out,
  160–162
Factitious behavior
  criterion of, 312
  descriptive summary of, 313, 385,
    386–388, 410–412
  diagnosis of, 409
  follow-up of, 409–410
  interview: factitious disorder by
    proxy, 400–401, 401–409
  vs. malingering, 386, 387, 410, 412
  mental status characteristics of,
    388–389
    affect double message, 389–390
    autonomic signs, 389
    cooperation with experts, 392–393
    detailed knowledge, 392
    facial expressions, 390
    gestures, 391
    goal-directed movements, 391
    grooming behavior, 390
    investigation defeat, 393
    mimicking, 393
    psychomotor movements, speech
      double message, 391–392
    reactive movements, 390
    speech, 392
    symbolic movements, 391

verbal strategies of, 392–393
victim role assumption, 392,
  405–406
voice, 390
steps to unravel fabrication, 399–400
voice-stress analysis technique,
  393–395, **395**
  detection instruments, 397–399
  question sequence, 396
  set the stage for lying, 396
  unrecorded trial interview, 396–397
  yes-or-no answers, 396
Falsifying, lying
  vs. concealing behavior, 353, 354
  cross-examination technique for,
    358–360
  steps of
    listen, 360–361
    tag, 361–362
    confront, 363–365
    solve, 365–366
    approve, 366
  descriptive summary of, 313, 349, 350
    to cover up, 351
    to divert responsibility, 351
    to slander, 351–352
  diagnosis of, 383
  interview: borderline personality
    disorder, conduct disorder,
    366–367
    listen, 367–369
    tag, 369–371
    confront, 371–372
    solve, 372–380
    approve, 380–383
    cross-examination, 370–383
    direct examination, 367–370
  mental status characteristics of
    affect double message, 352–355,
      353, 368–369
    autonomic response, 354
    contradictions, 357
    defensive attitude, 357